Athletic Training Student Primer

A Foundation For Success

Second Edition

ANDREW P. WINTERSTEIN, PhD, ATC

ASSOCIATE CLINICAL PROFESSOR

PROGRAM DIRECTOR—ATEP

DEPARTMENT OF KINESIOLOGY

UNIVERSITY OF WISCONSIN–MADISON

MADISON, WISCONSIN

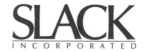

SLACK
INCORPORATED

ISBN: 978-1-55642-804-3

The procedures and practices described in this book should be implemented in a manner consistent with the professional standards set for the circumstances that apply in each specific situation. Every effort has been made to confirm the accuracy of the information presented and to correctly relate generally accepted practices. The authors, editor, and publisher cannot accept responsibility for errors or exclusions or for the outcome of the material presented herein. There is no expressed or implied warranty of this book or information imparted by it. Care has been taken to ensure that drug selection and dosages are in accordance with currently accepted/recommended practice. Due to continuing research, changes in government policy and regulations, and various effects of drug reactions and interactions, it is recommended that the reader carefully review all materials and literature provided for each drug, especially those that are new or not frequently used. Any review or mention of specific companies or products is not intended as an endorsement by the author or publisher.

SLACK Incorporated uses a review process to evaluate submitted material. Prior to publication, educators or clinicians provide important feedback on the content that we publish. We welcome feedback on this work.

Published by: SLACK Incorporated
6900 Grove Road
Thorofare, NJ 08086 USA
Telephone: 856-848-1000
Fax: 856-853-5991
www.slackbooks.com

Contact SLACK Incorporated for more information about other books in this field or about the availability of our books from distributors outside the United States.

Library of Congress Cataloging-in-Publication Data

Winterstein, Andrew P., 1962-
   Athletic training student primer : a foundation for success / Andrew P. Winterstein. -- 2nd ed.
      p. ; cm.
   Includes bibliographical references and index.
   ISBN 978-1-55642-804-3 (alk. paper)
   1. Athletic trainers--Training of--United States. 2. Sports injuries--Treatment. I. Title.
   [DNLM: 1. Athletic Injuries--therapy. 2. Allied Health Personnel--education. 3. Emergency Treatment. 4. Sports Medicine. QT 261 W788a 2009]
   GV223.W56 2009
   617.1'027--dc22
                                        2009018012

Last digit is print number: 10   9   8   7   6   5   4   3   2   1

DEDICATION

Middle age is clearer,
Now it dawns on you;
Now you hafta laugh at what you
Used to think you knew.
~Steve Forbert

This book is dedicated to all of my mentors from the University of Arizona, University of Oregon, and University of Wisconsin who showed both an interest and remarkable patience when I was a student and very young professional.
You know, back when I really knew a lot.
Thank you for showing me what really matters.
For Mom and Dad.
Of course, Barb

CONTENTS

VISIT THE COMPANION WEB SITE AT

HTTP://WWW.SLACKBOOKS.COM/ATPRIMER

PHOTO AND ILLUSTRATION CREDITS

ILLUSTRATIONS AND FIGURES

Original Medical Illustrations by Melissa Ebbe

Chapter 5: Figures 2 to 9, 11, and 12
Chapter 6: Figures 1 to 8, 10 to 12, and 18 and illustrations on pp. 98, 105, 107, 111, and 118
Chapter 7: Figures 1 to 10 and illustrations on pp. 129, 131, 134, 136, 137, 139
Chapter 8: Figures 1, 2, 10 to 16
Chapter 9: Figure 7
Chapter 10: Figure 1 and illustration on p. 202
Appendix D: Illustrations on pp. 311 and 312
All illustrations by Melissa Ebbe © 2003 Melissa Ebbe.

Figures Provided by Andrew P. Winterstein

Chapter 5: Figure 1
Chapter 6: Figures 9, 14 to 17, and 19 and figures on pp. 106, 115, and 119
Chapter 7: Figures 11 and 12 and figures on pp. 137, 143, 145
Chapter 8: Figures 3, 4, and 8
Chapter 9: Figures 4 to 6
Chapter 12: Figures 1 to 5
Chapter 13: Figures 3 to 5
Chapter 14: Figure 3
Chapter 15: Figure 1

Chapter 1 opening photo (p. 3) and photo Chapter 8 (p. 155) courtesy of UW Health.

Chapter 2 opening photo (p. 25) courtesy of the National Athletic Trainers' Association.

Chapter 5 opening photo (p. 77) courtesy of University of Wisconsin–Madison Athletic Communications.

Chapter 3 opening photo (p. 39), Chapter 14 opening photo (p. 257), Chapter 16 opening photo (p. 287), Figure 11-4, and images on pages 141, 220, and 260 used under license from iStockphoto.com.

ACKNOWLEDGMENTS

I often tell my athletic training students that taking on a large endeavor is like eating an elephant—you have to work slowly and take it "one bite at a time." It also helps if you do not start at the wrong end. I am not sure if completing this second edition qualifies as eating a second elephant—it just felt that way at times. Truth be told, you cannot eat an elephant by yourself so I have many people to thank.

Thank you to Scott Barker for continuing to be my multimedia guru and offering his generous talents to the Web components of this project. He is still the smartest athletic trainer I know (still tied with Sara Brown anyway). Thank you for your generosity but mostly for your friendship.

Sincere appreciation is extended to all the athletic trainers, physicians, and health care professionals at the University of Wisconsin–Madison, UW Health, and University Health Services. They are a wealth of knowledge and constant source of encouragement. Special thanks are reserved for Kathleen Carr for helping me become a better care provider as part of the best-kept sports medicine secret on campus. Thanks also to David Bernhardt for his constant support of the athletic training education program. A heartfelt thanks is reserved for Greg Landry for providing the Foreword to this text (not to mention over 20 years of guidance and friendship).

Thank you to Dr. Ken Schreibman for his assistance in obtaining images for the interactive anatomy program found on the companion Web site and for being a wonderful resource to our program.

Tim McGuine is a great friend and the most underrated athletic training research professional on the planet. Thanks for your encouragement and support and for making me look smart. We need to fish soon.

I am blessed to have great colleagues in the Department of Kinesiology, especially those who listen to my rants, drag me out for the occasional run, and join me for "research" days on the river (you know who you are). Thank you to Shari Clark, Jan Helwig, Pat Hills-Meyer, and Rebecca Nelson for your dedication to quality instruction in the athletic training education program.

I would be remiss if I did not show my sincere gratitude to the staff of SLACK Incorporated. Thank you for believing in the second edition of this project. Special thanks to Jennifer Briggs for her patience and encouragement. Sincere thanks to April Billick for her design and editing assistance.

I am blessed with love and support from my parents, siblings, and extended family. I hope I never take it for granted. Thanks for the inspiration and encouragement.

There are not enough ways to say thanks to my wife Barb for putting up with all the late nights and weekends spent on this and all my "projects." All husbands should be so lucky.

Lastly, I wish to thank my current and former athletic training students from the University of Wisconsin–Madison for teaching me far more then I could ever teach them.

ABOUT THE AUTHOR

Andrew P. Winterstein, PhD, ATC is an associate clinical professor in the Department of Kinesiology at the University of Wisconsin–Madison where he currently serves as the program director of their CAATE accredited undergraduate athletic training education program. He also maintains an affiliate appointment in the Department of Orthopedics and Rehabilitation in the School of Medicine and Public Health. Dr. Winterstein has coordinated the athletic training education efforts since 1999 and has been at the University of Wisconsin since 1986. He provided clinical care as part of the athletic training staff in the Division of Intercollegiate Athletics for 14 years before moving to direct the AT education program. A 1984 graduate of the University of Arizona with a Bachelor of Science degree in Secondary Education and Biology, Andy has had a variety of athletic training and educational experiences.

Prior to his appointment at the University of Wisconsin–Madison, Andy was a graduate assistant at the University of Oregon in Eugene. At the University of Oregon, he earned a Master's of Science in Applied Physiology and Athletic Training. In 1994, Andy received his Doctorate in Educational Administration with an emphasis in higher education and sports medicine-related issues from the University of Wisconsin–Madison. Dr. Winterstein's academic interests include studying emerging technologies and their use in teaching and learning, medical humanities and their application to athletic training education, and the scholarship of teaching and learning (SoTL). His papers and abstracts have appeared in the *Journal of Athletic Training, Athletic Therapy Today,* and *Athletic Training and Sports Health Care.* He has been privileged to make numerous professional presentations at the state, regional, and national level.

A certified member of the National Athletic Trainers' Association since 1985, and certified member of the Wisconsin Athletic Trainers' Association, Dr. Winterstein is active in many aspects of athletic training. He serves as a reviewer for the *Journal of Athletic Training;* is a reviewer and member of the editorial board for the *Journal of Athletic Training Education* and *Athletic Training and Sports Health Care;* and has served on several state, regional, and national committees. Dr. Winterstein has received numerous awards, including the 2008 Great Lakes Athletic Training Association Outstanding Educator Award, 2007 Wisconsin Athletic Trainers' Association Outstanding Educator Award, and the 2006 UW-Madison School of Education Distinguished Service Award. He and his colleagues are three-time winners of the NATA Educational Multimedia Committee award for educational innovations and have been awarded the MERLOT Classics Award for exemplary on-line learning objects. In addition to this text, he is the co-author of *Administrative Topics in Athletic Training: Concepts to Practice* published by SLACK Incorporated

In his spare time, Andy enjoys fly fishing, fly tying, reading, and writing. He resides in Madison, Wisconsin with his wife, Barb.

INTERVIEW PARTICIPANTS AND CONTRIBUTORS

I am once again indebted to the thoughtful professionals from around the country who provided insights into their athletic training lives so that I may provide students with a balanced view of this profession. Thank you for your honest and thoughtful contributions. Three cheers for the young professionals who reflected on their own student experiences in order to assist new students. I am excited that our profession continues to attract some of the best and brightest

These professionals listed below (young and not so young) represent the very best of what the profession has to offer. Learning from their experiences has been a highlight for me.

Thomas Abdenour
Marjorie Albohm
Scott Barker
Ronnie P. Barnes
Thomas B. Barr
Samuel F. Bell
Brianna Bennett
Sara Brown
Pepper Burruss
Beth Chorlton
Shari Clark
Leah J. Frommer
Ashleigh Gauvain
Lauren M. Germanowski
Christopher Gibbons
Mark Gildard
Neal Glaviano
Kevin Guskiewicz
Dawn Hammerschmidt
Regina Hash
Dennis Helwig
Jay Hertel
Juliet Huang
Robert Huggins
Geoff Kaplan

Shari Khaja
Scott Linaker
Danielle Lueck
Elisabeth Macrum
Tony Marek
Tim McGuine
Dennis Miller
Mike Nesbitt
Julie O'Connell
Denise O'Rand
David Perrin
Chris Pircher
David Pryor
René Revis Shingles
Paula Sammarone Turocy
Jessica Scott
Patrick Sexton
Brad Sherman
Sandra Shultz
Keith Skinner
Chad Starkey
Jennifer Street
Daniel G. Tampf
Sarah Vizza
Jaime A. Young

FOREWORD

It is no surprise that the first edition of *Athletic Training Student Primer: A Foundation for Success* enjoyed tremendous popularity amongst athletic training students. Now, by using feedback from students and certified athletic trainers, Dr. Andrew P. Winterstein has made it even better. He meticulously reviewed the entire text and improved every chapter.

This textbook is an amazingly thorough introductory book. It is rich in clinical information and helpful tips for the student. As the title implies, it provides an excellent foundation for the field of athletic training and does a great job of introducing the reader to the field. Dr. Winterstein has a knack for making this introductory material fun to learn and has written the book to encourage the student to think independently rather than just memorizing material.

Dr. Winterstein preserved the writing style from the first edition, making the text enjoyable to read and making the readers feel like they are in a conversation with him. He played off one of the strengths of the first edition and added more real-world career advice from athletic trainers. As with the first edition, he selected leaders in sports medicine and athletic training to ensure that the information would be valuable to any student. He also carefully selected feedback that is optimistic about the field of athletic training profession, revealing to the beginning student why athletic trainers find their work so enjoyable.

In the second edition, Dr. Winterstein has provided more information and details on sports medicine injuries and conditions, thus improving the content of those important chapters. He expanded the chapter on education requirements and strategies for success. There are new sections on planning, prevention, and initial care and a new chapter on taping, bracing, and basic skills. The accompanying Web site provides video instruction for these skills as well as interactive CT anatomy that is sure to get the readers' attention.

It is a privilege to write a forward to the second edition. I agree whole heartedly with Marjorie Albohm, MS, ATC/L, who wrote the forward to the first edition and stated, "Every athletic training student should read this book."

Gregory L. Landry, MD
Professor of Pediatrics and Sports Medicine
University of Wisconsin School of Medicine and Public Health
Madison, Wisconsin

PREFACE

Athletic Training Student Primer: A Foundation for Success
Prim • er *noun* 1) A book that covers the basic elements of a subject. 2) An introductory book.

RD Cummings said, "A good book has no ending." I certainly hope that is true. The *Athletic Training Student Primer* is more about beginnings than endings. My hope is that this text will help students establish a foundation for the study of athletic training and, most importantly, create a starting point for an academic and professional journey that does not end. The first edition of this text grew from my own desire to help students understand introductory athletic training content, educational requirements, and professional practice issues. At the center of this project has always been a desire to blend the technical elements of practicing athletic training with the human dimensions of being an athletic trainer. That is why core content is augmented by "real world" advice, historical tidbits, and feedback from students and professionals.

The *Athletic Training Student Primer* is designed to be the very first book in an athletic training curriculum. The second edition of the text has undergone an extensive revision. Changes include the following:

✓ A chapter-by-chapter review with more information and greater detail on specific sports medicine injuries and conditions

✓ Increased content on employment settings, including feedback from working athletic trainers

✓ Expanded resources and up-to-date information on educational requirements and strategies for success

✓ New section on planning, prevention, and initial care

✓ New chapter on taping, bracing, and basic skills that includes video instruction on the accompanying Web site

✓ Additional real-life case studies and points of historic interest

✓ Course Web site that includes basic taping skills and interactive CT anatomy

The second edition of the *Athletic Training Student Primer* is another step on my own professional journey. I liken the opportunity to share this information to having an ongoing conversation with prospective students about a topic I care about: athletic training. Thanks for joining me on this trail and I hope the information proves useful.

UNDERSTANDING ATHLETIC TRAINING

CHAPTER 1

ATHLETIC TRAINING
AN ALLIED HEALTH PROFESSION

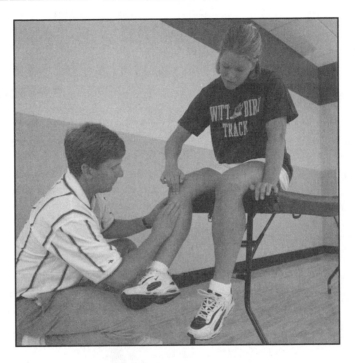

Athletic training enables one to apply a love for sport and physical activity with an expertise in health care.

David H. Perrin, PhD, ATC
Provost, University of North Carolina–Greensboro

Certified athletic trainers are unique health care providers who specialize in the prevention, assessment, treatment, and rehabilitation of injuries and illnesses. Whether certified athletic trainers are found at a high school, on the sidelines of a National Football League (NFL) contest, or working with a local sports medicine physician, the athletic trainer brings a unique perspective to the medical community. Certified athletic trainers work with more than just athletes and can be found anywhere that people are physically active.[1]

Upon completion of this chapter, the student will be able to:

✓ Be able to explain what an athletic trainer does

✓ Describe the common employment settings in which athletic trainers work

✓ Explain the value of athletic trainers to all physically active populations, not just competitive athletes

✓ Discuss how others view the athletic trainer as part of the health care community

✓ Distinguish the roles and responsibilities of an athletic trainer

✓ Describe the continuing education (CE) needs of the athletic trainer following certification

✓ Explain the various licensure and regulation standards for the practice of athletic training

✓ Identify the challenges facing athletic trainers in various work settings

✓ Appraise the demands created by balancing professional and personal obligations

AN ALLIED HEALTH PROFESSION

WHAT'S IN A NAME?

It can be trying at times. A certified athletic trainer must be in good standing with the Board of Certification (BOC) and, in most states, hold a state license to legally practice as an athletic trainer. Yet despite these requirements, when faced with the question of, "What do you do for a living?" the response of, "I'm a certified athletic trainer" is often met with a quizzical, "What's that?"

This can be bothersome; however, rather than being amazed that people know nothing about the profession, it is best to take the time to educate them. When someone says he or she is studying to be a nurse, everyone knows what that means. Athletic training, however, is fairly new and the name of the profession can be confusing for those who do not understand it. If faced with "What's that?" students (and professionals) need to be able to tell people exactly what an athletic trainer does, with whom athletic trainers work, and what it takes to become an athletic trainer. When it comes time to tell someone about athletic training, rely on the definition provided by the National Athletic Trainers' Association (NATA) (ie, the professional organization dedicated to the advancement of the profession of athletic training):

> Athletic training is practiced by athletic trainers, health care professionals who collaborate with physicians to optimize activity and participation of patients and clients. Athletic training encompasses the prevention, diagnosis, and intervention of emergency, acute, and chronic medical conditions involving impairment, functional limitations, and disabilities.[1]

The more people who understand the full dimension of an athletic trainer's role, how he or she fits into the health care picture, and the proper way to refer to this unique health care professional, the less we will hear the "What's that?" response. In fact, thanks to the growing ranks of the profession and the efforts of the NATA, *athletic training* and *certified athletic trainer* are becoming commonplace in the public lexicon.

The National Athletic Trainers' Association

The NATA is the professional membership association for certified athletic trainers and others who support the athletic training profession. Founded in 1950 (see Chapter 2), the NATA has grown to nearly 30,000 members worldwide today. While being a member of the NATA is not required (certification can be maintained with the BOC without paying NATA dues), the majority of certified athletic trainers choose to be members of the NATA to support their profession and to receive a broad array of membership benefits. The goal is to join together as a group to promote the profession of athletic training. NATA members can accomplish more for the athletic training profession through an organization than they can individually. The NATA national office currently has more than 40 full-time staff members who work to support NATA's mission:

> The mission of the NATA is to enhance the quality of health care provided by certified athletic trainers and to advance the athletic training profession.

Beyond being part of a nationwide group with the common goal of supporting athletic training, some of the individual benefits of NATA membership include the following:

✓ A subscription to the monthly *NATA News* magazine

✓ Access to the peer-reviewed, Medline-indexed *Journal of Athletic Training*

✓ Access to CE opportunities

✓ Discounted registration for the annual meeting and symposium

✓ Access to the NATA members-only section of the Web site, which includes the career center and on-line directories

✓ Various affinity programs that provide members with discounts on a range of professional services from insurance to financial planning

DEFINING OUR PROFESSION

Allied Health Professional

Athletic training is an allied health profession. When you analyze that phrase, the word that stands out is *profession*. A great deal has been written about the characteristics of a profession. By definition, a profession is an occupation that requires special academic and practical training. To "profess" implies that a profession openly declares its expertise and service for society.[2] Characteristics of athletic training as a profession include the following[3]:

Athletic Trainers—Not "Trainers"

This material was developed by the National Athletic Trainers' Association to educate the public on the difference between certified athletic trainers and personal trainers.

Look around you. The world today is on the move, and people are becoming more active, more interested, more educated. We're getting "trained" in fitness, sport, even in computers. As a result, the word *trainer* has lost its meaning. Let us see if you know the difference between a personal trainer and a certified athletic trainer.

Certified Athletic Trainer

An athletic trainer is a person who meets the qualifications set by a state regulatory board and/or the BOC Inc and practices athletic training under the direction of a physician.

Certified Athletic Trainers

- Must have at least a bachelor's degree in athletic training, which is an allied health profession
- Must pass a 3-part exam before earning the ATC credential
- Must keep their skills current by participating in CE
- Must adhere to practice guidelines set by one national certifying agency

Daily Duties

- Provide physical medicine and rehabilitation services
- Prevent, assess, and treat injuries (acute and chronic)
- Coordinate care with physicians and other allied health providers
- Work in schools, colleges, professional sports, clinics, hospitals, corporations, industry, military

Personal Trainer

A personal (fitness) trainer is a person who prescribes, monitors, and changes an individual's specific exercise program in a fitness or sport setting.

Personal Trainers

- May or may not have higher education in health sciences
- May or may not be required to obtain certification
- May or may not participate in CE
- May become certified by any one of numerous agencies that set varying education and practice requirements

Daily Duties

- Assess fitness needs and design appropriate exercise regimens
- Work with clients to achieve fitness goals
- Help educate the public about the importance of physical activity
- Work in health clubs, wellness centers, and various other locations where fitness activities take place

If you have questions about the person providing health care for you, for your student, or for a colleague, speak up! Be sure you are getting the right care for the right situation.

✓ Expertise in a body of knowledge and skills
✓ Trusteeship as guardians of this knowledge for society
✓ Professional training and certification
✓ Adherence to an ethical code of conduct
✓ Service and value of performance above reward

Certified athletic trainers are health care professionals who specialize in preventing, recognizing, managing, and rehabilitating injuries that result from physical activity. Athletic trainers are organized and, through the many activities of the NATA, serve to advance this knowledge for the general public. Athletic trainers adhere to clearly defined standards of care and follow an ethical code of conduct that places the care of their patients above their own reward. Copies of the BOC *Standards of Professional Practice* and the NATA *Code of Ethics* are provided in Appendices A and B. While it seems that athletic training easily fits the common characteristics of a profession, some elements were still missing as of the early 1990s. These include recognition from the larger medical community and an increased contribution to the body of knowledge through original research.

In June 1990, the American Medical Association (AMA) officially recognized athletic training as an allied health profession. As a young profession that only had its formal organized origins in the 1950s, AMA recognition was a historic achievement.

The need to increase the amount of original research in the profession was directly addressed by the formation of the National Athletic Trainers' Association-Research and Education Foundation (NATA-REF) in 1991. The primary aim of the foundation is encouraging scientific research among professionals such as certified athletic trainers who focus on improving the health care of the physically active population. The NATA-REF strategies to achieve this goal include the following[4]:

✓ Advance the knowledge base of the athletic training profession

✓ Encourage research among athletic trainers who can contribute to the athletic training knowledge base

✓ Provide forums for the exchange of ideas pertaining to the athletic training knowledge base

✓ Facilitate the presentation of programs and the production of materials, providing learning opportunities about athletic training topics

✓ Provide scholarships for undergraduate and graduate students of athletic training

✓ Plan and implement an ongoing total development program that establishes endowment funds, as well as restricted and unrestricted funds, that will support the research and educational goals of the Foundation

The NATA-REF has made a tremendous impact on building a research culture in athletic training. Since the first NATA-REF grants were funded in 1991, well over 2.25 million dollars of research funding has been awarded.[4] The growing presence of athletic training research scientists at top-tier institutions allows the next generation of scientists to take athletic training research to new heights. Athletic trainers are competing for and landing federal dollars to examine a range of research questions. Continued advancements of athletic training research are essential for further recognition of the profession across the scientific and health care communities.

Physical Activity

Physical activity has always been a cornerstone in helping define the athletic training profession. Athletic trainers can apply their expertise to all active people, not just the traditional competitive athlete. Athletic trainers are valuable health care providers and defining their scope of practice is essential to establishing their place in the broader health care picture. Words like *athlete* and *physical activity* are present in many laws that dictate athletic training practice at the state level and therefore, the NATA has issued a position on the definition of physical activity. That position states that physical activity consists of athletic, recreational, or occupational activities that require physical skills and utilize strength, power, endurance, speed, flexibility, range of motion (ROM), or agility.[5] This definition clearly addresses the evolving role of the athletic trainer as a care provider who works with more than just athletes.

In 2007, the NATA Board of Directors voted to remove "physical activity" from the mission statement and updated the definition of athletic training to include broader terminology in the description of the athletic trainer's role as part of a health care team. The athletic trainer's level of state regulation (see Regulation of Athletic Training Practice on p. 15) will continue to guide the boundaries of professional practice. While athletes and physically active people have been the cornerstone of our practice and expertise, new generations of athletic trainers should challenge these traditional definitions and provide their expertise to a broader range of practice. Change can be a bit painful and other professions may view the growing role of the athletic trainer with skepticism. However, if a professional is well educated, has a market for his or her skills, practices within the law and in an ethical manner, he or she will be on solid footing. Athletic training is such a profession.

THE BOARD OF CERTIFICATION

The BOC has been responsible for the certification of athletic trainers since 1969. Upon its inception, the BOC was an entity of the NATA. However, in 1989, the BOC became an independent, nonprofit corporation. The mission of the BOC is, "To certify athletic trainers and to identify, for the public, quality health care professionals through a system of certification, adjudication, standards of practice and continuing competency programs."

The BOC provides a certification program for the entry-level athletic trainer and establishes requirements for maintaining status as a Certified Athletic Trainer (AT). A 9-member Board of Directors governs the BOC. There are 6 athletic trainer directors, 1 physician director, 1 public director, and 1 corporate/educational director.

Describing Athletic Training

Describing athletic training to someone who is unfamiliar with the profession can be challenging. The comments below address this very issue.

Q: How do you describe athletic training to a prospective student or someone who does not know what athletic trainers do?

A: I make sure that students understand athletic training is a health care profession. I talk to students to try and understand why they're interested in the profession. Students often give me a standard response of "I like athletics." I want them to understand it's more than that; this is a health care profession that is academically challenging. Students who enter this profession, like any other health profession, must be able to use and apply what they learn in the classroom and laboratory in order to provide the highest quality professional health care to their patients. Athletic training is not simply a job, it is a profession, and like any profession it takes dedication and commitment in order to achieve and maintain the knowledge and skill your patients expect.

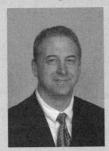

Patrick J. Sexton, EdD, ATC/R, CSCS

Associate Professor and Director of Athletic Training Education

Minnesota State University, Mankato

Mankato, MN

A: An athletic trainer is a health care professional who is skilled in the techniques of prevention, assessment, treatment, and rehabilitation of musculoskeletal conditions and related problems. Athletic trainers are employed throughout health care, providing services to physically active people of all ages. They are the primary health care providers for athletes at the secondary school level, college and university, and professional sports level. They work closely with physicians and bring a team approach to injury and illness management. Athletic trainers are known for their aggressive approach to injury management and rehabilitation, returning people quickly and safely to full preinjury functional levels.

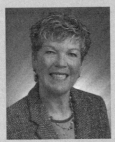

Marjorie Albohm, MS ATC/L

President, National Athletic Trainers' Association

Sports Medicine Consultant

Indianapolis, IN

A certified athletic trainer must pass a comprehensive examination administered by the BOC. The certification exam is composed of multiple choice as well as hybrid-style questions. Hybrid questions may include scenarios, images, and/or video to assess the candidate's knowledge and clinical decision-making and application abilities. The BOC exam assesses a candidate's knowledge of athletic training within the framework of the 6 domains of athletic training as defined by the *Role Delineation Study*. The *Role Delineation Study* is a survey of entry-level athletic trainers' professional duties and responsibilities. The results define the content areas and skills needed in the practice of athletic training. This study provides the framework for the certification examination.

Developing a fair and comprehensive examination is no small task. The questions are written, validated, and reviewed by a panel of content experts in coordination with psychometricians (those who specialize in the design, administration, and interpretation of quantitative tests for the measurement of specific variables). Each question is referenced to at least 2 textbooks that can be found in the BOC listing of exam references (available for viewing at the BOC Web site at www.bocatc.org). The exam items are repeatedly edited by the item writing teams for clarity and content.[6]

The 6 domains of athletic training identified in the *Role Delineation Study* and the percentage of exam questions dedicated to each domain are as follows[7]:

1. Prevention and risk management (15.72%)
2. Clinical evaluation and diagnosis (22.91%)
3. Immediate care (17.5%)
4. Treatment, rehabilitation, and reconditioning (23.31%)
5. Organization and administration (11.29%)
6. Professional development responsibility (9.27%)

The certification process assures that entry-level professionals have met a standard of minimum competency. Only those who pass can call themselves certified athletic trainers and use the "ATC" or "CAT" designation. A detailed discussion of the educational preparation that allows students to sit for the certification exam and a greater discussion of the exam process is provided in Chapter 3.

Domains and Competencies

These is sometimes confusion between the "domains" of athletic training and the content areas that make up the Athletic Training Educational Competencies. There are 12 content areas (outlined in Chapter 3) that make up the educational competencies presented in accredited athletic training education programs. The 6 domains of athletic training are the areas covered in the *Role Delineation Study*. Students should think of the content areas and educational competencies as foundational knowledge while the role delineation domains are practice areas.

PROFESSIONAL PRACTICE DOMAINS AND WORK ENVIRONMENTS

Athletic trainers can be found in a variety of employment settings (see p. 11) that will require them to provide health care particular to the needs of their patients in that setting. One constant for athletic trainers in all settings is the supervision and guidance provided by physicians (Figure 1-1). Athletic trainers, like other allied health professionals, work under the direction of a licensed physician. Practice domains for the athletic trainer cross all employment boundaries, outline the general roles and responsibilities the athletic trainer fulfills as a health care provider, and are reflective of the scope of the athletic trainer's duties. Each domain outlined next has been identified from the *Role Delineation Study*.[7]

Prevention and Risk Management

It is appropriate that the domain of prevention falls at the top of the list since a large portion of what athletic trainers do involves working to prevent or minimize injury. Prevention and risk management can take several forms. Communicating and educating patients, parents, administrators, coaches, and other health care providers about the risk associated with activity are key components of prevention. Athletic trainers must understand the pre-participation screening process to help identify the conditions that place participants at risk. The athletic trainer must be able to fit and use protective equipment, develop and apply taping and bracing techniques, design and implement conditioning programs, and promote nutritional practices to help maintain a healthy lifestyle. Athletic trainers must identify environmental risk factors and properly maintain the environment in which they practice. All of these tasks are examples of how athletic trainers work to deter injury in their daily duties.

Clinical Evaluation and Diagnosis

The athletic trainer must possess the ability to recognize, evaluate, and diagnose injuries and illnesses. These clinical skills allow the practitioner to fulfill a variety of essential functions. Determining appropriate referral, establishing immediate treatment needs, and monitoring the progress of rehabilitation programs all require the use of evaluative skills. Physical examination skills require a strong working knowledge of anatomy, the mechanics of injury, and the appropriate use of "hands-on" skills. An athletic trainer must be able to take a medical history, observe for signs of injury and illness, use his or her hands to feel for structural abnormalities, evaluate joint stability and muscle function, and apply specific functional tests to determine the status of a patient.

Students often find learning the steps involved in clinical assessment and the hands-on practice of these skills one of the highlights of an athletic training education program (see Chapter 4).

Immediate Care

The immediate care of injuries requires the athletic trainer to be able to quickly and calmly activate an established emergency action plan, initiate life-saving procedures like cardiopulmonary resuscitation (CPR), use appropriate emergency equipment, and communicate effectively with others in emergency situations. The athletic trainer must be prepared to take a leadership role in an emergency or act as a member of a response team in carrying out an emergency action plan. Athletic health care professionals must maintain

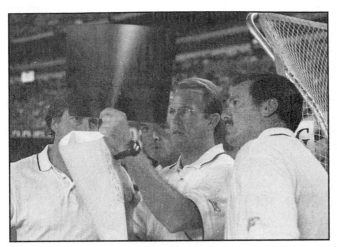

Figure 1-1. The relationship between the team physician and the athletic trainer is the cornerstone of the sports medicine team. (Courtesy of Jim Beiver and the Green Bay Packers Football Club.)

current certification in emergency skills and be prepared to activate those skills at a moment's notice.

Treatment, Rehabilitation, and Reconditioning

Athletic trainers must use their skills and knowledge to determine the best course of treatment for specific injuries and illnesses. The athletic trainer, working under the direction of a physician, can administer therapeutic exercises and modalities in the interest of facilitating his or her patient's recovery and return to function. The athletic trainer must work closely with the physician to determine when the patient can return to activity. In many employment settings, the athletic trainer will work alongside other allied health professionals, such as a physical therapist, over the course of treatment and rehabilitation. A significant portion of the athletic trainer's expertise lies in his or her ability to understand the demands of the patient's physical activity or competitive sport. The athletic trainer is the only health care professional in a position to deal with the athlete from the time of the initial injury throughout the period of rehabilitation until the athlete's complete, unrestricted return to practice or competition.

Organization and Administration

The role of the athletic trainer has been likened to a gatekeeper. The athletic trainer must interact with a wide variety of individuals, organizations, and health care personnel in providing care for his or her patients. This gatekeeper role includes managing information, developing procedures, understanding insurance guidelines, communicating effectively, adhering to state regulations, and maintaining medical records. These are just some of the organizational and administrative tasks associated with athletic training. The ability to delegate responsibilities, communicate, and manage multiple tasks while at the same time provide the best possible patient care requires exceptional organizational skills.

Professional Development and Responsibility

As a professional, an athletic trainer must be dedicated to improving his or her knowledge over the course of his or her career and practicing in a responsible fashion. Once a student becomes a certified athletic trainer, he or she must meet specific CE requirements set forth by the BOC in order to maintain his or her credential. An athletic trainer who participates in CE, adheres to the *Standards of Professional Practice*, follows the NATA *Code of Ethics*, and obeys state regulations serves the profession and the interests of the public. The public is entitled to the protection that comes with highly educated and ethical health care providers. It is possible to have your certification revoked. Appendix C outlines the items that may cause an athletic trainer to lose his or her certification standing with the BOC.

It is also the professional responsibility of an Athletic trainer to serve as a guardian to the knowledge unique to his or her profession.[3] In this role, the athletic trainer must be an educator. He or she must educate patients, employers, other health care professionals, and the greater public to the domains and practices of the athletic trainer. It is the responsibility of the athletic trainer to provide stewardship to the profession and advance it for the next generation of health care providers. This can only be achieved through responsible professional practice.

Continuing Education

CE requirements are meant to insure that Athletic trainers stay current in the field of athletic training. The purpose of CE is to insure Athletic trainers:

- ✓ Obtain current professional development information
- ✓ Explore new knowledge in specific content areas
- ✓ Master new athletic training-related skills and techniques
- ✓ Expand approaches to effective athletic training
- ✓ Further develop professional judgment
- ✓ Conduct professional practice in an ethical and appropriate manner

Recertification Requirements

All certified athletic trainers (ATs) must complete the following recertification requirements to maintain their certified athletic trainer credential. The requirements for recertification include the following:

Adherence to the BOC *Standards of Professional Practice*

Certified ATs are expected to comply with the BOC *Standards of Professional Practice* at all times. A copy of the document is available on the BOC Web site at www.bocatc.org.

Submission of the BOC Annual Certification Fee

Every AT is required to pay an annual certification fee to the BOC. The annual certification fee is an administrative fee that supports the activities required of the BOC. Fee payments are collected by one of the following methods:

- NATA members: If membership dues are current, the certification fee is included in your membership dues (ie, the NATA pays the fee to the BOC)
- Nonmembers of the NATA: Invoice is mailed directly to each nonmember by October 31st for the current year's fee

Maintenance of Emergency Cardiac Care

ATs must be able to demonstrate ongoing certification in the competencies outlined in the BOC emergency cardiac care (ECC) guidelines throughout the reporting period. Continuing education units (CEUs) are not awarded for maintaining ECC.

NOTE: ECC certification must be current each year. Depending on the ECC provider, ECC recertification may not be required each year.

ECC must include the following:

- Adult CPR
- Automated external defibrillation (AED)
- Pediatric CPR
- Airway obstruction
- 2nd rescuer CPR
- Barrier devices (eg, pocket mask, bag valve mask)

Acceptable ECC providers are those adhering to the most current *International Guidelines for Cardiopulmonary Resuscitation and Emergency Cardiac Care*.

Examples of courses that provide the above requirements include, but are not limited to:

- CPR/AED for the Professional Rescuer through the American Red Cross
- BLS Health care Provider through the American Heart Association

NOTE: Online courses are only acceptable if the practical portion is tested with an instructor.

The BOC reserves the right to request ECC documentation at any time; this includes, but is not limited to, the BOC audit. The only acceptable documentation is the original certification card(s) OR a photocopy (front and back) of the certification card(s) obtained upon successful completion of the ECC course. The card(s) must be signed by the instructor and the card holder. Letters provided by instructors are not acceptable forms of documentation. Instructor cards are not acceptable.

Completion and Reporting of Continuing Education Units

ATs must complete a predetermined number of CEUs within a given time period. CE requirements are intended to promote continued competence, development of current knowledge and skills, and enhancement of professional skills and judgment beyond the levels required for entry-level practice. CE activities must focus on increasing knowledge, skills, and abilities related to the practice of athletic training.

a. CEUs/Contact Hours—CEUs are based on contact hours. Contact hours are defined as the number of actual clock hours spent in direct participation in a structured education format as a learner. One (1) CEU is equivalent to one (1) contact hour. CEUs will be awarded only for activities that are completed within your reporting period. CEUs in excess of the amount required cannot be carried over for credit in subsequent reporting periods. CEUs cannot be earned prior to certification.
(continued)

Recertification Requirements (continued)

b. Documentation—Original documentation confirming participation in an activity must be kept for one (1) year after the reporting period has ended (see category description for documentation specifics).

c. Mandatory Audit—A percentage of individuals submitting the CE Reporting Sheet will be randomly chosen for audit. Audited individuals will be required to submit their original documentation to the BOC for review. Detailed instructions pertaining to the auditing process will be provided to audited individuals. A response to the audit notification is due within 45 days of the receipt of notification. The BOC reserves the right to audit any individual at any time.

d. Change of Address—Changes in mailing address must be provided to the BOC. Failure to keep the mailing address current can result in suspension or revocation of certification. You can keep your address updated by logging onto www.bocatc.org.

e. *Role Delineation Study, Fifth Edition*—The *Role Delineation Study, Fifth Edition* defines the current entry-level knowledge, skills, and abilities required for practice in the profession of athletic training. It contains the entry-level standards of practice, the domains of athletic training, an entry-level job analysis, and a review of literature containing over 450 publications. In addition to serving as the blueprint for the BOC exam, it serves as a guide in determining relevant content areas for CE activities. Copies of the *Role Delineation Study, Fifth Edition* may be ordered online at www.bocatc.org.

Recording Continuing Education Information
It is the responsibility of each AT to document CE activities.

There are 2 methods to report CE:

- Submit CE on the BOC Web site using ATC Online at www.bocatc.org. There is no cost to use ATC Online.
- Report CE via mail. The CE Reporting Sheet can be used to record and submit documentation of activities. However, there is a $25 processing charge for all paper submissions. The reporting sheet can be found at www.bocatc.org.

BOC Recertification Requirements updated February 2008. Adapted with permission from the Board of Certification. Available at http://www.bocatc.org/images/stories/athletic_trainers/recertificationrequirements2006-2011.pdf. Accessed March 1, 2008

Certified athletic trainers are required to obtain 75 CEUs every 3 years. One CEU unit equals 1 hour of CE contact. Athletic trainers can obtain CE by attending symposiums, taking courses, and participating in a variety of professional endeavors. At the conclusion of each 3-year term, Athletic trainers must meet requirements that include the following:

- ✓ Completion of a predetermined number of CEUs including recertification in CPR at least once in the 3 years. CPR must be current at the time the CEU report is submitted.
- ✓ Adherence to the NATA-BOC *Standards of Professional Practice*.
- ✓ Submission of annual NATA-BOC certification fee or payment of NATA annual dues.
- ✓ Maintenance of the CE folder.

See Appendix C for information on obtaining CE in athletic training.

EMPLOYMENT SETTINGS FOR THE ATHLETIC TRAINER

Athletic trainers can be found in a range of employment settings. While the profession has its origins in the intercollegiate settings (see Chapter 2), the past 25 years have seen tremendous growth into all areas of health care where patients can benefit from the unique skills athletic trainers offer. The NATA keeps up-to-date data on salaries for athletic trainers. Results of recent salary survey results are available to members through the NATA at www.nata.org. An overview of salary information for athletic training is also provided by the Bureau of Labor Statistics in the *Occupational Outlook Handbook* available at www.bls.gov/oco. Many factors can influence salary Figures and some data presented are not representative of full-time employment. Students must keep these facts in mind when reviewing this data.

> ℹ️ Descriptions of athletic training work settings are provided below. To supplement this material, a number of Career Boxes are sprinkled throughout the text. These boxes provide insight into a variety of athletic training employment settings from practicing athletic trainers.

PROFESSIONAL SPORTS

One of the highest profile positions in the profession of athletic training is with a professional sports team. However, there are only a small number of professional sports teams available that hire athletic trainers. The various major professional sports leagues have athletic training organizations with a rich history of supporting education. Athletic training students may have the opportunity to experience the professional setting through an internship program offered by the Professional Baseball Athletic Trainers Society (PBATS). It is common for professional teams in the NFL to provide internship opportunities during summer training camps, and the National Basketball Association (NBA) athletic trainers host educational sessions for students at the NATA's annual symposium.

Athletic trainers also provide their expertise to the Association of Tennis Professionals (ATP), Professional Golf Association (PGA), Ladies Professional Golf Association (LPGA), the Professional Rodeo Tour, Women's National Basketball Association (WNBA), professional soccer, and automobile racing.

COLLEGES AND UNIVERSITIES

The origin of the NATA rests with a collection of athletic trainers who provided care in the collegiate setting. It was in this setting that the profession began to be recognized as an integral part of the sports medicine team (see Chapter 2). There are a wide range of positions available in the collegiate and university environment. From the small liberal arts college with a nonscholarship athletic program to the National Collegiate Athletic Association (NCAA) Division 1 major-college sports programs, a wide variety of sports medicine programs employ athletic trainers. It is commonplace for a head athletic trainer or director of athletic training services to lead such a program and assistants to round out the sports medicine staff providing health care services to the student-athlete.

A growing number of colleges and universities also provide athletic training services to the general student population through an intramural sports program or through the university health center. This care is provided in the spirit of extending health care to all individuals involved in physical activity, not just the student-athlete.

Colleges and universities make up the most common clinical education and field experience settings for athletic training students. It is important that universities do not view the athletic training student as a replacement for qualified staff. Increased attention to medical coverage issues and an emphasis on the proper role of the athletic training student may lead to the creation of more athletic training employment opportunities in the college and university setting.

SECONDARY SCHOOLS

The number of high schools that have the services of an athletic trainer has grown considerably. Despite this growth, there is still a recognized need to improve the daily availability of the athletic trainer in this setting. There are several models to place an Athletic trainer into the high school environment. Some high schools hire a full-time athletic trainer not unlike the model used in a college. In fact, some high schools have expanded programs to include assistant athletic trainers. Some high schools will hire a teacher/athletic trainer. This model requires the athletic trainer to teach specific courses and provide athletic training services. This model can be very time intensive. It is best to negotiate a reduced teaching load to make the workload more manageable. A common model to provide care to the intercollegiate athlete is for an individual school or school district to contract with a sports medicine clinic to provide athletic training coverage. These contracts may vary from an athletic trainer who visits a school a few times a week to an athletic trainer who provides daily health care services.

In 1996, the American Academy of Pediatrics (AAP) asked the AMA to support activities and efforts to place certified athletic trainers in all secondary schools. This resolution was amended in 1998. It supports the establishment of athletic medicine units in any school supporting a sports program; a physician and an allied health coordinator, preferably a certified athletic trainer, should lead these units.

ATHLETIC TRAINING EDUCATOR

The role of the athletic training educator can take on many dimensions. Athletic trainers employed in various clinical settings may serve as supervisors or clinical instructors as part of an athletic training education program. It is not uncommon for smaller schools to have positions that are split between clinical care and instruction in an athletic training program. Teaching, research, coordination of clinical education, and program administration are common duties of the athletic trainer in an academic appointment position. It is also not uncommon for athletic trainers to gather clinical experience prior to making a transition to the academic environment. Qualifications for such

Athletic Training "In the Spotlight"

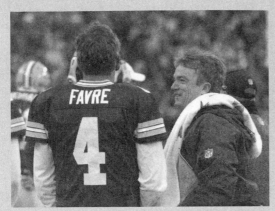

Photo courtesy of Jim Beiver and the Green Bay Packers Football Club.

Q & A with Pepper Burruss

Head Athletic Trainer

Green Bay Packers—NFL

Pepper Burruss, a certified athletic trainer and physical therapist, joined the Green Bay Packers in 1993 following 16 seasons with the New York Jets as an assistant athletic trainer. Burruss was hired by the Jets in 1977 after receiving his bachelor of science degree in physical therapy from Northwestern University Medical School. One year earlier, he had graduated with honors from Purdue University, where he earned a bachelor of arts degree in health and safety education.

He has served 2 terms on the executive committee of the Professional Football Athletic Trainers Society (PFATS), first as an AFC assistant athletic trainer representative, then as the NFC head athletic trainer representative. He was one of two NFL athletic trainers appointed to join a distinguished group of physicians serving on the NFL Cervical Spine Committee. Their goal was to review current research and recommend state-of-the-art cervical spine emergency response procedures in the NFL arena. Previously, he has served as the PFATS representative to the NATA Inter-Association Spine Task Force, which has created guidelines for the appropriate care of the spine-injured athlete and distributed that information across the country in the form of published guidelines, a videotape series, and numerous educational seminars.

A gifted public speaker, Burruss has lectured at 7 NATA Clinical Symposia; multiple state, district, and college meetings; as well as numerous service organizations throughout Wisconsin.

A product of Wappingers Falls, NY, where he attended Ketcham High School, he was inducted into the school's hall of fame in 2000. Born Thomas Pepper Burruss in Beacon, NY, he and his wife, Nancy, have one son, Shane, and one daughter, Christina. Also a medical practitioner, Nancy is an Associate Professor and Director of the Undergraduate Program at the Bellin College of Nursing in Green Bay.

Q: As a head athletic trainer in the NFL, describe some of the general duties you are responsible for in the course of your job.

A: Certainly, the every day care of sports injuries from preparticipation evaluations to being present on the field, through the acute care and evaluation of an injury to the eventual rehabilitation phase. Some of the misunderstood aspects of the NFL sports medicine environment are the responsibilities that make it a "year round" job. Our involvement in the college draft evaluations, the Free Agency physicals, the off-season conditioning program coupled with the customary off-season rehabilitation, mini camps, and administrative duties such as staff evaluations, budget preparation, and injury analysis all make for a busy "nonseason."

Q: In your 30+ years in the league, what are some of the biggest advancements in sports medicine that you have observed? Which of these do you feel has had the greatest impact in assisting the athletic trainer in providing care to his or her patients?

A: The "scope" (arthroscopy) and magnetic resonance imaging (MRI) are now a part of everyday sports talk, but 30 years ago they were not; in fact, the words *sports medicine* did not ring out as they do today. The exponential growth in quality education and research have borne advances in all facets of sports medicine. Certainly, the impact of the computer, not only in everyday life, but in the athletic training room cannot be over looked. The future of computer and video-aided analysis is endless and beyond what we might comprehend at this time.

Q: You were an assistant with the New York Jets when Dennis Byrd had a spinal cord injury in 1992. His recovery is well documented as he was able to walk unassisted onto the field for the opening day ceremonies in 1993. Dennis Byrd publicly credited the sports medicine team with helping to save his life through their swift and efficient emergency response. Explain how that situation influenced you as a professional and how it influences your preparation today.

(continued)

Athletic Training "In the Spotlight" (continued)

A: It made me feel blessed as the outcome was so positive but could have turned out totally different with virtually the same exact care. He was both lucky and blessed as his injury was incomplete, he had excellent care, and was a motivated patient. How did it influence me? There is not a football game since that I do not give thanks for his recovery and I ask that should a like situation present itself, I remain calm, trust my education, and make good decisions. It also reinforced the adage, "You hope for the best but prepare for the worst."

Q: In the state of Wisconsin, there was no bigger sports icon than Brett Favre. The recently retired-returned-and retired again quarterback has started 269 consecutive regular season games. What was it like for you and your medical team to deal with the spotlight that was cast on him anytime he was injured? To what do you credit his longevity in a sport with so many injuries?

A: Early on in his career, it was like any other "valuable player" on your team whereas there was some perceived extra pressure to "get him well." As his career progressed and his legend grew, we grew accustomed to his toughness and will to play, almost to a fault, thinking, "No matter what we do, he will play." He was a special teammate, "one of a kind" and our staff only accepts a small amount of credit for his well being. He was not afforded any special care that would not be given to any other teammate.

Q: What injuries or conditions that you encounter are still in need of further study? Which ones do you feel we still do not understand well enough? What areas would you like to see more research, specific to the athletes you care for?

A: There are the rote answers like nutrition, supplements, visual and cognitive training that all can be studied. It is hard to tell what injury today might be the "ACL of yesteryear" (whereas 30 years ago the ligament was either ignored or augmented with extra-articular support). Certainly, central nervous system (CNS) injuries (brain and spinal cord) remain "mysterious" and are hot topics. Likewise, the hip/groin/abdominal research is burgeoning with all of the "core" attention. To me, the award-winning product or technique will be when a functional evaluation, to objectively evaluate one's sports-specific functional capability (or rehabilitation status), is discovered and perfected.

positions range from possession of a master's degree to doctoral requirements for faculty positions.

The research, publication, teaching, and administration requirements of holding a faculty position vary greatly by institution. The demands of administering an athletic training education program may present unique challenges to faculty seeking tenure at the university level. It is imperative for prospective athletic training educators to understand the mission and expectations of their institution prior to committing to a faculty position.

CLINICS AND HOSPITALS

The clinical setting now represents the largest employment segment for athletic trainers. Thirty-two percent of certified athletic trainers work in a clinical environment or a clinic/high school combined environment.[8] Many Athletic trainers in the clinical setting contract outreach services to local high schools. Sports medicine clinics may be affiliated with educational institutions or be completely private and owned by an athletic trainer, physical therapist, or physician. The practice regulations in the clinical setting may require the Athletic trainer to work under the supervision of a physical therapist for the purpose of billing for service. However, significant progress has been made in establishing AMA Current Protocol Terminology

(CPT) billing codes for athletic training services.[9] As regulations and billing practices change, the role of the Athletic trainer in this environment will continue to grow. Several states are working with models for reimbursement by a third-party payer (ie, insurance company) for athletic training services. This topic is of such importance that the NATA maintains an advisory council on reimbursement issues.

The athletic trainer in the clinical setting often takes on the role of physician extender. Physicians often hire athletic trainers to provide patient intake and triage, exercise prescription, rehabilitation, and patient education.[10] Athletic trainers often enjoy the positive professional relationships found working with a variety of health care personnel in the clinical environment. In addition, some clinical employment settings may offer work hours and duties that adhere to a more consistent schedule than other settings.

CORPORATE INDUSTRIAL SETTINGS

One of the newest employment settings to utilize the expertise of the athletic trainer is the corporate industrial clinical setting. These positions provide Athletic trainers the opportunity to work with employees in physically active job environments. Corporations often have on-site workplace clinics that deal with injuries and rehabilitation associated with

Salaries

Salaries for athletic trainers vary by job setting, region, rural versus metropolitan, and a host of personal factors. Students should carefully investigate a range of job settings and a variety of geographic locations to get an accurate reflection of current salaries. Similar positions may vary by as much as $5000 to $10,000 from state to state. However, money is not always the largest determinant of job satisfaction. Athletic training salaries have shown steady improvement. However, athletic training is like many areas of health care and education where motivators other than money attract students to the field. Athletic trainers deserve, and must demand, competitive salaries. A job that pays too low will only improve if people will not accept an unfair wage.

Consult the following resources to learn more about wages in your geographic area:

- NATA (www.nata.org): The NATA routinely performs salary surveys for all settings and areas of the country.

- United States Department of Labor Bureau of Labor Statistics (www.bls.gov): This government agency has wage information available for multiple health care professions (the athletic training code is 299091). Users can create their own search parameters to create national or state profiles for any profession.

the physical nature of some jobs. An emphasis is also placed on preventing injury and promoting healthy lifestyles among employees. The athletic trainer as a skilled practitioner in this area is well suited to apply his or her skills to this unique population. Automobile companies, manufacturing, and other occupations that require physically active employees have been some of the first to recognize the value of the athletic trainer.

MILITARY AND LAW ENFORCEMENT

Athletic trainers can now be found utilizing their skills in providing care for individuals in physically demanding professions like the military and law enforcement. Both areas involve demanding training periods and injuries are common. If fact, long before athletic trainers were present in military settings, injury data was often collected in "boot camp" environments. In the Armed Forces, athletic trainers work on and off base in fitness and wellness centers, new recruit readiness programs, pre-enlistment readiness programs, initial entry training, and advanced initial

training. They work as part of a health care team and generally are part of the civilian workforce. Athletic trainers are currently working for the Marines, Navy SEALS, US Coast Guard, US Army, the Federal Law Enforcement Training Center, and the Fairfax County Police Department.[11]

AN EVOLVING ROLE FOR THE ATHLETIC TRAINER

The profession of athletic training may have originated in settings that focused on team sports and educational settings, yet recent data demonstrate that has changed. Only 34% of certified members of the NATA currently work in the university, college, junior college, or high school setting. Sixty-three percent are employed in a clinic, hospital, industrial, corporate, or private setting.[8] The next generation of athletic trainers will need to be prepared to work in settings outside of the traditional athletic environment. The growing acceptance and understanding of physical activity as a cornerstone to a healthy lifestyle places the athletic trainer in a position to provide expertise to a larger segment of the health care community.

What will be the next employment setting to benefit from the expertise of the Athletic trainer? The answer is only limited by the creativity and entrepreneurship of the individual. Providing practitioners practice within the boundaries of their state regulation, the possibilities are endless. Growing numbers of athletic trainers can currently be found working with the arts in the areas of music and dance. Athletic trainers have provided care and technical information to performers in many environments, including television and motion pictures. Some Athletic trainers are applying their skills to professional auto racing teams. Many athletic trainers have used their allied health background and interpersonal skills to carve out successful careers in medical and pharmaceutical sales. Wherever people can benefit from a skilled and versatile health care practitioner, there is promise for the athletic trainer.

REGULATION OF ATHLETIC TRAINING PRACTICE

The completion of the certification exam alone does not fully define the right to practice athletic training. The regulation of the practice of any allied health profession is the responsibility of the state. Athletic trainers are subject to practice acts that vary from state to state regarding the scope and allowable practice of athletic training. Forty-six states currently regulate the practice of athletic training (Table 1-1). Athletic

Table 1-1
Athletic Training Regulation by State

Licensure

Arizona	Kansas	North Dakota	Washington	Alabama	Maine
Arkansas	Massachusetts	Connecticut	Michigan	Rhode Island	Delaware
Mississippi	Tennessee	South Dakota	Missouri	Texas	Florida
Nebraska	Montana	Florida	Georgia	New Hampshire	Vermont
Florida	New Mexico	Virginia	Idaho	Oklahoma	New Jersey
Illinois	Wisconsin	Indiana	Nevada	Iowa	North Carolina

Certification

Kentucky	Louisiana	New York	Pennsylvania	South Carolina

Registration

Minnesota	Oregon

Exemption

Colorado	Hawaii	Wyoming

No Regulation

Alaska	California	Maryland	West Virginia

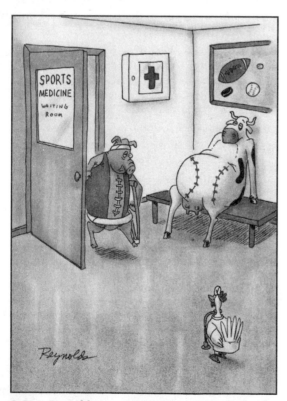

© **Dan Reynolds.** www.cartoonstock.com

The purpose of regulation is two-fold. It is designed to protect the public by insuring that professionals who practice athletic training have met a minimum level of preparation. Regulation also protects the profession by insuring that only properly trained and credentialed practitioners may use the title of athletic trainer or certified athletic trainer (ATC or CAT). The 4 most common forms of regulation are licensure, certification, registration, and exemption.

LICENSURE

States that license athletic training have established regulations that define the scope of professional practice for Athletic trainers. These laws, overseen by a state licensing board, prohibit the practice of athletic training by individuals who do not hold a license. Despite similarities that may exist from state to state, it is the individual licensing board that carries the greatest influence on the interpretation rules and the practice of athletic training in a given state with a licensure law.[12] While most adhere to the same minimum requirements established by the NATA-BOC, some states have established their own certification examination and their own CE requirements. The fee for a license can also vary from under $50 in some states to a few hundred dollars in others.

trainers and new graduates should be familiar with state regulations before practicing in a new state. This includes graduate assistants.

CERTIFICATION

Certification is a form of title protection that certifies that an Athletic trainer has met the basic requirements to perform the duties of an athletic trainer. The BOC is a certifying agency most commonly associated with these requirements. A state may pass a practice act that requires a form of credentialing much like a licensure law must be passed. Certification laws are considered less stringent than licensure in that they only protect the title and minimum requirements to hold a credential. They do not help define the duties that can be carried out in the practice of the profession.[4]

REGISTRATION

Registration laws require that qualified athletic trainers register with the state in order to practice athletic training. This registration is a form of title protection. Only qualified professionals may register, call themselves athletic trainers, and therefore practice in that state. Registration laws usually outline the minimum educational requirements to qualify for registration (ie, BOC certification). Like certification, the law does not define the scope of practice for the profession and is therefore not restrictive.

EXEMPTION

Exemption laws allow athletic trainers to practice the profession without violating the practice act of other medical and health professions. These laws are designed to prevent conflict with the existing practice acts of physicians, physical therapists, physician assistants, and other allied health professionals. Athletic trainers practicing in states with exemption laws are still subject to standards and qualifications designed to qualify for the exemption.

CHALLENGES FACING ATHLETIC TRAINING

Athletic training, like any profession, faces many challenges as it grows and moves forward. What was once a small profession with approximately 125 members attending the first meeting in 1950 is now a complex group of health care providers that numbers in excess of 30,000. There are issues unique to individual work settings that center on hours, salary, and working relationships. There are broader questions that are of concern to the profession as a whole (eg, reimbursement for services, regulation and licensure, education reform, the athletic trainer's scope

Regulation and the Athletic Training Student

The practice acts enacted in 46 states are designed to preserve and promote health and safety for the public by regulating the profession of athletic training. The majority of these acts exempt athletic training students from compliance, thus allowing them to carry out specific tasks in an educational setting as part of a program preparing them for certification. Athletic training students may be required to identify themselves as a student to meet the requirements of the law (ie, a nametag). Examples include the following:

- Anyone following a supervised course of study leading to a degree or registration as an athletic trainer in an accredited or approved educational program if the person is identified by a title that clearly indicates student or trainee status is exempt from the registration law in the state of Oregon.[1]
- The subchapter of the athletic trainers affiliated credentialing board does not require a license under this subchapter for any of the following:
  - An athletic training student practicing athletic training within the scope of the student's education or training, if he or she clearly indicates that he or she is an athletic training student.[2]

References

1. Oregon Health Licensing Agency (OHLA) Board of Athletic Trainers. www.oregon.gov/OHLA/AT/ Accessed March 2008.
2. Wisconsin State Statute Chapter 448 Medical Practices: Subchapter VI Athletic Trainers Affiliated Credentialing Board.

of practice, and many others). Students can make better decisions regarding their course of study and their career goals by understanding these issues.

PROFESSIONAL QUALITY OF LIFE ISSUES

The issue of burnout among athletic trainers has long been a concern in some employment settings. In a 1996 report by the NATA College/University Athletic Trainers Committee, more than 60% reported work overload. The volume of the work is not the only issue; the nature of the Athletic trainer's job is also a factor in his or her satisfaction. The 1996 report also noted that job responsibilities were varied and sometimes in conflict with written job descriptions. Burnout has

Challenges Facing Athletic Training

Q: What are the challenges facing the athletic training profession?

A: One of the greatest challenges that continues to face our profession is professional recognition and credibility. Unfortunately, for those who are not familiar with the qualifications and skills of an athletic trainer, the title "athletic trainer" can be somewhat misleading. As a profession, we need to continually strive to educate the public, schools, and legislators regarding the unique skills and knowledge base of certified athletic trainers, and the critical role they play in the health care of the physically active. As many high schools around the country do not have the services of a certified athletic trainer, this is an area that I believe it is particularly important for us to focus on. Advancing the knowledge base within the athletic training profession through research and education is another important avenue for raising our professional recognition and stature. As the research culture within the athletic training profession continues to grow, so will our national and international recognition, which is already moving athletic trainers to the forefront of the recognition, management, and care of injuries to the physically active.

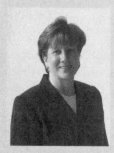

Sandra J. Shultz, PhD, ATC, CSCS

Associate Professor and Director of Graduate Study

Department of Exercise and Sport Science

University of North Carolina at Greensboro

A: The challenges facing the athletic training profession are very similar to those being faced by all allied health professions in the United States: distinguishing entry-level practice from advanced practice, educating future professionals in the knowledge and skills that they will need to practice as entry-level and advanced practitioners, and then marketing that practice in an appropriate and consistent manner that will ensure employment and a salary that is commensurate with the education, preparation, and contribution of the professional. In regard to the distinguishing of entry-level practice, the profession needs to determine where those practice boundaries lie, acknowledge that not all job settings are appropriate for entry-level practitioners, and then ensure that the educational requirements of those different levels are appropriate and consistent with the employment needs. This delineation may require athletic training to determine that the knowledge and skills required in some new and emerging practice settings are beyond entry level and should be developed through advanced graduate education or specialty certification.

Once this practice level distinction is determined, the profession of athletic training then must "sell" athletic training's role in the highly competitive arena of health care in a manner that highlights the professional preparation of the athletic trainer, as well as the uniqueness of the skill sets that athletic trainers possess. Too often when describing our scope of practice, we compare ourselves to other health care professionals and talk about how we are similar or different to/from that profession. In my opinion, this is the wrong approach. Athletic trainers have a comprehensive and unique skill set that is both taught through accredited educational programs, but also that are acquired through the required clinical education experiences. This skill set goes well beyond what is required by CAATE and delineated in the NATA Educational Competencies. The skill set includes highly evolved interpersonal skills, case management strategies, and highly efficient coordination of personnel, materials, and schedules at a level not typically developed in the other allied health disciplines; there is a significant difference between the provision of care for 4 patients every 15 minutes in a clinic or physician's office as compared to managing the care of 100 patients in a 1-hour time block and successfully returning those patients back to a high level of functional ability, and we need to "sell" the benefit of those differences. Athletic training must market our services to those patients and physicians who may be able to benefit from those services; we cannot assume that they understand our value. Finally, athletic trainers need to "sell" their value to organizations, as well as their skill set, and demand salaries that are commensurate with that value.

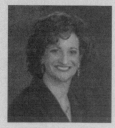

Paula Sammarone Turocy, EdD, ATC

Rangos Rizakus Endowed Chair and Department Chair

Duquesne University

been described as a syndrome of inappropriate attitudes toward clients and self. In the 1980s, the topic had garnered a great deal of attention in the athletic training literature with inconclusive results. Campbell et al[13] reported 40% of survey respondents "burned out" while Capel's study[14] of 332 athletic trainers concluded that although burnout exists, her sample reflected only average burnout scores. Quality of work life and achieving balance between professional pursuits and personal life is a hot topic among athletic training professionals. The degree of job satisfaction and potential to avoid burnout are specific to individual work settings and personal characteristics.

More recent attention has been given to professional socialization and various quality of life issues among athletic trainers in high school and intercollegiate settings.[15,16] These studies describe athletic trainer's roles in these settings as rewarding but also challenging. The rewards are found in the patient care duties and developing interpersonal relationships, while the challenges deal with the sometimes bureaucratic nature of the work environment and the ability to balance professional and personal lives to prevent burnout. Dr. Pitney interviewed active athletic trainers about these quality-of-life issues. When asked what advice they would give to an athletic trainer taking a position with Division I intercollegiate athletics, unequivocally their statements pertained to preventing burnout and finding a balance between their professional and personal lives. One study participant commented:

> I guess the advice or recommendations that I would give would be to find a way to realize that there is life outside of intercollegiate athletics. I think that one of the faults, I guess in the way I see it, in that type of a setting is that you, the person, become so wrapped up and involved in the institution, the athletic department, the teams that are associated with the department, the travel with those teams, everything that goes on within that department, that you sometimes lose a sense that there's life outside the department.

Additional research is needed to better understand these important athletic training work setting issues. It should be noted that the studies mentioned above explore only intercollegiate and high school settings; investigation of other work settings would be a welcome addition to the literature. It is also noteworthy that this issue is not unique to athletic training; role stress issues are commonplace for the caregiver. No matter the work environment, the athletic training professional who can achieve a healthy balance between caring for others and caring for him- or herself and his or her loved ones will be well positioned to avoid the professional pitfall of burnout.

SUMMARY

Athletic training is a rewarding allied health career that can be practiced in a wide variety of employment settings. Students who understand the full scope of the athletic training profession will be better prepared to make choices regarding their course of study and career goals. The influence of the NATA on the promotion of the athletic training profession is central to understanding the growth of the broader profession into the current work settings available today. The role of the BOC on the practice of the profession cannot be understated. The BOC preserves the standards of professional practice by insuring that only qualified professionals can be identified as certified athletic trainers.

The laws of the state where you choose to practice will dictate the scope of your professional activities as athletic trainer. The athletic training profession is constantly evolving to provide practice opportunities in a variety of new settings. As these venues change, the athletic trainer must stay in tune with the regulation and standards that will guide their professional practice. As athletic trainers exercise the domains of the profession and extend themselves to provide care to their patients, they should be aware of potential burnout and job stress. The ability to achieve personal and professional balance is one of the keys to a fulfilling career and personal life.

REFERENCES

1. National Athletic Trainers' Association. Athletic training: a unique health care profession. Available at www.nata.org. Accessed August 9, 2008.
2. Cruess SR, Cruess RL. Professionalism can be taught. *BMJ.* 1997;315:1674-1677.
3. Hannam SE. *Professional Behaviors in Athletic Training.* Thorofare, NJ: SLACK Incorporated; 2000.
4. National Athletic Trainers Association Research and Education Foundation. Available at www.natafoundation.org. Accessed August 9, 2008.
5. National Athletic Trainers' Association. Athletic training: statement on physical activity. Available at www.nata.org. Accessed August 9, 2008.
6. Board of Certification Inc. What is the BOC? Available at www.bocatc.org. Accessed August 9, 2008
7. Board of Certification Inc. *Role Delineation Study.* 5th ed. Omaha, NE: Author; 2004.
8. National Athletic Trainers' Association. 2008 membership statistics. Available at www.nata.org. Accessed July 25, 2008.
9. Matney M. CPT codes take effect in January. *NATA News.* 2002:46.
10. National Athletic Trainers' Association. Work settings for athletic trainers: hospitals, clinics, and physician offices. Available at www.nata.org/about_AT/worksettings/hosp-clinic.htm. Accessed January 27, 2008.

Work and Family Issues for the Athletic Trainer

Athletic training jobs in all settings can be rewarding, but they require time and effort. Planning for a family, achieving a healthy balance between your career and personal life, and not burning out are issues to be thought of in advance.

Q: How do you balance family and work as an ATC?

A: Someone said to me once, "No one dies saying that they wished they would have worked more." Realizing the truth in this, I try to work smarter by setting priorities with regard to family, work, and self. My own work environment as an educator is flexible and tolerates a varied schedule. For many athletic trainers, though, flexible thinking with regard to division of labor and questioning the traditional delivery of services are both critical. For example, is it really so bad for one athletic trainer to simultaneously cover 2 collegiate basketball teams who are practicing in adjacent gyms at the same time?

I try to impress upon our students that, once they are employed it is up to them to make a desirable work environment. We stress priorities and the need to have open communication regarding acceptable and unacceptable working parameters.

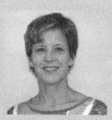

Sara D. Brown, MS, ATC

Director, Programs in Athletic Training

Boston University

A: Finding a balance between family and career is not an easy task. It requires careful thought about your priorities and continual review of these priorities as they will change throughout your career and family life. First and foremost, if you have the ability to plan ahead, I recommend waiting to start a family until after you have finished your schooling and have established your career on an initial level. This is the most sane option and one in which you will be most likely to excel.

Secondly, I recommend you explore your maternity/paternity leave options and do not be afraid to look outside the box. While not predominantly evident, some employers will honor family leave, personal leave, part-time work, or medical leave for situations centered around child birth and early infant care. This may be a time that family needs to take a priority and you make adjustments with your career to support that. Usually, once children are in school full-time it is easier to return the focus to your career. Once your children leave the nest, it may again be time to really excel with your career.

Finally, it is always helpful to have a spouse or significant other who understands the demands of your career and is willing to be a support and share the family workload. Whatever the situation, I always advise my students to put their health and family's well-being first. Work will always be there, and it should be a life-long process for attaining your career goals.

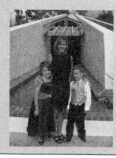

Denise O'Rand, PhD, ATC

Associate Professor

Athletic Training Education Program Clinical Coordinator

San Diego State University

11. National Athletic Trainers' Association. Work settings for athletic trainers: military and law enforcement. Available at www.nata.org/about_AT/worksettings.htm. Accessed July 25, 2008.

12. Richard R. Management strategies in athletic training. In: Perrin DH, ed. *Athletic Training Education Series.* 3rd ed. Champaign, IL: Human Kinetics; 2005.

13. Campbell D, Miller MH, Robinson WR. The prevalence of burnout among athletic trainers. *Athl Train J Natl Athl Train Assoc.* 1985;20(2):110-113.

14. Capel SA. Psychological and organizational factors related to burnout in athletic trainers. *Athl Train J Natl Athl Train Assoc.* 1986;21(4):322-327.

15. Pitney WA. Organizational influences and quality-of-life issues during the professional socialization of certified athletic trainers working in the National Collegiate Athletic Association Division I setting. *J Athl Train*. 2006;41(2):189-195.

16. Pitney WA. The professional socialization of certified athletic trainers in high school settings: a grounded theory investigation. *J Athl Train*. 2002;37(3):286-292.

🌐 WEB RESOURCES

National Athletic Trainers Association
www.nata.org
This site offers links to NATA committees, publications, position statements, and all aspects of the professional organization. A special section reserved for members allows access to employment listings and other member benefits.

Board of Certification, Inc
www. bocatc.org
The BOC Web site provides the most up-to-date information for certification candidates and CE information for current professionals.

National Athletic Trainers' Association Research and Education Foundation
www.natafoundation.org
The NATA-REF site provides details on previous research funded by the foundation, details on upcoming calls for research proposals, information on education opportunities, and scholarship information for students.

United States Department of Labor Bureau of Labor Statistics
www.bls.gov
Government resource for wage information on health care professions. Users can create their own search parameters to create national or state profiles for any profession.

What Others Say About Athletic Trainers

Throughout my career, from high school to the Olympic Games, athletic trainers have been an invaluable resource and huge contributors to my success and longevity. Always there when I need them, they are there to get me ready for practice and competition, and there to take care of me afterwards. However, it's those times when I'm injured, and need to get back on the track, that I consider them most important.

Suzy Favor Hamilton

Track and Field Champion

Seven-Time US National Champion

Three-Time Olympian

Nine NCAA Titles

It's important to have a good relationship with your athletic trainer because you're a partner with them, really. The better they know you, the better they know your body. You know your body best, but the athletic trainer serves as a second opinion for you. Once you get to know them, you feel like they know you as well as you do. Their advice and experience is invaluable. When you go to them with something, they've already experienced it. They can ease your mind and get you on the road to recovery quickly. Trust is the most important thing.

Craig Counsell

Major League Baseball Player (1995-Present)

Infielder, Milwaukee Brewers

Member Two World Series Championship Teams (Florida '97, Arizona '01)

The players I observe on the PGA TOUR while commentating for ESPN benefit greatly from the availability of sports medicine professionals at every tour stop. During my own career, I endured many injuries and surgeries that brought me in contact with athletic trainers. I enjoyed the interaction with athletic trainers because they understand the athlete's mind and body, along with the demands that go with competing at a very high level. Athletic training and sports medicine in general are terrific and rewarding fields.

Andy North

ESPN Golf Commentator/ Professional Golfer

Two-Time US Open Champion

My experience with athletic trainers was shaped in college. Our athletic trainer was great to work with during my 4 years at the University of Wisconsin. He was always professional and treated me with great respect and care as a student-athlete. He was highly respected and a great asset to UW Basketball.

Michael Finley

San Antonio Spurs

13-Year Veteran, Two-Time NBA All Star

Member of 2006-2007 NBA Champions

Job Description: Head Athletic Trainer

So you want to apply for the position of head athletic trainer? Here is a look at a job description from a medium-sized Division II Intercollegiate Athletics Department. Do you have what it takes?

General Description and Duties

The head athletic trainer typically has ongoing responsibility for the development, organization, and administration of the sports medicine program, including providing work direction to other athletic trainers. The following examples of typical work activities are meant to illustrate the general range of work functions performed by the head athletic trainers.

The head athletic trainer typically performs the following:

- Prevent, recognize, and assess athletic injuries. Implement preventive and rehabilitation programs to treat athletic injuries using the appropriate therapeutic modalities and treatments.
- Inform coaching staff and other health professionals on the status of injuries and treatment plans.
- Use a variety of therapeutic modalities in accordance with physician orders, including, but not limited to, heat, cold, light, sound, electricity and rehabilitation and exercise equipment, and apply bandages, tapes, and braces to prevent and treat injuries.
- Advise student-athletes on how to prevent injuries and maintain their physical condition. Regularly evaluate the physical condition of student-athletes.
- Educate and counsel athletes and staff regarding conditioning, athletic training, and rehabilitation.
- May attend practices and athletic events and provide medical emergency coverage to student-athletes. Travel with sports teams to away games as needed.
- May provide access to over-the-counter medication for student-athletes in accordance with physician directions, applicable university policy, and legal guidelines and ensure required documentation.
- Maintain equipment and cleanliness of the athletic training and rehabilitation facilities.
- Maintain appropriate medical records of injuries, treatment plans, and progress.
- Develop and administer rehabilitation programs for athletic injuries, including assisting in scheduling and assigning students for therapy.
- Coordinate athletic training programs and program development, including coordinating facility operations.
- Coordinate or assign other athletic trainers and provide direction and training to less experienced athletic trainers or athletic training students.
- Assist coaches in designing and implementing conditioning programs.
- Provide support to the athletic training curriculum by providing academic or clinical instruction to students enrolled in such classes.
- Maintaining insurance records and monitoring and verifying insurance billings.
- Provide work direction to other athletic trainers, including assisting in employee selection, scheduling and assigning work, reviewing work of other athletic trainers, and providing input to performance evaluations.
- Assign athletic trainers to students, athletes, and/or sports programs, and ensure needed coverage for practices, home events, and team travel.
- Develop and recommend program policies and procedures to the athletic administration for implementation, ensuring compliance with provisions of the applicable national collegiate athletic association, Occupational Safety and Health Administration (OSHA) and Health Insurance Portability and Accountability Act (HIPAA).
- Monitor all injury reports and rehabilitation plans and progress. Advise and consult athletic administration on all major injuries and treatment not covered by student-athlete's insurance.
- Develop and monitor athletic training program budget, including equipment and supplies for the athletic training facility.
- Monitor, review, and verify injury reports and medical records and take appropriate action as required. Ensure proper maintenance and confidentiality of all medical records and follow insurance processing and procedures.

(continued)

Job Description: Head Athletic Trainer (continued)

Qualifications

Education and Experience—The head athletic trainer must demonstrate sufficient experience to be able to oversee athletic training operations for intercollegiate athletics and provide work direction to other professionals. Typically, incumbents must possess 3 to 4 years of experience as a certified athletic trainer with progressive responsibility, including at least 1 year of experience in a lead capacity with some responsibility for program administration. Some experience must have been at the college level. Additionally, a master's degree in athletic training or related field of study is preferred.

License/Certification Requirements—Incumbents must possess and maintain NATA-BOC certification. In addition, incumbents are required to possess and maintain certification in CPR/AED for the professional rescuer and first aid.

Knowledge—Incumbents must possess a general knowledge of the principles and practices of athletic training, including conditioning and injury prevention, as well as injury assessment and rehabilitation; the full range of therapeutic modalities and their practical use and physiological basis; other therapeutic preventions and treatments such as taping, bracing, and massage; effective use of rehabilitation and exercise equipment; rules, regulations, and guidelines established by the campuses' governing national collegiate athletic association (eg, NCAA or National Association of Intercollegiate Athletics) pertaining to student-athletes, their training, sports medicine care, and health and safety; OSHA standards for handling blood-borne pathogens (BBP); maintaining medical records, including HIPAA standards; and following insurance procedures. In addition, head athletic trainers must possess a demonstrated knowledge of effective lead techniques and practices and a working knowledge of campus human resource practices, payroll procedures, and campus budget and related administrative processes and procedures.

Abilities—Incumbents must be able to effectively assess and evaluate injuries and their severity; develop conditioning and rehabilitation programs and manage and treat injuries; use the full range of appropriate therapeutic modalities, treatments, and rehabilitation and exercise equipment to treat and prevent injuries; determine the appropriate referrals for athletes to other health care professionals; recognize life-threatening situations and administer the appropriate emergency aid; use a computer to perform medical, insurance, and other recordkeeping functions; and work in an environment with competing priorities. In addition, incumbents must possess strong interpersonal and communications skills to develop effective working relationships with athletes and to serve as a liaison among athletes, coaching staff, parents, physicians, and other health professionals. In addition, incumbents must exhibit the organizational and administrative abilities necessary to develop and coordinate a sports medicine program and must be skilled in establishing program priorities; providing work direction and training to other athletic trainers; promoting teamwork to optimize effectiveness; developing and implementing policies and procedures to ensure compliance with applicable regulating agencies; developing and monitoring the program budget; ensuring rehabilitation objectives are achieved and medical records are secured as confidential, accurate, and complete; and ensuring accurate maintenance of insurance records and billings.

CHAPTER 2

HISTORICAL PERSPECTIVES

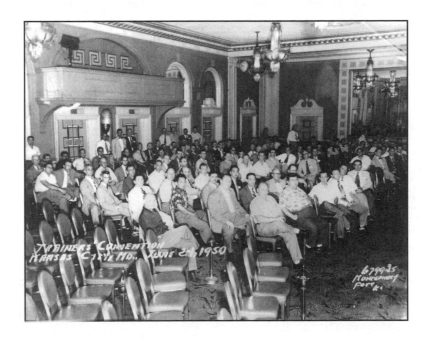

The pioneers in this profession were visionaries. I think they were willing to take a chance or risk. I mean this in a positive way, willing to venture out and try things. Maybe even fail, but the fear of failure did not prevent them from moving forward.

René Revis Shingles, PhD, ATC
Associate Professor, Athletic Training Education Program
Central Michigan University

A RICH HISTORY

When reflecting on the origins of the athletic training profession, you may have to reach well back into the history of civilization to choose a starting point. Some have tried to associate the origins of the profession back to the 5th century BC and the ancient Greeks where athletics was central to the culture. The presence of paidotribes or "boy rubbers" assisting athletes and soldiers has been suggested as the beginnings of athletic training.[1,2] It is possible I suppose. However, outside of the Greeks, the remainder of the world viewed what we would call fitness only as a tool for war and survival. It would take centuries to see a logical link between historic events and present-day athletic training. The genuine origin of something that resembles the profession of athletic training likely lies in the 19th century. The evolution of physical activity and organized sport combined with a need to rehabilitate soldiers returning from the wars is where I choose to place the beginnings of our profession. Table 2-1 outlines some of the earliest activities that served as precursors to modern athletic training.

25

Table 2-1
Historic Precursors to the Athletic Training Profession

5th century BC	Paidotribes serve as assistants to Greek athletes
19th century	Interest in physical activity increases with the development of gymnastics in Germany
1860s	Gymnastics is taught in American universities at the time of the Civil War
1881	Harvard hires James Robinson to fulfill the role of athletic trainer
1905	President Roosevelt threatens to abolish football due to the number of deaths and serious injuries
1918	Dr. Samuel Bilik publishes *The Trainers Bible*, believed by many to be the first book dedicated to athletic training
1932	US Olympic team has athletic trainers as part of the staff
1938	Dr. Augustus Throndike publishes text on the medical problems of athletes, the first devoted to the topic
1938	The first NATA founded at the Drake relays. The organization would struggle with lack of funding and the United States entrance into WWII
1944	NATA no longer in existence as WWII draws to a close

Adapted from Ebel RG. *Far Beyond the Shoe Box: Fifty Years of the NATA.* New York, NY: Forbes Custom Publishing; 1999.

The late 1800s brought the sport of football to American college campuses. By 1905, President Theodore Roosevelt threatened to abolish football due to a number of deaths and serious injuries. At the time, treatment of injuries was the responsibility of the coach or maybe a physician. However, Harvard and Yale are credited with having two of the first individuals hired to fulfill the role of athletic trainer: James Robinson at Harvard and Michael C. Murphy at Yale and later Penn.[2] The early athletic training profession had no shape or structure. There were no formal requirements and no organizations to support the craft. The men who entered the profession to render care, train, and condition athletes often had minimal competence and no education. However, many of these early practitioners have been described as responding to their labors with an abundance of character, a passion for service, and a nobility of selflessness.[2] The journey from a group of poorly educated bucket-and-sponge practitioners to a modern allied health profession is directly linked to the development of a professional organization and the establishment of educational and professional criteria.

Upon completion of this chapter, the student will be able to:

✓ Summarize the origins of the NATA

✓ Describe the key pioneers in the development and advancement of the athletic training profession

✓ Identify key dates and historic events in the advancement of athletic training

✓ Discuss the role women and minorities have played in the profession and the common obstacles they have encountered

A PROFESSIONAL ORGANIZATION

STARTS AND STOPS: PROFESSIONAL BEGINNINGS

The first NATA was organized in 1938 in conjunction with the Drake relays in Iowa. William Frey from the University of Iowa and Charles Cramer from the Cramer Chemical Company of Gardner, Kansas formed the original organization. The organization was divided into western and eastern regions. They would hold 2 annual meetings a year, one at the Drake relays and another at the Penn relays. The tradition of athletic trainers gathering at common athletic events and forming organizations was a common event. Many state organizations that are thriving today evolved in this same fashion.

The first NATA was not meant to be. The nation had to contend with larger issues. The entrance into World War II limited any chance of true professional growth for the organization. Many of the young men serving as athletic trainers were called to, or enlisted for, military service. By 1942, the original organization had 142 members and a financial shortfall. The organization was no longer in existence once the war ended in 1945.[2]

A STRONG FOUNDATION

Many soldiers who returned from the war were in need of physical rehabilitation. This time period saw a rapid acceleration of rehabilitation techniques and an expansion of the allied health concept. By the late 1940s, there were several universities that had the services of an athletic trainer. Organizations began to emerge based upon logical regional alignments. Groups would often meet in conjunction with a track meet or other event. By 1950, the Southern Conference, Eastern Conference, Pacific Coast Conference, and Southwest Conference all had formed Athletic Trainers' Associations. However, at this point in time, athletic training was a confederation of individuals doing roughly the same job. There were no guidelines, education requirements, or standards. To be a true profession, there would need to be a national organization to address such issues. It would begin in June 1950 in Kansas City, Missouri, thanks largely to the sponsorship of the Cramer Chemical Company.

Charles and Frank Cramer were brothers who in 1922 formed the company that would later become Cramer Products. Charles was a pharmacist who had developed a liniment that was used by athletic trainers, and the brothers were part of the first group of athletic trainers who traveled with the US Olympic team in 1932. June 24 to 25, 1950 would be the date of the first National Training Clinic. Over 100 attendees took part in the original meeting. During this clinic, a group held a meeting and outlined what would become a formal organization, the NATA. The new group capitalized on the loyalty members had to their regional groups and developed 9 districts that would be self-governing, and one representative from each would make up the Board of Directors. Charles Cramer would serve as the secretary, a post he held until 1954.

The NATA would meet again in Kansas City in both 1951 and 1952. With each passing year, new changes would further give shape to the fledgling organization: the board established a chair, a constitution and by-laws were enacted, the organization extended beyond the college ranks to include athletic trainers from professional sports, and a logo was adopted to give identity to the organization. By the time the NATA held its annual meeting in Bloomington, Indiana in 1955, several important goals had been achieved. The most important goal was the NATA had survived. Now it was time for the NATA to stand on its own. The organization would need to break away from its dependence on a specific company in order to be viewed as a true professional group. The Cramer family had supported the organization during its formative years, but now the NATA needed to move forward on its own. In this spirit, the young organization selected its own "executive secretary." William "Pinky" Newell from Purdue University became the first active athletic trainer to hold the position.[2,3]

During the years that Pinky led the organization (1955 to 1968), monumental changes took effect that continue to influence the profession of athletic training to this day. Promoting professional recognition, developing educational standards, creating a professional journal, and instituting a code of ethics are some of the organizational highlights that took place during the 1950s and 1960s. In 1959, the first undergraduate curriculum for athletic trainers was developed and approved by the Board of Directors and by 1968, a committee was formed to confirm the preparation of athletic trainers by a process of certification. As the 1960s drew to a close, the AMA had acknowledged the NATA as an organization worthy of support by the medical community. The times indeed were changing for the men of the NATA. For one thing, they were not all men anymore.

PROFESSIONAL ADVANCEMENT: EDUCATION AND CERTIFICATION

If you look at the underlying principles that shaped every dramatic change in our profession, they can be linked to educational reform and the evolution of our educational standards. There are obviously many items in the history of our profession that are extremely important, several milestones (AMA recognition, certification, etc) but few are as central to what we do and what we can do as the educational evolution has been.

Marjorie Albohm, MS, ATC/L
President, NATA

Educational Preparation

Two central themes have dominated the preparation of athletic training professionals: education and certification. Many of the original members of the NATA envisioned the organization as a place for athletic trainers to exchange ideas and knowledge. Education would dominate much of the association's activities, both continuing educational opportunities for current athletic trainers and the question of appropriate preparation of new athletic trainers. Education was not a subject that some of the original athletic trainers embraced outright. Many of these men learned their skills through hands-on apprenticeship as opposed to formal education. However, the pioneers of the NATA had the vision to see that recognition in the medical community could only come through an appropriate path of professional preparation.

Not For Men Only

The title for this sidebar is taken from a column that appeared in the *NATA Journal* in the 1970s that was written by Holly Wilson from Indiana State University. The original column dealt with the entry of women into the field of athletic training. Holly, like many pioneering women in athletic training, saw that as competition increased for women athletes, the need to provide them with competent care would also increase. Women were taking their rightful place in the athletic training profession. The passage of Title IX in 1972 provided increased opportunities for women in intercollegiate athletics and a concurrent growth in opportunities for women in athletic training.

The first wave of women in athletic training did meet some resistance and had obstacles to overcome; however, we often found support from our male counterparts in the profession that helped women get a foothold and allowed for the growth we have seen in the past 30 years.

I don't feel the early women in athletic training have been properly recognized for the role they played in determining that women can compete at a very high level without suffering long-term consequences. You have to remember that in the beginnings of competition for women, we were asked many questions that seem absurd today: Will widespread competition cause injury to the reproductive system? How can we best protect the breast tissue? All sorts of things were wondered about. It was often the ATC through care and documentation who showed that yes, women can compete without secondary problems.

Marjorie Albohm, Current President, NATA

Selected Key Dates:
- 1950—The NATA is founded in Kansas City with no female members.
- 1966—Dorothy "Dot" Cohen, a graduate student, becomes the first woman to join the NATA.
- 1972—Sherry Bagagian is the first woman to sit for the NATA certification examination.
- 1972—Title IX of the Higher Education Act that prohibits sex discrimination in school and college athletic programs is signed into law.
- 1974—Ad Hoc Committee on Women established by NATA.
- 1976—Gail Weldon is the first woman athletic trainer selected to US Olympic team medical staff.
- 1984—Janice Daniels, the District Eight director, is the first woman elected to the NATA Board.
- 1992—Eve Becker-Doyle is hired as executive director of the NATA, the first woman to hold the position.
- 1995—Gail Weldon is the first woman elected to the NATA Hall of Fame.
- 1996—The Women in Athletic Training Task Force is recognized as on official NATA committee.
- 2000—Julie Max is elected president of the NATA; she is the first woman to hold this position.
- 2002—Ariko Iso is hired by the Pittsburgh Steelers organization, making her the first woman to be hired as a permanent full-time staff athletic trainer in the NFL.
- 2003—Sandra J. Shultz is awarded the NATA-REF New Investigator award, the first woman to receive an NATA-REF award.
- 2007—Marjorie Albohm is elected president of NATA, the second woman to hold this position.

There have been several "firsts" and remarkable change since the first women entered the athletic training profession. Facilities that once were obstacles are now largely gender neutral. Women have assumed leadership roles throughout the organization, including the very top. It is hoped that as move deeper into this new century, the issues of gender will focus not on the care provider but instead on how athletic training contributes to answering questions about health care problems unique to women.

Adapted in part from Graham C, Schlabach G. The women of athletic training—women in athletic training committee update. *NATA News*, October 2001.

In 1955, William "Pinky" Newell as the National Secretary of the NATA established the Committee on Gaining Recognition. The committees for education and certification would evolve from this early effort. The development of a model curriculum for the preparation of athletic trainers was a top prior-ity of this early committee. In 1959, the NATA Board of Directors approved an educational model reflective of the athletic training environment at the time. There was an emphasis on preparation that would allow employment in the secondary school setting. The model also included courses that represented the

National Athletic Trainers' Association Governing Structure

NATA Board of Directors

- President
- One representative from each of the 10 districts:
  - District One (Eastern Athletic Trainers' Association): Connecticut, Maine, Massachusetts, New Hampshire, Rhode Island, Vermont, Quebec, New Brunswick, and Nova Scotia
  - District Two (Eastern Athletic Trainers' Association): Delaware, New Jersey, New York, and Pennsylvania
  - District Three (Mid Atlantic Athletic Trainers' Association): Maryland, North Carolina, South Carolina, Virginia, West Virginia, and District of Columbia
  - District Four (Great Lakes Athletic Trainers' Association): Illinois, Indiana, Michigan, Minnesota, Ohio, Wisconsin, Manitoba, and Ontario
  - District Five (Mid America Athletic Trainers' Association): Iowa, Kansas, Missouri, Nebraska, North Dakota, Oklahoma, and South Dakota
  - District Six (Southwest Athletic Trainers' Association): Arkansas and Texas
  - District Seven (Rocky Mountain Athletic Trainers' Association): Arizona, Colorado, New Mexico, Utah, and Wyoming
  - District Eight (Far West Athletic Trainers' Association): California, Hawaii, and Nevada
  - District Nine (Southeast Athletic Trainers' Association): Alabama, Florida, Georgia, Kentucky, Louisiana, Mississippi, and Tennessee
  - District Ten (Northwest Athletic Trainers' Association): Alaska, Idaho, Montana, Oregon, Washington, Alberta, British Columbia, and Saskatchewan

NATA Committees, Councils, Think Tanks, and Project Teams

NATA's various committees and councils have many purposes, but they all share a common goal: to help carry out the work of the NATA Board of Directors. Each committee, council, and project team has an NATA member as chairperson. The chairs work with committee, council, and work group members and NATA staff liaisons to accomplish goals. These groups represent a major evolution in the governance structure in the NATA. This new structure is designed to foster more member involvement and to be responsive to member needs.

Committees

Clinical & Emerging Practices Athletic Trainers' Committee

Purpose: The mission of CEPAT is to develop and promote new areas for athletic training employment and address employment issues, such as working conditions, for athletic trainers in existing settings. The committee will support staff in research as it relates to job development and improvement as well as serve as a liaison to athletic training educators in order to translate changes in professional education standards and emerging employment issues.

College/University Athletic Trainers' Committee

Purpose: Identify and address issues of concern to athletic trainers in the college and university setting.

Convention Program Committee

Purpose: Oversee the planning and implementation of the NATA Annual Meeting and Clinical Symposia.

District Secretaries/Treasurers Committee

Purpose: Assist NATA and the districts by exchanging information about membership procedures, common needs and goals, and related matters.

Education Council Executive Committee

Purpose: Oversee matters related to athletic training education.

Continuing Education Committee

Purpose: Provide leadership in the creation, development, implementation, delivery, and evaluation of CE.

(continued)

National Athletic Trainers' Association Governing Structure (continued)

Postprofessional Education Review Committee

Purpose: Responsible for developing standards for postcertification education, coordinating accreditation through the Graduate Review Committee, and promoting the quality of master's and doctoral level education. Responsible for overseeing the development, implementation, and evaluation of specialty certifications.

Ethnic Diversity Advisory Committee

Purpose: Identify and address issues relevant to American Indian/Alaskan Natives, Asian/Pacific Islanders, Black, non-Hispanic, and Hispanic members. Additionally, address health care concerns affecting physically active individuals in these ethnic groups. Advocate sensitivity and understanding toward ethnic and cultural diversity throughout the profession and the association.

Finance Committee

Purpose: Oversee and review NATA financial matters and investment program.

Honors and Awards Committee

Purpose: Oversee and administer the NATA's honors and awards program.

National Athletic Training Students' Committee

Purpose: Facilitate communication with and issues of athletic training students.

Postprofessional Education Review Committee

Purpose: Review postcertification graduate education programs.

Secondary School Athletic Trainers' Committee

Purpose: To address those employment issues impacting athletic trainers related to existing and emerging employment markets through a coordinated effort with internal and external entities.

Strategic Implementation Team

Purpose: Keep the NATA strategic plan up-to-date through the process of strategic thinking. Monitor internal and external conditions and trends affecting the NATA and the athletic training profession.

Young Professionals Committee

Purpose: To identify and address the interests, needs, and concerns of young athletic training professionals (<35 years of age).

Councils

Council of Revenue

Purpose: To pursue third-party reimbursement for athletic training services.

Ethics Council

Purpose: Ensure that the NATA *Code of Ethics* and the membership standards, eligibility requirements, and membership sanctions and procedures are enforced.

Governmental Affairs Council

Purpose: Oversee the NATA's governmental relations and regulatory efforts. Advocate for regulation favorable to athletic training.

International Council

Purpose: Advocate for members who are living, working, or stationed outside the United States.

Journal Council

Purpose: To oversee the operations of the *Journal of Athletic Training*.

(continued)

National Athletic Trainers' Association Governing Structure (continued)

National Legal Review Group

Purpose: The NATA National Legal Review Program is a system of reviewing, prioritizing, and funding legal issues that impact the profession of athletic training on a national basis. The goal of this program is to protect and advance the profession of athletic training through the legal system.

Outcomes Advisory Panel

Purpose: Support the marketing and legislative efforts of the NATA by providing professional expertise to evaluate research and propose outcomes research development and implementation.

Postprofessional Education Council

Purpose: Oversee and promote NATA accredited and postprofessional graduate athletic training education and residency programs. Oversee and develop athletic training specialty board certification.

Professional Education Council

Purpose: Act as an advocate and resource for students and educators associated with accredited baccalaureate and entry-level athletic training education programs.

Pronouncements Council

Purpose: To develop and/or review position statements, pronouncements, and other documents on behalf of NATA.

Public Relations Council

Purpose: Provide input and direction to NATA's public relations program.

Think Tanks

Think tanks provide a forum for members to exchange information and network with colleagues who share similar interests and goals. The think tanks also serve as a pool for project teams. Members can sign up for specific think tanks and participate in exchanges in a web forum. Project teams work on specific targeted projects.

Current think tanks:

- Clinical and emerging practice
- College and university
- Communications
- Diversity and gender issues
- Education
- Ethics
- Fundraising
- International
- Legislative/regulatory/revenue reimbursement
- Life balancing
- Meeting planning
- Membership
- Public relations
- Students
- Urgent information
- Young professionals

Adapted from National Athletic Trainers' Association. Involve evolve. *NATA News.* 2008.

prerequisites for schools of physical therapy. This is likely due to the influence of Pinky Newell, himself a physical therapist and athletic trainer. Athletic training students were encouraged to pursue physical therapy as a means to expand their employability.[4]

The initial curriculum drew heavily from existing courses in various academic areas. Few courses distinguished the curriculum from existing physical education programs.[4] Since athletic training was a new profession, it is understandable that this would happen. In time, there would be a new kind of athletic trainer. The athletic training educator would emerge to develop courses and define the content that would distinguish athletic training as a distinctive subject area. Despite this early development of the curriculum model, only a few colleges and universities developed athletic training curriculums. During the late 1960s, the Committee on Gaining Recognition was officially divided into 2 subcommittees: Professional Education and the Subcommittee on Certification.

Sayers "Bud" Miller from the University of Washington was the first chair of the Professional Education subcommittee. It was the responsibility of the committee to evaluate and recommend NATA recognition of the education programs. This marked the beginning of curriculum review for athletic training education. Dr. Miller was a visionary educator; his leadership of the Professional Education subcommittee helped develop specific behavioral and skill objectives that began to shape the body of knowledge in athletic training. In 1969, the first undergraduate athletic training education programs were recognized by the NATA. These programs included Mankato State University, Indiana State University, Lamar University, and the University of New Mexico. Later in 1972, the first graduate programs would be approved at Indiana State University and the University of Arizona.

The 1970s saw significant growth in the number of athletic training education programs. By 1982, there were 62 undergraduate and 9 graduate programs approved by the NATA. The evolution of the curricular and clinical requirements saw greater emphasis on content specific to athletic training. While still encouraged, physical therapy prerequisites were given less emphasis as athletic training continued to evolve as a unique and specific allied health area. The 1970s also saw a declining emphasis on physical education as a teaching certification companion to athletic training. The availability of the teaching credential remained a part of the NATA-approved program until 1980. After that time, students could determine for themselves whether to complete the teaching credential.

In the 1980s, the athletic training curriculum evolved to further establish its place alongside established academic areas. An emphasis was placed on establishing an athletic training major or an academic equivalent to a major. The policy allowing for NATA approval of an equivalent major allowed programs to pursue major status while implementing new changes in the athletic training curriculum. In 1983, the *Guidelines for NATA Approval* specified subject matter requirements rather than specific courses. Also at this time, the *Athletic Training Educational Competencies* replaced specific behavioral objectives previously developed in the 1970s. The new competencies were based on the "performance domains" identified in the first role delineation study conducted by the NATA-BOC in 1982. These changes helped establish a competency base for athletic training education programs. These early efforts in athletic training education set the foundation for a landmark event in the evolution of athletic training, recognition as an allied health profession.

In 1990, the AMA officially recognized athletic training as an allied health profession. Table 2-2 outlines key dates in athletic training education history. This recognition grew from the NATA Professional Education Committee's urging to seek an outside agency to accredit professional preparation programs in athletic training. The NATA sought accreditation by the AMA's Committee on Allied Health Education Accreditation (CAHEA). The AMA House of Delegates voted to recognize athletic training as an allied health profession. This allowed the current accreditation model to be put into place. Following this watershed event, the Joint Review Committee for Athletic Training Education (JRC-AT) was formed and co-sponsored by the AMA, NATA, and other professional groups representing family physicians, pediatricians, and orthopedic surgeons. The JRC-AT sits as a separate entity from the professional organization much like the BOC. CAHEA was disbanded in 1994 and replaced by the Commission on Accreditation of Allied Health Programs (CAAHEP). CAAHEP is recognized by the United States Department of Education as an accreditation agency for allied health programs. The JRC-AT continued to be responsible for the review of programs under the *Standards and Guidelines for Athletic Training Education*.

Further evolution was to come in June 2006 when the JRC-AT became independent from CAAHEP and changed its name to the Commission on Accreditation of Athletic Training Education (CAATE). CAATE is the agency responsible for the accreditation of over 350 professional (entry-level) athletic training educational programs. The American Academy of Family Physicians (AAFP), the AAP, the American Orthopaedic Society for Sports Medicine (AOSSM), and the NATA cooperate to sponsor CAATE and to collaboratively develop the *Standards for Entry-Level Athletic Training Educational Programs*.

Table 2-2
Key Dates in Athletic Training Education

1959	First athletic training curriculum model approved by NATA
1969	NATA Professional Education Committee (PEC) and NATA Certification Committee developed (former subcommittees of Committee on Gaining Recognition)
	First undergraduate athletic training curriculums approved by NATA
1970	First national certification examination administered by NATA Certification Committee
1972	First graduate athletic training curriculum approved by the NATA
1980	NATA resolution requiring athletic training curriculum major, or equivalent, approved by NATA Board of Directors
1983	First edition of *Athletic Training Educational Competencies* developed
1990	Athletic training recognized as an allied health profession by the AMA
	Joint Review Committee for Athletic Training Education (JRC-AT) was formed and cosponsored by the AMA, NATA, and other professional groups representing family physicians, pediatricians, and orthopedic surgeons. Free-standing group separate from the NATA
1991	Essentials and Guidelines for an Accredited Educational Program for the Athletic Trainer approved by the AMA Council on Medical Education
1994	First entry-level athletic training educational programs accredited by AMA Committee on Allied Health Education and Accreditation (CAHEA)
	Commission on Accreditation of Allied Health Education Programs (CAAHEP) formed (replaced CAHEA as entry-level athletic training education program accreditation agency)
	NATA Education Task Force appointed
1996	NATA Education Task Force recommendations approved by the NATA Board of Directors, paving way for elimination of internship route to certification
	NATA Education Council formed
2004	All BOC exam candidates graduates of accredited programs
2006	Commission on Accreditation of Athletic Training Education (CAATE) formed
	Degree Task Force Recommends all athletic training programs offer a degree in athletic training by 2014 to 2015

Adapted in part from Delforge GD, Behnke RS. The history and evolution of athletic training education in the United States. *Journal of Athletic Training.* 1999;34(1):53-61.

The academic preparation of highly skilled care providers will take another step in 2014-2015 when all entry-level athletic training programs must offer a degree in athletic training. This recommendation was born from an Education Council task force that explored the question of what type of degree should be offered in athletic training. While the current system allows for both undergraduate and graduate entry-level degrees, it was a consensus that all programs must offer a degree—not just a major. This step will allow athletic training to continue to evolve as a health care profession. If history is an indicator, the discussion on entry-level education will continue to be a focal point of discussion for the profession.

A full discussion of current educational requirements for athletic training students can be found in Chapter 3.

 Board of Certification

The proper name of the organization responsible for the certification of athletic trainers is the Board of Certification, Inc (BOC). Any reference to the BOC by any other name is strictly based on the historical context at any given point in time.

The History of Athletic Training Certification

In 1968, the NATA's Professional Advancement Committee put forward a proposal that a certification examination be developed for athletic trainers. A 1969 article by Lindsay McLean titled *Does the NATA Need a Certification Examination?* took the discussion to the full membership.[5,6] The article discussed employment opportunities, working conditions, and limited programs offering athletic training education as problems that did not reflect a truly mature profession. One possible solution was for the NATA to develop a written and practical examination to address professional preparation issues facing the profession and NATA. Lindsay McLean headed up the subcommittee on certification and was the first chair of the NATA-BOC.[6]

In June 1969 upon recommendation from the Professional Advancement Committee, the NATA Board allowed those qualified by experience to apply for active membership, leading to certification by the grandfather clause. It was mandatory that they apply for active membership classification. The board also passed that the grandfather clause be closed for this type of membership December 31, 1969. New members would have to sit for the certification exam. The Certification Examination Subcommittee would develop the new examination.

The content of the first certification examination was developed by surveying members on what areas should be included on the examination within the following categories: basic science, theory of athletic training, and practical application of athletic training. Respondents indicated whether a particular area should be included and in what percentage should each area be represented. The Certification Examination Subcommittee made the following recommendation[6]:

- ✓ Seventy-five written questions assessing the candidate's knowledge of anatomy, physiology, mechanics and pathology of athletic injury, and the principles of injury prevention

- ✓ Seventy-five written questions on the theory and practical application of athletic training

- ✓ Five oral-practical questions to assess the candidate's skill in recognizing specific injury conditions, demonstrating adhesive strapping, and evaluating and fitting of protective equipment

It was determined that active members and associate members who met the educational and apprenticeship requirements should be eligible to take the examination. There were 4 original routes to sit for the certification exam:

1. Graduation from an NATA-approved athletic training education program.

2. Completion of an apprenticeship program.

3. Graduation from a school physical therapy degree with a minimum of 2 years athletic training experience beyond the student athletic trainer level.

4. Special consideration route (minimum 5 years as an "actively engaged" athletic trainer).

The committee also surveyed the membership to determine what title should be granted to those successfully completing the certification process. It was determined that those who passed the certification examination should be called "athletic trainer, certified." This nomenclature was selected rather than "athletic therapist, certified."[6] Several professionals feel this would have been a good time to change the name to something more descriptive of the athletic trainer's duties. The debate still continues today.

The hard work of the committee came to fruition when the first certification examination was offered in Waco, Texas in August 1970 with 15 candidates. Additional milestones included the following:

- ✓ In January 1971, midyear examinations were held in 4 cities

- ✓ In June 1971, twenty-four candidates took the examination at the NATA annual meeting in Baltimore, Maryland

- ✓ The first female candidate took the examination in June 1972

Since those early days, thousands of athletic trainers have been certified. There are currently over 26,000 certified members in the NATA.[7]

It may seem that the decision to develop and carry out the certification process was the largest milestone for the Certification Committee and the NATA-BOC. In fact, 2 important events would follow to help solidify and protect the credential of athletic training professionals. Recognition of the BOC as a certifying agency and full incorporation of the NATA-BOC are of equal importance.

In response to the increasing variety of certifications offered by various organizations in the late 1970s, the federal government sought to develop an organization that would accredit these certifying organizations. The National Commission for Health Certifying Agencies (NCHCA) was established for this purpose. The NCHCA ensures that the certification, credential, and program uses acceptable testing, psychometric, and legal principles.[6] Extensive criteria are required for an organization to be granted NCHCA accreditation. Several positive steps were taken to meet these criteria, including creating a well-defined independent governance structure for the NATA-BOC and the implementation of the *Role Delineation Study for the Entry-Level Athletic Trainer.* This study became the blueprint for the certification examination and helps insure that the test is a reliable measure of the required skills for the profession. In 1982, the NATA-BOC was granted NCHCA accreditation. The NATA-BOC was the first allied health sports medicine organization to be so recognized.

In June 1989, an equally important step was taken to distance the NATA from the BOC. Potential conflicts of interest could be alleged if an organization that provides membership is also a certifying agency. In 1989, the NATA Board of Directors elected to create an independent separate organization, the NATA-BOC, Inc. This independence alleviated any potential concern based on the structure of the organization. The NATA-BOC has the sole power and authority to certify athletic trainers. Visionary leadership and hard work has provided athletic trainers with an entry-level credential that is recognized and respected in the health care community. A testament to the value of the credential and the role of the athletic trainer in delivering health care to active populations is the number of employers who request that their athletic health care be provided by an NATA-BOC athletic trainer, certified.[6] In recent years, the certifying agency for athletic trainers is no longer called the NATA-BOC and is now formally the Board of Certification, Inc (BOC).

In 1994 in response to concerns over the preparation of athletic trainers for a changing health care landscape, the NATA Board of Directors appointed Richard Ray of Hope College and John Schrader of Indiana University as co-chairs of the Education Task Force. Their charge was to examine all aspects of the professional preparation of athletic trainers. In 1996, they submitted a report to the NATA Board with 18 recommendations. These recommendations have largely been referred to as "educational reform." The most significant recommendation was that there be only one route to certification as an athletic trainer. This called for the elimination of the internship route to certification and by 2004, all candidates for BOC certification were graduates of an accredited educational program in athletic training.

The NATA Board adopted all 18 recommendations put forth by the Education Task Force. While unifying the educational requirements of the athletic trainer, the recommendations also included the development of the Education Council to serve as a clearinghouse for educational policy regarding all aspects of entry-level preparation for the athletic trainer, including entry-level postgraduate programs. CAATE currently accredits both undergraduate and graduate entry-level programs.

The actual certification examination took another step in its continual evolution in 2008—the test is now longer conducted on-line. The examination is a mix of knowledge-based multiple choice questions and scenario-based or "hybrid" questions that require knowledge and clinical decision-making skills. In order to attain certification, an individual must complete an entry-level athletic training education program accredited by CAATE and pass the BOC certification exam. In order to qualify as a candidate for the BOC certification exam, an individual must meet the following requirements[8]:

✓ Endorsement of the exam application by the recognized Program Director (PD) of the CAATE-accredited education program

✓ Proof of current certification in ECC

THE MODERN ERA OF ATHLETIC TRAINING: GROWTH AND CHANGE

As evidenced in the previous sections, certification and education was a significant focus throughout the past 20 years of the NATA. In addition to the huge strides made in these important areas, the 1980s and 1990s saw many other changes. In 1983, the NATA was incorporated, which opened the door for greater financial growth of the organization. In 1972, the organization had $2000 in assets and by the end of the 1980s, those assets would exceed $2 million.[2] In 1988, NATA went through significant professional growth. The NATA Board approved the purchase of a national headquarters in Dallas, Texas. The building was named in honor of Otho Davis who stepped down after 19 years as the organization's executive director. This move cleared the way for the largely volunteer organization to hire a professional executive director and staff. The mid 1980s also saw the NATA obtain its first corporate sponsorship. While controversial at the time, corporate sponsorship has provided revenue for the growing organization and has allowed for the development of a variety of programs. In 1985, Quaker Oats/Gatorade became the first corporate sponsor of the NATA.

1990 saw the hiring of Alan A. Smith, Jr as the first full-time executive director of the NATA. Mr. Smith would serve in that capacity until 1992 when he resigned and was replaced by Eve Becker-Doyle in 1993. During the 1980s and 1990s, the NATA saw tremendous growth in membership. The organization that had approximately 100 members in 1950 has now grown to a current membership of over 28,000 with 79% of those members certified by the NATA-BOC.[7] In 1992, the athletic training profession took another major step with the establishment of the NATA-REF. The mission of the NATA-REF is to advance the athletic training profession through education and research. As of 2008, the NATA-REF had awarded over $2.25 million in funding for original research.[9]

A More Diverse Future?

The history of the NATA is well represented by persons of diverse backgrounds. Athletic trainers like Naseby Rhinehart, Henry "Buddy" Taylor, Frank Medina, and Marsha Grant Ford (the first African American woman to become certified) hold a special place among the other pioneers that make up the rich history of our professional organization. However, in contrast to the populations we serve, the athletic training profession is under-represented in terms of people of color. The NATA reported in 2007 that 83% of its members were white (see table below).[1]

All Members by Ethnicity	
Unspecified	5.8%
Asian or Pacific Islander	3.5%
Black (not Hispanic origin)	0.5%
Hispanic	0%
Other	1.3%
Mixed ethnicity	22%
White	83%

To better respond to these issues, the NATA maintains the Ethnic Diversity Advisory Council. This council maintains the following mission:

The Ethnic Diversity Advisory Council is dedicated to service, devoted to advocacy and committed to unity. We want to identify and address issues relevant to American Indian/Alaskan Natives, Asian/Pacific Islanders, Blacks (non-Hispanic), and Hispanics both in the health care arena and in the NATA. We advocate sensitivity and understanding towards ethnic and cultural diversity throughout the profession and the association. We strive to enhance the growth and development of the NATA, and our objectives are designed to unify the association. So, join us in our efforts to promote service, advocacy and unity.

The important topic of improving diversity and creating environments that are welcoming to all people will continue to receive attention through the work of the Ethic Diversity Advisory Council and through efforts of all athletic trainers. In an editorial in the *Journal of Athletic Training*, then-editor Dr. David Perrin commented, *"Preconceived notions about those who are different with regard to race, ethnicity, religion, and sexual orientation "go out the window" when we learn and work in a diverse environment."*[2]

The profession of athletic training is open to everyone.

References

1. National Athletic Trainers' Association. Ethnic diversity advisory council. Available at www.nata.org. Accessed March 17, 2008.
2. Perrin DH. Promoting diversity in athletic training. *Journal of Athletic Training.* 2000;35:131.

THE FUTURE IS NOW!

Where does the NATA go from here? A look at the most recent strategic planning documents shows 4 areas of focus and 2 overriding strategic dimensions.
- ✓ Areas of focus
  - ○ Favorable state regulation
  - ○ Revenue for athletic training services
  - ○ Marketing and public relations
  - ○ Job development
- ✓ Strategic directions
  - ○ Increasing member personal satisfaction and professional stature
    - ■ Action areas
      - ❑ Fostering emerging leadership
      - ❑ Communicating with members
      - ❑ Refined education
      - ❑ Providing strategies for life balance
  - ○ Empowering members to utilize their skills, expertise, and full scope of practice
    - ■ Action areas
      - ❑ Maximizing legislative influence
      - ❑ Demonstrating the value of athletic trainers
      - ❑ Marketing the profession
      - ❑ Guaranteeing financial responsibility

If history serves well, the professional organization will serve as a vehicle to move these issues forward on behalf of the greater profession. At the time of this

NATA Hall of Fame

The NATA recognizes outstanding members who have demonstrated service and dedication to the profession with a variety of awards. Key awards categories include the NATA Educators' Award, Service Award, and Most Distinguished Athletic Trainer Award. The pinnacle award presented by the NATA is the induction into the NATA Hall of Fame. Most of the historical pioneers mentioned in this chapter are members of the NATA Hall of Fame.

Award Description

The NATA Hall of Fame was created to recognize members who have demonstrated career excellence in the athletic training profession. It is the highest honor that may be bestowed upon a member. Therefore, individuals inducted into the Hall of Fame must exemplify the mission statement of the NATA by enhancing the quality of health care provided by athletic trainers and advance the athletic training profession with such qualities as leadership, service, dedication, scholarly activities, promotion, and professionalism.

Examples of activities that are considered include the following:

- Leadership and service at the national, district, and state levels
- Scholarly activities
- Honors and awards received
- Volunteerism at the national, district, and state levels
- Presentations, educational activities, and other activities that build awareness of athletic training

Qualifications

- These elite candidates must have a minimum of 25 years as a certified member of the NATA in good standing
- Individuals may be nominated no more than every other year

they treat. Their goal is to enhance health care, both for those who practice and those who receive care. Like all political action committees, NATAPAC will work to effect change by supporting candidates for public office whose views and intentions mesh with their own goals.[10]

SUMMARY

The NATA and the profession of athletic training are both quite young. Our brief history can teach us a great deal about the value of service, the dedication of professionals to advance our cause, and the need for continued participation by members. The pioneering men and women of athletic training have advanced the profession by leaps and bounds in less than 65 years. It serves us well as individuals and members of a larger group to learn about the deeds of those who have come before us as we strive not to make the same mistakes and to set our sights ever higher as a profession.

The NATA (and the profession it promotes) has quite a bit on its plate for the future: political action, greater efforts to improve job settings, and attention to education. Continued advancement will require active professionals with the same level of dedication, participation, and service that has brought the organization to where it is today. As athletic training moves further into the 21st century, it is remarkable to look back and see where it came from; the future is indeed bright.

REFERENCES

1. Arnheim DD, Prentice WE. *Principles of Athletic Training*. 13th ed. New York, NY: McGraw-Hill Higher Education; 2009.
2. Ebel RG. *Far Beyond the Shoe Box: Fifty Years of the NATA*. New York, NY: Forbes Custom Publishing; 1999.
3. Hillman SK. Introduction to athletic training. In: Perrin DH, ed. *Athletic Training Education Series*. Champaign, IL: Human Kinetics; 2000.
4. Delforge GD, Behnke RS. The history and evolution of athletic training education in the United States. *Journal of Athletic Training*. 1999;34:53-61.
5. McLean JL. Does the NATA need a certification examination? *Journal of Athletic Training*. 1999;34:292-293.
6. Grace P. Milestones in athletic trainer certification. *Journal of Athletic Training*. 1999;34:285-291.
7. NATA. 2008 Membership statistics. Available at www.nata.org. Accessed July 25, 2008.
8. Board of Certification Inc. Exam eligibility. Available at www.bocatc.org. Accessed August 12, 2008
9. NATA-REF. NATA Research and Education Foundation. Available at www.natafoundation.org. Accessed July 25, 2008.
10. NATA-PAC. NATA political action committee. Available at www.natapac.org. Accessed August 12, 2008.

writing, many of these strategic initiatives are shaping up. Changes in the NATA committee structure and targeted programming to increase the involvement of younger members have already taken place. The NATA has recently increased its political activism on behalf of the profession through several sponsored legislative awareness events and the formation of the NATA Political Action Committee (NATAPAC). The NATAPAC was established in 2005 and works on behalf of all certified athletic trainers and the people

🌐 WEB RESOURCES

National Athletic Trainers' Association
www.nata.org

This site offers links to NATA committees, publications, position stands, and all aspects of the professional organization. Special section reserved for members allows access to employment listings and other member benefits.

Board of Certification, Inc
www.bocatc.org

The BOC Web site provides the most up-to-date information for certification candidates and CE information for current professionals.

NATA Political Action Committee
www.natapac.org

NATAPAC, established in 2005, is working on behalf of all certified athletic trainers and the people they treat. Like all political action committees, NATAPAC hopes to effect change by supporting candidates for public office whose views and intentions mesh with their own goals.

CHAPTER 3

GETTING STARTED
EDUCATIONAL REQUIREMENTS
FOR ATHLETIC TRAINING

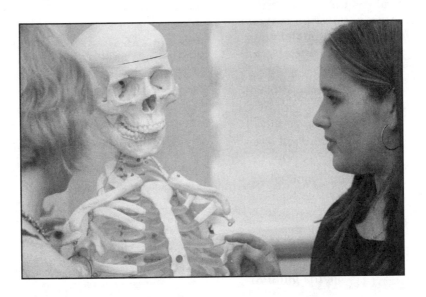

A good athletic trainer is someone who promotes the profession in everything they do. Someone who stays very current tries to learn new skills through continuing education, and most of all enjoys the profession of athletic training.

Kevin Guskiewicz, PhD, ATC
Professor, Department of Exercise and Sport Science/Director,
Sports Medicine Research Laboratory
University of North Carolina–Chapel Hill

If you have found your way to this chapter, chances are that you have enrolled in an introductory course to help you decide if athletic training is the right choice for you. It is imperative that students explore and understand their desired course of study, specifically the rigor and clinical demand and the professional opportunities that await them upon graduation. To sit for the BOC examination to become a certified athletic trainer, you must graduate from an athletic training education program that is accredited by CAATE. There is only one mechanism for professional preparation in athletic training.

The mission of CAATE is to provide comprehensive accreditation services to institutions that offer athletic training degree programs and verify that all CAATE-accredited programs meet the acceptable educational standards for professional (entry-level) athletic training education.[1] Universities and colleges that offer athletic training education programs must be dedicated to supporting the educational program, put forth the appropriate faculty and resources, and undergo an extensive self-evaluation followed by an on-site review in order to be an accredited program. Athletic training programs utilize a combination of formal classroom instruction and clinical experience to prepare athletic trainers to apply a wide variety of specific health care skills and knowledge within each domain that comprises athletic training.

Upon the completion of this chapter, the student will be able to:

- ✓ Explain how to obtain information on educational programs in athletic training
- ✓ Identify the organizations that work cooperatively to establish, maintain, and promote appropriate standards of quality for athletic training education programs
- ✓ Describe the content requirements of an athletic training education program
- ✓ Discuss the clinical requirements associated with an athletic training education program
- ✓ Identify qualities and characteristics that will contribute to success as an athletic trainer
- ✓ Describe the varied learning opportunities associated with clinical education
- ✓ Explain the guidelines for appropriate clinical supervision
- ✓ Discuss strategies to maximize the clinical learning experience
- ✓ Identify ethical issues that commonly face the athletic training student

Is Athletic Training Right for Me?

Making Contact: Finding an Athletic Training Education Program

A listing of accredited entry-level athletic training education programs can be found on-line at the CAATE Web site at www.caate.net. There are 2 kinds of entry-level education programs: undergraduate and entry-level master's. While there are fewer entry-level master's programs, it is anticipated that a growing number will pursue accreditation in the future. Entry-level master's programs may be more appropriate for prospective students who already hold a degree in a related field and would like to pursue athletic training without getting a second undergraduate degree. Students in this situation may be able to finish a program in 2 or 3 years rather than the typical 4-year degree. The NATA Task Force on Degrees in 2005 explored whether athletic training should require all programs to offer degrees in athletic training and what level should that degree be offered. The task force recommended (and the NATA board approved) that all athletic training programs offer a degree in athletic training and that this degree should be in place by 2014 to 2015. At this time, programs can be offered at either the undergraduate level or entry-level master's. A survey of other professions shows a trend of allied health programs moving to the graduate level for entry-level participation. This will be a topic of much discussion for the profession in the future. For now, the overwhelming majority of program offerings are undergraduate degree programs.

Some students will select their college or university choice based on the athletic training education program, some will find the program after they are on campus, and some may seek out a program as a transfer from a 2-year college or another institution. In any case, the best place to start is with both the program's and university's Web site. It is important to look closely at all aspects of the college or university. Athletic training programs can be found at small liberal arts colleges, major research universities, and every where in between. It is important to find both the program and school that best fits you. Interested students should speak to as many program personnel as possible. Making contact with the program director is usually the first step. Students may also try to speak with faculty, clinical instructors (CIs), and current students in the program. Speaking to current students is essential to get a feel for the program. Prospective students are encouraged to gather a range of inputs and never accept just one view on a program's strengths or weaknesses. Some athletic training programs will offer interest classes to help students get an overview of the program and profession (likely the kind of class that put this very book into your hands). Some campuses will offer formal athletic training interest programs to help students get small amounts of observational and hands-on experiences as they explore their desire for an athletic training course of study. Students are strongly encouraged to take advantage of any and all mechanisms to explore a program prior to applying for admission. The NATA Web site (www.nata.org) maintains an information section for prospective students that contains a wealth of information. Some topics include the following:

- ✓ Preparing for certification
- ✓ Information on joining the NATA
- ✓ Tools to locate athletic training programs
- ✓ Specific resources for college and secondary school students
- ✓ Videos from current student members of the NATA

Students will notice that the NATA Web site also lists advanced graduate programs in athletic training. Graduate education is commonplace among

Who's Who in the Athletic Training Education Program

Program Director

The program director is responsible for the day-to-day operation, coordination, supervision, and evaluation of all aspects of the athletic training educational program.

Clinical Coordinator

Clinical coordinators oversee the clinical field experiences for athletic training students. This may involve training CIs, evaluating clinical sites, and insuring that all guidelines are followed in the clinical settings and students are protected.

Faculty

Faculty teach required subject matter in the program and, depending on the type of institution, carry out a research agenda related to athletic training.

Approved Clinical Instructor

An approved clinical instructor (ACI) is a faculty, staff, or adjunct allied health or medical community member who provides formal instruction and/or evaluation of clinical proficiencies in the athletic training education program.

Clinical Instructor

A CI provides direct supervision of student in athletic training and other health care settings during clinical and field experiences.

Medical Director

The medical director serves as a resource to the program director and ATEP faculty regarding the medical content of the curriculum.

Clerical and Support Staff

Clerical and other support staff provide support to the overall athletic training education program.

Adapted from Commission on Accreditation of Allied Health Education Programs. *Standards and Guidelines for the Athletic Trainer.* 2001:1-12.

a desire to expand the depth of their athletic training knowledge. It is still a widespread practice for universities to fund graduate assistant positions that allow graduate students to get additional clinical experience while providing service to the intercollegiate athletic program. In exchange for this service, students are provided with a stipend and often full tuition remission. Students must then find an area of study to pursue a master's degree. While some degree programs are particularly useful, the downside of such an assistantship is that there is no guarantee of a meaningful connection between the clinical and academic programs. Students must explore these graduate options with care. Master's and doctoral level education is discussed further in Chapter 16.

Do Not Just Listen— Go and See!

Most athletic training education programs will require a period of observation in conjunction with an introductory class. The process of "job shadowing" is an excellent way to learn about a specific employment setting or gain an overview of the athletic training profession. Students who have had little exposure to the profession may wish to shadow an athletic trainer prior to enrolling in an introductory course. Current athletic training students may wish to shadow a professional in a work environment that they have not been exposed to within their program. These experiences will only assist the student in making an informed decision about his or her future. Do not just listen—go and see for yourself.

COLLEGE PREPARATION

As more and more high schools have the services of an athletic trainer, a greater number of high school students will identify an interest in the profession prior to attending college. In fact, many high schools have programs that allow students the opportunity to job shadow athletic trainers or develop basic skills. It is not uncommon for secondary schools to offer classes in basic athletic injuries or for advanced biology or health classes to have units on sports medicine.

While participating in a high school athletic training environment may be helpful, it should not be considered essential to collegiate study. The most important preparation prior to college is a successful academic program. Students with an interest in athletic training would be well served by a high school college preparatory program that includes an adequate amount of math and science. This should include both a broad range of sciences, including chemistry,

athletic trainers, with approximately 70% holding an advanced degree.[2] These advanced programs have been reviewed and approved by the NATA. These programs are designed for students who have completed entry-level preparation in athletic training, are already certified or eligible for certification, and have

---

Table 3-1

Common Admission Criteria for Athletic Training Education Programs

- Overall grade point average (GPA)
- Grades in specific courses
  - Introductory athletic training classes
  - Specific prerequisites
  - Core science classes
- Required observational hours
  - Many programs require observations in athletic training settings while the specific number of hours may vary; students should use the observation time to learn as much about the student experience as possible
- Essay
  - Professional and academic goals
  - Statement of interest
- Letter of recommendation
  - A letter from an instructor or athletic trainer that speaks to the student's academic potential and interest in athletic training
- Interview

The items listed above are common examples. Students should investigate the specific criteria for the program they are interested in attending.

---

physics, and biology. Health and human biology are also solid preparatory classes, and anatomy is a wonderful preparatory class if it is available. Individual programs and universities will look at different factors regarding admission. Grades, class rank, Scholastic Aptitude Test (SAT) or ACT scores, and interviews and recommendations are all key components. High school students with an interest in studying athletic training in college should work with their high school guidance counselor to plan an appropriate program.

program has a limited enrollment, it is paramount that prospective students gather appropriate data regarding the admissions process. No program that offers limited enrollment can guarantee entrance to students, so make sure you understand the admission requirements before you pursue the program. Students are entitled to make an informed decision regarding their desire to enroll and their realistic opportunity for admission. Table 3-1 lists typical admission criteria for an athletic training education program.

ATHLETIC TRAINING EDUCATION PROGRAM REQUIREMENTS

A COMPETITIVE COURSE OF STUDY

While each educational program is unique, the accreditation process is in place to insure that all programs meet essential standards for the preparation of athletic training students. Students should be aware that most athletic training education programs are competitive and require an admissions process. Limits in classroom and lab space, limited numbers of CIs (an 8:1 ratio of students to CI is recommended), and limited clinical experience opportunities may guide the available space in any given program. If a

THE ATHLETIC TRAINING CURRICULUM: CONTENT, COMPETENCIES, AND CLINICAL PROFICIENCY

CONTENT AREAS FOR ATHLETIC TRAINING EDUCATION

Each content area contains competencies that are a collection of knowledge, skills, and clinical abilities that an athletic training student completing an entry-level athletic training education program must master in order to be prepared to sit for the BOC certification examination. The 12 content areas as outlined in the NATA Educational Competencies are as follows[3]:

Desirable Qualities and Characteristics for Athletic Trainers

Groups of practicing athletic training professionals were asked, "If you had to pick specific qualities or character traits essential to success in our profession, what would they be?" The list below is a summary of their responses:

- Passion for their chosen field
- Intelligence
- Common sense
- Compassion/empathy
- Creativity
- Balanced and well rounded person
- Adaptability
- Curiosity
- Desire for lifelong learning
- Professionalism
- Work ethic
- Self-motivated
- Forward thinker
- Loyalty
- Ethics
- Even temperament
- Sense of humor
- Honesty
- Communicator
- Objective

1. Risk management and injury prevention: Injury and illness risk factors that may be encountered and the requisite planning and implementation of risk management and prevention programs

2. Pathology of injuries and illnesses: The physiological responses of human growth and development and the progression of injuries, illnesses, and diseases

3. Orthopedic clinical examination and diagnosis: The assessment of injuries and illnesses to determine proper management and referral

4. Medical conditions and disabilities: Recognition, treatment, and appropriate referral of the general medical conditions and disabilities of athletes and others involved in physical activity

5. Acute care of injury and illness: Recognition, assessment, treatment, and appropriate referral of acute injuries and illnesses

6. Therapeutic modalities: Planning, implementation, documentation, and evaluation of the efficacy of therapeutic modalities in the treatment of injuries and illnesses

7. Conditioning and rehabilitative exercise: Planning, implementation, documentation, and evaluation of the efficacy of therapeutic exercise programs for the rehabilitation and reconditioning of injuries and illnesses

8. Pharmacology: Pharmacologic applications, including awareness of the indications, contraindications, precautions, and interactions of medications and the governing regulations relevant to the treatment of injuries and illnesses

9. Psychosocial interventions and referral: Recognition, intervention, and appropriate referral of sociocultural, mental, emotional, and physical behaviors

10. Nutritional aspects of injury and illness: Understanding and recognition of the nutritional aspects of athletics and physical activity and to provide appropriate referral

11. Health care administration: Development, administration, and management of health care facilities and associated venues that provide care to athletes and others involved in physical activity

12. Professional development and responsibilities: Understanding professional responsibilities, avenues of professional development, and national and state regulatory agencies and standards in order to promote athletic training as a professional discipline and to educate athletes, athletic training students, the general public, the physically active, and associated individuals

The professional content areas outlined above are required content for all athletic training educational programs. In addition, programs can require a range of prerequisites or complimentary courses that go above and beyond the listed requirements. The number and structure of such courses will vary by program. Examples of courses that may serve as prerequisite courses or provide complimentary content in an athletic training education program include the following:

- ✓ Exercise physiology
- ✓ First aid and emergency care
- ✓ Human anatomy
- ✓ Human physiology
- ✓ Kinesiology/biomechanics
- ✓ Statistics and research design
- ✓ Strength training and reconditioning
- ✓ Chemistry
- ✓ Physics
- ✓ Biochemistry

Table 3-2

Commonly Identified Educational Needs

The items below were gleaned from multiple interviews with practicing athletic trainers in response to the question, "As a practicing ATC, in which specific areas do you wish you could have gathered more preparation?"

- Applied physiology
- Basic sciences
- Biomechanics
- Gait analysis
- Health care systems
- Nonorthopedic injury/illness
- Organization and administrative issues
- Pharmacology
- Physical and manual medicine
- Postural evaluation and a more holistic (versus segmental) approach
- Psychological aspects of care
- Technology applications
- Third-party payer and reimbursement issues

Many of these desired areas of preparation are now core aspects of the athletic training curriculum. Students should be aware that newly minted professionals must be committed to CE as they explore greater depth in any given area and pursue additional desired skills.

✓ Psychology
✓ Neurophysiology

These areas will comprise the core of the athletic training curriculum. Programs have great freedom to determine how these topics are presented and what the courses will be named. Programs will vary in how they sequence their courses and how they distribute the information. For example, a course entitled "Medical Aspects of Exercise and Sport" may focus primarily on the medical conditions and disabilities area but could also include content on risk management or administration. A course titled "Recognition and Diagnosis of Injuries and Illnesses" is pretty straight forward on what content area it is addressing, while "Advanced Athletic Training" could address, in part, multiple areas. Students can be assured that if a program has met the standards of CAATE accreditation, these content areas will be covered.

Sequencing of courses insures that students obtain the information in a logical fashion and that the necessary foundation is in place prior to learning specific information in the athletic training core program. It is also important that courses be sequenced so that athletic training students can acquire specific clinical skills prior to putting the skills into practice. A greater discussion of clinical requirements appears on p. 46.

Professions are constantly evolving. Athletic training has evolved to its current place among allied health professions through research, educational preparation, and advancements in clinical practice. Despite these advancements, it is not uncommon for athletic trainers to find themselves wishing they had gathered more skill in a specific area. Table 3-2 outlines areas in which practicing athletic trainers wish they had more preparation. Practicing athletic trainers comment that they have addressed these areas through CE and many have become enhanced in recent years by expanding the NATA Educational Competencies for athletic training education. Despite the strength of the athletic training curriculum, the need for successful professionals to be lifelong learners cannot be overstated.

EDUCATIONAL COMPETENCIES AND CLINICAL PROFICIENCIES

Competence and Proficiency

com•pe•tence *noun*

- The state or quality of being adequately or well qualified; ability.
- A specific range of skill, knowledge, or ability.

pro•fi•cien•cy *noun*

- The state or quality of being proficient; competence.

The NATA Education Council has identified the *Athletic Training Educational Competencies* and clinical proficiencies for the health care of athletes and others involved in physical activity. The *Athletic Training Educational Competencies* are designed to assist in identifying the knowledge and skills to be mastered within an entry-level educational program.[3] Athletic training education programs must use the competencies for curriculum development and the education of students enrolled in their program. Students in an athletic training education program can expect to have access to a master list of how the competencies are being met in their program. Some programs offer these with each syllabus, some distribute a master list annually, and some print the master list of competencies in the student handbook or make them available on-line.

Competencies are outlined within each of the previously discussed content areas and the practice domains that make up the role of the certified athletic trainer. Each competency is classified by behavioral objectives as follows[3]:

✓ Cognitive domain (knowledge and intellectual skills)

✓ Psychomotor domain (manipulative and motor skills)

✓ Clinical proficiencies (decision making and skill integration)

Below are some specific examples of each type of competency[3]:

✓ Content area: Risk management and injury prevention

   o Cognitive: Identify and explain the epidemiology data related to the risk of injury and illness related to participation in physical activity.

   o Psychomotor: Instruct a patient regarding fitness exercises and the use of weight-training equipment to include correction or modification of inappropriate, unsafe, or dangerous lifting techniques.

   o Clinical proficiency: Select, apply, evaluate, and modify appropriate standard protective equipment and other custom devices for the patient in order to prevent and/or minimize the risk of injury to the head, torso, spine, and extremities for safe participation in sport and/or physical activity. Effective lines of communication shall be established to elicit and convey information about the patient's situation and the importance of protective devices to prevent and/or minimize injury.

✓ Content area: Acute care of injuries and illnesses

   o Cognitive: Determine what emergency care supplies and equipment are necessary for circumstances in which the athletic trainer is the responsible first responder.

   o Psychomotor: Perform a secondary assessment and employ the appropriate management techniques for nonlife-threatening situations, including but not limited to environmental illness.

   o Clinical proficiency: Demonstrate the ability to manage acute injuries and illnesses. This will include surveying the scene, conducting an initial assessment, utilizing universal precautions, activating the emergency action plan, implementing appropriate emergency techniques and procedures, conducting a secondary assessment, and implementing appropriate first-aid techniques and procedures for nonlife-threatening situations. Effective lines of communication should be established and the results of the assessment, management, and treatment should be documented.

Educational content and specific competencies will be met through traditional classes, labs, and clinical opportunities. It is the clinical opportunities that help set athletic training programs apart from other endeavors. Putting new knowledge into practice in a controlled supervised setting is the essence of experiential learning.

In addition to competencies and clinical proficiencies, the *Athletic Training Educational Competencies* includes foundational behaviors of professional practice. These represent basic behaviors that permeate every aspect of professional practice. Programs should incorporate them into instruction across the curriculum. The behaviors comprise the application of common values in athletic training and are as follows:

✓ Primacy of the patient

✓ Teamed approach to practice

✓ Legal practice

✓ Ethical practice

✓ Advancing knowledge

✓ Cultural competence

✓ Professionalism

CLINICAL EXPERIENCE AND FIELDWORK IN ATHLETIC TRAINING

Clinical experience is a vital element to the educational preparation of the athletic trainer. Athletic training has long provided hands-on opportunities for students to practice skills. These clinical opportunities link the theory of the classroom to the practice of the clinical environment. Clinical education is based on the student's ability to demonstrate mastery of clinical proficiencies. The required clinical components of an athletic training education program will allow students the opportunity to see a variety of settings, interact with an array of sports medicine professionals, and develop needed athletic training skills. However, clinical proficiency extends beyond the simple mastery of skills—it requires an integration of cognitive, psychomotor, and affective components to form an appropriate clinical outcome. The clinical education experience provides students with technical skills as well as the opportunity to see how athletic trainers utilize interpersonal skills, work with diverse patient populations, and collaborate with other professionals. Through a structured and varied clinical program, students can learn both the art and the science of athletic training.

CLINICAL REQUIREMENTS

The CAATE *Standard for the Accreditation of Entry-Level Athletic Training Programs* outlines the requirements for a college or university to offer an accredited athletic training education program. This guide provides the following highlights for the clinical education of athletic training students:

✓ The content of the curriculum must include formal instruction in the expanded subject matter as identified in the *Athletic Training Educational Competencies*. Formal instruction must involve teaching of required subject matter with instructional emphasis in structured classroom and laboratory environments.

✓ Clinical experiences must follow a logical progression that allows for increasing amounts of clinically supervised responsibility. The clinical education plan must follow and reinforce the sequence of formal classroom and psychomotor skill learning.

✓ Clinical experiences must provide students with opportunities to practice and integrate the cognitive learning, with the associated psychomotor skills requirements of the profession, to develop entry-level clinical proficiency and professional behavior as an athletic trainer as defined by the *Athletic Training Educational Competencies*.[3]

These guidelines provide the link from the classroom to the real world of athletic training. This divide can be crossed in many ways. The most common method of obtaining clinical experiences is with the intercollegiate sports teams at your college or university. However, programs are required to offer a variety of experiences. Programs must provide opportunities

for students to gain clinical experiences with a variety of different populations, including genders, varying levels of risk, protective equipment (to minimally include helmets and shoulder pads), and medical experiences that address the continuum of care that would prepare a student to function in a variety of settings and meet the domains of practice delineated for a certified athletic trainer in the profession.[1] Many athletic training education programs offer clinical rotations in high schools, sports medicine clinics, recreational sport programs, clinic/industrial environments, and an assortment of related allied health settings. Each program will differ and prospective students should inquire about the number and variety of clinical experiences over the course of the program. Students should also gather information on the number of CIs and the students to CI ratio.

 Supervision of Clinical Experiences

Supervised clinical experiences shall involve daily personal contact and supervision between the CI and the student in the same clinical setting. The instructor shall be physically present in order to intervene on behalf of the individual being treated.[1]

Reference

1. Commission on Accreditation of Athletic Training Education. Standards for the Accreditation of Entry-Level Athletic Training Education Programs. Available at http://caate.net/documents/standards.6.30.08.pdf. Accessed April 19, 2009.

The CAATE standards also state that:

The athletic training curriculum must include provision for clinical experiences under the direct supervision of a qualified approved clinical instructor (ACI) or CI in an appropriate clinical setting.

✓ *The ACI or CI must be physically present and have the ability to intervene on behalf of the athletic training student to provide on-going and consistent education.*

✓ *The ACI or CI must consistently and physically interact with the athletic training student at the site of the clinical experience.*

✓ *There must be regular planned communication between the Athletic training education program and the ACI or CI.*

✓ *The number of students assigned to an ACI or CI in the clinical experience component must be of a ratio that will ensure effective education and should not exceed a ratio of 8 students to 1 ACI or CI in the clinical setting.*

Several provisions allow for the protection of the athletic training student. The student's clinical experience requirements must be carefully monitored.

✓ The length of clinical experiences should be consistent with other comparable academic programs requiring a clinical or supervised practice component. Such policies must be consistent with federal or state student work-study guidelines as applicable to the campus setting.

✓ Consideration must be given to allow students comparable relief (days off) from clinical experiences during the academic year as compared to other student academic and student activities offered by the institution (eg, other health care programs, athletics, clubs).

Under the supervision of a CI, students can learn and practice specific clinical proficiencies as they progress through their program. The above guidelines and strict supervision requirements are important to protect the welfare of the patient and to provide feedback to the student. Students may progress to a point in their program where they can carry out specific field experiences on their own within a set of established guidelines.

Experience

ex•pe•ri•ence *noun*

- Active participation in events or activities, leading to the accumulation of knowledge or skill: a lesson taught by experience; a carpenter with experience in roof repair. The knowledge or skill so derived.
- An event or a series of events participated in or lived through.
- The totality of such events in the past of an individual or group.

EXPERIENTIAL LEARNING

The essence of experiential learning is doing things. The only way to really learn the skills required to be an athletic trainer is by doing. Clinical experiences will provide students with the chance to perform the skills learned in an academic setting. Students also learn the day-to-day practice of athletic training that cannot be duplicated in an academic exercise. The clinical setting is a very different learning environment when compared to the confines of the classroom or laboratory. In an academic program, the goal is to provide students with knowledge and to facilitate creative thinking, while the clinical setting is designed to serve the needs of patients.[4] The academic program serves the needs of the students while clinical settings provide service delivery. Clinical settings are wonderful learning environments. Research shows that student learning ranks alongside patient care as a factor of job commitment.[5] However, students must be aware that the expectations for clinical settings will vary; the needs of patients come first. Creative instructors and appropriate supervision will allow students to meet their learning goals, but there will be a time when getting the job done in the interest of the patient is the priority. An intercollegiate athletic training setting has responsibilities to student-athletes and the local sports medicine clinic must serve the needs of its patients. However, it is the fact that these settings serve patients that makes them appropriate sources of clinical education.

In clinical environments, the workload, pace, and demands of a particular setting may cause students to feel these settings are less flexible than the academic structure to which they are accustomed. In addition, when athletic training students first spend time in the clinical environment, the ratio of instructors to students is rather low. This is a tremendous advantage over the long haul, but initially it can give the feeling of closer scrutiny than commonly found in the classroom setting.[4] This scrutiny is essential since the tasks you perform as part of a clinical experience have direct impact on the patients served in that setting. Students adjust rather easily to this type of supervision since the availability of the athletic training clinical supervisor is an invaluable learning resource. Supervision is key to clinical education. While experiences will vary from program to program, the presence of a supervisor is required for specific learning activities that involve patients. There can be other related experiences in your program that may allow for differing levels of supervisory interaction. Students should always make sure they communicate with their director and clinical supervisor to make sure they are adhering to the requirements of the program.

Clinical learning is situational and, at times, self-directed. It requires interaction, observation, practice, and problem solving.[2] Clinical learning must be an active process. Clinical or "real world" environments do not always provide situations in which there is a "right" answer. Students must adapt to this uncertainty and learn that there can be many ways to approach the same problem. Athletic training students who bring genuine curiosity and adaptability to the learning environment will be well positioned to succeed.

THE CLASSROOM— CLINICAL CONNECTION

Ideally, clinical education serves to link athletic training theory to practice. However, this is not always

Part of a Health Care Team: Working With Patients

The items below were gleaned from multiple interviews with practicing athletic trainers in response to the question, "As learners in a health care setting, students may find themselves assisting with patient care. What items must be explained or stressed to students about this learning environment?"

- Do not ever lose sight that you are dealing with a person not just an injury.
- Medical confidentiality is central to any discussion of patient care.
  - This is stressed as a standard of care and then as a matter of ethical behavior.
- Never forget that this is a "health care environment."
  - The fact that it takes place often in an athletic setting should not diminish this point.
- Patients come from all walks of life, with a range of differences (eg, socio-economic, religious, ethnic). Students have to be able to deal with these differences and be aware of the unique needs of all patients.
  - Students have to handle each patient carefully and learn about any situation that may influence how they are able to provide care for them.
- Proper professional behavior is essential.
  - This can be difficult when the patient is also a peer.
- Remember you are dealing with patients.
- Students cannot be afraid to ask for help when they are outside their limitations; this is something they are bound to do (ethically) as a professional.
- Students need to understand the emotional side of working with athletes, things like compassion, empathy, toughness, understanding, and all the different challenges facing that patient.
- Students need to understand the medical-legal issues related to their roles.
  - Do not do things that you have not been properly trained to do.
  - Know the boundaries of your skills.

 ## The Clinical Experience: A Student Perspective

Graduate students from a variety of athletic training postcertification programs were asked to outline what advice they would give to a new athletic training student about how to make the most of their clinical experiences. They provided the following insights:

- Always remember that you are a student—it is a learning experience. Do not be afraid to make mistakes; sometimes it is the best way to learn.
- Ask questions and do not be afraid to try new things. Everyone was once in your shoes and the only way to learn is to try it. Ask questions of the CIs, other athletic trainers, as well as other students in the program.
- Athletic trainers are very busy, but they love to share their knowledge when asked. You learn best by hearing, seeing, and doing. Use the time to do all three and gain confidence.
- Be open to all clinical experiences. Sometimes something you think will not be appealing ends up being the most rewarding.
- Bring a topic from class to each day of your clinical rotation to discuss with your ACI. The down time at practices can allow for some good clinical discussion.
- Do not think that because you are doing what seems like a meaningless task that you aren't appreciated. Your work as part of a team of medical professionals and picking up slack does not go unnoticed.
- Have a positive attitude.
- If you do not know something, you have to be willing to ask. Observe the things around you and try to understand the reasoning behind why things are done.
- Jump in as much as possible. Do everything that you are comfortable with and have been properly trained to do.
- Learn everything you can from each supervisor you have because they all have a different take on athletic training.
- Take all the information you learned in class and get your hands dirty... put your skills to use.

(continued)

The Clinical Experience: A Student Perspective (continued)

- When working with a CI, ask him or her WHY he or she is doing something, but be sure that it is at the appropriate time. Then take that answer and find it in your classroom experience to see if the academic theory and research evidence supports such a practice.
- When you learn something, try to apply it right away in the clinical setting or even try things out on your classmates or yourself to get a feel for it.
- Work within your boundaries but do not be afraid to try things on your own. That is the way you learn. Always ask questions and gain knowledge from everyone you can. Everyone has something for you to learn.
- Your CIs are there for you to learn from and they have experiences outside of text books that are very valuable. Asking them questions will also challenge them to improve as CIs.
- Your supervisors are there to protect you. As a student, you should experience everything that your setting has to offer.

<u>Table 3-3</u>

Examples of Helpful Behaviors as Perceived by Athletic Training Students

Mentoring

Explains—"ATC answered all my questions in great detail."
Demonstrates—"ATC asked me to come over and watch the evaluation of the athlete."
Constructive feedback—"ATC suggested some things that I might have done differently."

Professional Acceptance

Respect for student knowledge—"ATC assigned me to design the athlete's post-op shoulder rehab program."
Supportive—"ATC stuck up for me to the coach and agreed with my decision."

Nurturing

Supportive—"ATC makes a note to ask me how things are going and if he could be of any help."
Confidence building—"ATC stated that he thought I would be a very good athletic trainer."

Modeling

Good decision making—"ATC showed intelligence when removing an athlete from practice."

These items were taken from critical incident information provided by athletic training students. Incidents that were not helpful have also been identified. Students can recognize these helpful behaviors and reflect on how their role as students can influence these positive outcomes.

Adapted from Curtis N, Helion JG, Domsohn M. Student athletic trainers perceptions of clinical supervisor behaviors: a critical incident study. J Athl Train. 1998;33(3):249-253.

---

an easy connection. This link is sometimes complicated by the fact that students may see practices in the clinical setting that differ from current interpretations of research presented in the classroom environment. The classroom and clinical environment must not be viewed as program components that are independent of one another. The more students can connect them as learning elements that complement one another, they can maximize their learning and will be better prepared to recognize and learn from the occasional differences that may arise.

Athletic training clinical education research has identified specific characteristics that contribute to a positive clinical education experience for the athletic training student.[6,7] These studies outline student perceptions of supervisor behaviors[8] as well as student and instructor perceptions of helpful clinical characteristics.[7] Tables 3-3 and 3-4 delineate specific characteristics of CIs identified by previous research. While research has identified specific desirable characteristics of CIs, the approach taken by the athletic training student in the clinical educational process

---

Table 3-4

Helpful Characteristics of Clinical Instructors

Helpful characteristics identified by both students and clinical instructors:

- Displays confidence
- Demonstrates respect for the student
- Manages clinical emergencies well
- Provides opportunities for students to practice both technical and problem-solving skills
- Demonstrates skills for the students
- Is willing to admit when he or she does not know something
- Discusses the practical application of knowledge and skills
- Remains accessible to students
- Listens attentively to students and athletes

Adapted from Laurent T, Weidner T. Clinical instructors' and student athletic trainers' perception of helpful clinical instructor characteristics. *J Athl Train.* 2001;36(1):58-61.

 ## Classroom-Clinical Connections: Making the Most of Clinical Experiences

The items below were gleaned from multiple interviews with practicing athletic trainers in response to the questions, "What advice do you give students for making the connection from between the classroom and the clinical setting? How can students make the most of the clinical experience?"

- Ask lots of "why" questions.
- Be proactive.
  - ○ CIs have patient care responsibilities that come first (true for all health care settings) so you may need to take the lead on some learning opportunities.
- Consult your textbooks often and "on the spot" if necessary.
- Do not just ask questions—ask for feedback and areas for improvement.
- Practice new skills as soon as possible in the clinical setting.
- Recognize differences between underlying principles and differences in application.
  - ○ Sometimes theory can be well grounded but students may see differences in application—explore these differences.
- Share information, questions, and discussion points with your peers.
  - ○ Peer-to-peer learning is significant in clinical settings.
- Use the skills you learn and try to get out of your "comfort zone."
  - ○ The clinical environments are designed to protect students (via supervision) from making an injurious mistake, so you can feel comfortable making suggestions and posing hypotheses.
- View your classroom and clinical experience as extensions of each other and study appropriately for both.
  - ○ When in clinical settings discuss items from the classroom.
  - ○ When in the classroom discuss items from the clinical setting.

Making The Most of The Clinical Experience
- Be an active learner.
- Come ready to learn each and every day.
- Do not watch something and assume you know how to do it.
- Get past the observation mode and get your "hands on" as quickly as possible.
- It takes time to develop clinical skills and it takes practice to become proficient. You might get a skill "checked off a list" and know how to do it; however, it takes lots of practice to use the skill.

(continued)

Classroom-Clinical Connections: Making the Most of Clinical Experiences (continued)

- Learn to be a clinician not the technician.
- Remember, too, that learning extends far beyond psychomotor skills. You learn when you interact with people (or watch your CI do this); you learn when you talk to a patient about how he or she is feeling about an injury. Seek opportunity.
- Students need to see the psychological and emotional components that go along with the physical. I do not think you can recreate that in the clinical environment. Students need to be at lots of practices and competitions to see as much as possible.
- Students should try to see as many settings as possible and try to understand the roles of all the people in those settings beyond the athletic trainer.
- Take advantage and seek out every learning opportunity possible.
- You cannot be a wallflower and just sit back; you will miss out on a lot.

Note: Asking questions, practicing skills, and being a proactive learner were the most common responses to both of these questions.

Table 3-5

Ethical Behavior: Points of Emphasis for Athletic Training Students

The items below were gleaned from multiple interviews with practicing athletic trainers in response to the question, "What ethical issues do you feel students may be faced with in the course of their clinical education and how would you help them address them?"

- Act in a professional manner.
- Avoid getting caught up in the profile of the athletic setting—keep the patient's needs in focus.
- Avoid potentially difficult social situations.
- Avoid relationships that can compromise your professionalism.
- Be aware of sexual harassment issues.
- It is difficult to combine a social relationship with one where you want to be perceived as a health care professional.
- Maintain confidentiality.
- Place the health and welfare of the patient (athlete) over the pressure that might be exerted by parents, coaches, or outside influences.
- Students need to understand they're not excused from any ethical considerations just because they are a student.

Note: Maintaining medical confidentiality and professional social boundaries were the two most common ethical behavior responses

---

will greatly impact the quality of the experience. See the box on Clinical-Classroom Connections to identify strategies for maximizing the clinical learning experience portion of an athletic training program. These recommendations were identified by practicing athletic trainers.

ETHICAL BEHAVIOR

The word *ethics* has its origin from the Greek word *ethos*, which means the essence of your character. The word refers to a person's values or principles. In athletic training, the NATA's *Code of Ethics* is designed to make athletic trainers aware of the principles of ethical behavior and to assure quality patient care.[6] A copy of the NATA *Code of Ethics* is provided in Appendix B. Students are not exempt from ethical behavior; issues of professionalism, proper conduct, and confidentiality are commonly encountered through the course of a student's educational program. Gaining an understanding of common ethical situations coupled with an understanding of the NATA *Code of Ethics* will assist students in resolving dilemmas they may encounter as athletic training students. Table 3-5 presents ethical points of emphasis for the athletic training student.

SUMMARY

Athletic training education programs adhere to a stringent process of review and accreditation that insures that the minimum standards in quality are achieved by programs preparing entry-level athletic trainers. These programs must present the required competencies and clinical proficiencies in the 12 content domains that make up the responsibilities of the athletic trainer. Athletic training programs are competitive, and students should avail themselves to the admission guidelines of the program they seek to enter. Prospective students should gather information about both the didactic (class room) and clinical portions of the program while making an informed decision regarding application.

The opportunity for athletic training students to learn, practice, and refine skills in a clinical environment is the bridge that links the classroom to the "real world" of athletic training. Some of the information contained within this chapter is gleaned from professionals with years of experience assisting students in reaching their full potential. The clinical and field experience can provide the "big picture" connections and insights into the various professional practice settings. Students must approach every clinical rotation experience as both an opportunity to develop skills and an opportunity to learn about their future. They must ask themselves, "What settings do I enjoy the most? What skills do I need to work on? What are my strengths? What are my weaknesses? How can I build upon my cumulative experiences to become the best athletic trainer I can become?" The fact that clinical experiences are initiated early in athletic training education programs is a unique learning component not found in all other allied health areas. Students are urged to take full advantage of these learning opportunities.

REFERENCES

1. Commission on Accreditation of Athletic Training Education. *Standards for the Accreditation of Entry-Level Athletic Training Education Programs*. Available at http://caate.net/documents/standards.6.30.08.pdf. Accessed April 19, 2009.
2. National Athletic Trainers' Association. 2008 membership statistics. Available at www.nata.org. Accessed July 25, 2008.
3. National Athletic Trainers' Association. *Athletic Training Educational Competencies*. 4th ed. Dallas, TX: Author; 2006.
4. Barnes MA, Evenson ME. Fieldwork Challenges. In: Sladyk K, ed. *OT Student Primer: A Guide to College Success*. Thorofare, NJ: SLACK Incorporated; 1997:271-288.
5. Winterstein AP. Organizational commitment among intercollegiate head athletic trainers: examining our work environment. *Journal of Athletic Training*. 1998;33:54-61.
6. Curtis N, Helion JG, Domsohn M. Student athletic trainer perceptions of clinical supervisor behaviors: a critical incident study. *Journal of Athletic Training*. 1998;33:249-253.
7. Laurent T, Weidner TG. Clinical instructors' and student athletic trainers' perceptions of helpful clinical instructor characteristics. *Journal of Athletic Training*. 2001;36:58-61.
8. Hannam SE. *Professional Behaviors in Athletic Training*. Thorofare, NJ: SLACK Incorporated; 2000.

WEB RESOURCES

National Athletic Trainers' Association
www.nata.org
This site offers links to NATA committees, publications, position stands, and all aspects of the professional organization. A special section reserved for members allows access to employment listings and other member benefits.

Commission on Accreditation of Athletic Training Education
www.caate.net
Provides a listing of CAATE-accredited programs. Serves as a resource for program directors and posts public information about the role of CAATE.

The NATA Education Council
www.nataec.org
A resource for information regarding all aspects of athletic training education.

Career Spotlight: Head Athletic Trainer

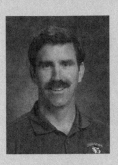

Scott Barker, MS, ATC

Head Athletic Trainer

California State University, Chico

My Position

The head athletic trainer is responsible for the development, organization, and administration of the sports medicine program, including providing work direction to other athletic trainers. As the head athletic trainer I am responsible for all elements of the athletic training services that are part of our sports medicine program.

Unique or Desired Qualifications

The head athletic trainer must demonstrate sufficient experience to be able to oversee athletic training operations for intercollegiate athletics and provide work direction to other professionals. People in this position must possess 3 to 4 years of experience as a certified athletic trainer with progressive responsibility, including at least one year of experience in program administration. A master's degree in athletic training or related field of study is preferred. The head athletic trainer must possess BOC certification and possess and maintain certification in CPR/AED (cardio pulmonary resuscitation and automated external defibrillation) for the professional rescuer and first aid.

Favorite Aspect of My Job

The day in and day out contact with student-athletes. As an athletic trainer, we see our student's athletes at extremes, from their highest highs to their lowest lows when injury presents. As athletic trainers we have the unique opportunity to be a significant influence in this person's life.

Advice

Always maintain your passion about what we do as athletic trainers. Never allow the job to become routine. Every time a student-athlete walks through your door, they are asking for your help. Whether they articulate this or not we have the opportunity to be a positive influence in their lives.

Note: For a complete overview of the job duties for a head athletic trainer, see the job description provided in Chapter 1.

CHAPTER 4

EDUCATIONAL RESOURCES FOR ATHLETIC TRAINING STUDENTS

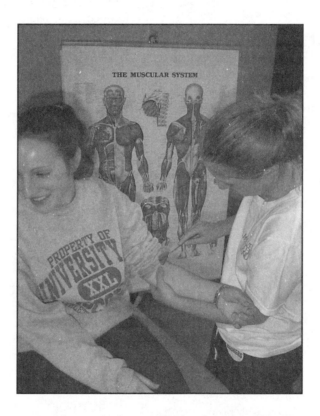

Students must strive to act in a professional manner. You are assisting with patient care in a medical facility, you need to maintain confidentiality, and keep your working relationships on a professional level.

Tony Marek, MS, ATC
Athletic Trainer
Peter Barbieri Manual Therapy–Reno Nevada

The decision to pursue athletic training as an academic major represents an exciting time for a prospective athletic training student. The opportunity to study an allied health profession that offers such a wide variety of learning opportunities should be exciting. Athletic atmospheres allow for stimulating clinical experiences. Sports can provide an enjoyable backdrop to accompany learning, and the opportunity to work with goal-oriented, physically active people is often a motivating factor for pursuing an athletic training program. However, athletic training is a rigorous academic endeavor. The very nature of combining traditional didactic coursework with clinical and field experiences creates a time demand that is different from many other academic programs. To be successful, athletic training students must understand their own learning preferences, recognize the need for strong study skills, and take advantage of the many resources available to assist them.

Upon completion of this chapter, the student will be able to:

✓ Identify his or her learning style

✓ Discuss specific study strategies to assist him or her in his or her academic program

✓ Describe methods of test taking that can improve performance

✓ Identify approaches to presentations and projects commonly found in athletic curriculums

✓ Outline potential sources of financial aid and scholarships available to the athletic training students

LEARNING PREFERENCES

Would you rather read information or listen to someone? Do you prefer a hands-on exercise or one that relies on paper and pencil? How you answer these questions is based on your own learning preferences or learning style. A learning preference addresses how a particular learner interacts with and responds to his or her learning environment.[1] Determining your learning style is usually accomplished by taking a learning styles inventory. Students who can identify their learning style can develop sound strategies for studying in college; the more effective the study strategies are, the more success the student will experience. Several tools are available to assess your preferred learning style. Table 4-1 provides a simple test to determine if your sensory learning preference is visual, auditory, or kinesthetic.

If you are a visual learner, you learn best by picturing information in your head. Visual learners tend to "see" a page of information. Visualizing colors, shapes, and size of objects assists in the recall of information for the visual learner. Visual learners can use study strategies that allow them to highlight notes using different color pens and shapes as visual cues.[1] Visual learners can benefit from associating images with specific concepts. This can be helpful in athletic training as students learn to associate anatomical images with various injuries and common injury mechanisms.

Auditory learners rely on their listening skills. Written notes and projects are often messy and writing during lecture activities sometimes can distract auditory learners. Auditory learners may benefit from studying in groups where they can hear what other students have to say. These students may wish to tape lectures and review sessions in order to listen to them again with care. Athletic training students who are auditory learners can take in a great deal of information while participating in their clinical setting. Following instruction from clinical supervisors

and taking patient histories rely heavily on auditory skills.

The kinesthetic or tactile sensory learning modality is most often associated with athletic training skill development. This is the classic "learning by doing" modality. This is sometimes thought of only in the context of learning the skill that is currently being studied. While this may be true, kinesthetic learners like to be active while they are learning. Using flashcards while riding an exercise bike, discussing concepts while jogging or walking with a friend, or drawing diagrams of concepts are all examples of kinesthetic learning.

While it can be helpful to determine your sensory preference to assist with your study strategies, it is best to develop study skills that involve a variety of learning styles. It is best to begin with study habits that are best suited to your preference and then gradually incorporate other styles.[1] Learning preferences are individual so do not be surprised if habits that work for your roommate do not work for you. Exploring your individual learning preference and adjusting your habits accordingly is the sign of a responsible student.

The literature on learning styles among allied health professionals does not indicate a clear preference of learning style for students in athletic training.[2,3] However, some studies have indicated that a high percentage of athletic training students are kinesthetic or tactile learners with a trend toward independent learning. Since athletic training students demonstrate great diversity in learning styles,[3] CAATE-accredited athletic training education programs will need to incorporate a wide variety of teaching methods in order to appeal to a broad range of student learning preferences. Hands-on clinical experiences, group activities, presentations, and student-centered learning projects are just a few examples.

STUDY SKILLS FOR ATHLETIC TRAINING STUDENTS

New college students can sometimes fall prey to the myth and folklore that surround studying. Some of my favorites include:

✓ "You do not have to go to class, just get the notes."

✓ "A little cramming is good right before the exam."

✓ "The caffeine edge will help you stay sharp."

✓ "Everyone pulls the all-nighter."

Table 4-1

Learning Preferences

This chart helps you determine your learning style. Read the word in the left column and then answer the questions in the successive 3 columns to see how you respond to each situation. Your answers may fall into all 3 columns, but one column will likely contain the most answers. The dominant column indicates your primary learning style.

When you..	Visual	Auditory	Kinesthetic and Tactile
Spell	Do you try to see the word?	Do you sound out the word or use a phonetic approach?	Do you write the word down to find if it feels right?
Talk	Do you dislike listening for too long? Do you favor words such as see, picture, and imagine?	Do you enjoy listening but are impatient to talk? Do you use words such as hear, tune, and think?	Do you gesture and use expressive movements? Do you use words such as feel, touch, and hold?
Concentrate	Do you become distracted by untidiness or movement?	Do you become distracted by sounds or noises?	Do you become distracted by activity around you?
Meet someone again	Do you forget names but remember faces or remember where you met?	Do you forget faces but remember names or remember what you talked about?	Do you remember best what you did together?
Contact people on business	Do you prefer direct, face-to-face, personal meetings?	Do you prefer the telephone?	Do you talk with them while walking or participating in an activity?
Read	Do you like descriptive scenes or pause to imagine the actions?	Do you enjoy dialog and conversation or hear the characters talk?	Do you prefer action stories or are not a keen reader?
Do something new at work	Do you like to see demonstrations, diagrams, slides, or posters?	Do you prefer verbal instructions or talking about it with someone else?	Do you prefer to jump right in and try it?
Put something together	Do you look at the directions and the picture?		Do you ignore the directions and figure it out as you go along?
Need help with a computer application	Do you seek out pictures or diagrams?	Do you call the help desk, ask a neighbor, or growl at the computer?	Do you keep trying to do it or try it on another computer?

Adapted from Rose C. *Accelerated Learning for the 21st Century.* New York: Delacorte Press; 1997.

✓ "Do not worry about the sources, the professor will never check."

These myths and legends rank right up there with the urban legends that circulate on college campuses everywhere. Table 4-2 (p. 61) presents effective strategies suggested by college students themselves.

The sections that follow are study skills that are appropriate for all aspects of your college experience. Most college and university campuses have resource centers to assist with the skills discussed in this chapter. Successful students often are those who make the most of the resources available to them. Seek out support to make the most of the learning experience.

NOTE TAKING

Most students develop a system for taking notes that "works best for them." It is important to use a consistent system for taking class notes in a way that allows you to refer to back to them as useful study tools. The following list includes suggestions for improving your note-taking system[4]:

✓ Listen actively. Think about the subject matter but try not to get behind.

✓ Be open minded about items you may disagree on. Do not let arguing hinder your note taking.

✓ Use symbols and abbreviations. Using common medical abbreviations can be a helpful tool.

Learning Preference Inventory—Information Processing

Assign the appropriate score for each of the statements below:

(3) Often

(2) Sometimes

(1) Seldom/Never

Visual Modality

_____ I remember information better if I write it down.

_____ Looking at the person helps keep me focused.

_____ I need a quiet place to get my work done.

_____ When I take a test, I can see the textbook page in my head.

_____ I need to write down directions, not just take them verbally.

_____ Music or background noise distracts my attention from the task at hand.

_____ I do not always get the meaning of a joke.

_____ I doodle and draw pictures on the margins of my notebook pages.

_____ I have trouble following lectures.

_____ I react very strongly to colors.

_____ Total

Auditory Modality

_____ My papers and notebooks always seem messy.

_____ When I read, I need to use my index finger to track my place on the line.

_____ I do not follow written directions well.

_____ If I hear something, I will remember it.

_____ Writing has always been difficult for me.

_____ I often misread words from the text (ie, "them" for "then").

_____ I would rather listen and learn than read and learn.

_____ I am not very good at interpreting an individual's body language.

_____ Pages with small print or poor quality copies are difficult for me to read.

_____ My eyes tire quickly, even though my vision check-up is always fine.

_____ Total

Kinesthetic/Tactile Modality

_____ I start a project before reading the directions.

_____ I hate to sit at a desk for long periods of time.

_____ I prefer first to see something done and then to do it myself.

_____ I use the trial-and-error approach to problem solving.

_____ I like to read my textbook while riding an exercise bike.

_____ I take frequent study breaks.

_____ I have a difficult time giving step-by-step instructions.

_____ I enjoy sports and so well at several different types of sports.

_____ I use my hands when describing things.   (continued)

Learning Preference Inventory—Information Processing (continued)

_____ I have to rewrite or type my class notes to reinforce the material.

_____ Total

Total the score for each section. A score of 21 points or more in a modality indicates a strength in that area. The highest of the 3 scores indicates the most efficient method of information intake.

Adapted from the Barsch Learning Style Inventory by Jeffrey Barsch, EdD and the Sensory Modality Checklist by Nancy A. Haynie.

Learning Style Characteristics: Evaluating Your Learning Preference
Check all of the characteristics that apply to you.

1. ( ) When I have a problem, I usually tell someone right away.

2. ( ) I keep a journal.

3. ( ) I often take notes, although I do not always refer to them.

4. ( ) I take good notes and then rewrite them at a later time.

5. ( ) I read in my free time.

6. ( ) I have the TV on even when I am not watching it.

7. ( ) I have good intentions of writing to people but usually call instead.

8. ( ) I often shut my eyes to help me concentrate.

9. ( ) When studying or solving a problem, I pace back and forth.

10. ( ) I would rather hear a book on audiocassette than read it myself.

11. ( ) Forget the cassette, I would rather wait until it comes out on film.

12. ( ) I prefer reading the newspaper to watching the news on TV.

13. ( ) I prefer to study in a quiet environment.

14. ( ) To remember a spelling, I see the word in my mind.

15. ( ) I prefer an oral exam to a written one.

16. ( ) I prefer a multiple-choice format on a test.

17. ( ) I would rather do a project than write a paper.

18. ( ) I would rather give an oral report than a written one.

19. ( ) I remember better what I read rather than what I hear.

20. ( ) I keep a personal organizer.

21. ( ) I reread my notes several times.

22. ( ) I would rather take notes from the text than attend a lecture on the material.

23. ( ) I often "talk to myself."

24. ( ) I learn best when studying with a partner.

25. ( ) I can locate a passage that I have read by "seeing it."

26. ( ) I find it hard to sit still when I study.

27. ( ) If I forget why I walked in the kitchen, I retrace my steps from the bedroom.

28. ( ) Once in bed for the night, I shut my eyes and plan the next day.

29. ( ) I cannot clean unless the music is on.

30. ( ) I would rather read directions than have someone tell me about them.   (continued)

Learning Preference Inventory—Information Processing (continued)

31. ( ) I can put something together as long as the directions are written.

Scoring

Compare your answers to the list below. Circle the number/letter combinations that correspond to your answers.

1. S	6. L	11. V	16. V	21. R	26. D
2. W	7. S	12. R	17. D	22. W	27. D
3. D	8. V	13. L	18. S	23. S	28. V
4. W	9. D	14. V	19. R	24. S	29. L
5. R	10. L	15. S	20. W	25. V	30. R
					31. R

Tally the number of S, W, D, L, and V Responses and record the totals:

S: W: D: R: L: V:

Three or more responses of one letter indicates you likely have a preference for that learning style. Most people have at least one preference and many have more than one.

Learning Preference Descriptions

Speaking (S): Indicates you have a preference for learning information by saying it. Talking about information helps you learn it. Strategies for these learners may include reading notes aloud, having a study partner, asking people to listen to your explanations, or anything that requires speaking of the material.

Writing (W): If your learning preference is writing, then any activity that involves writing will help you learn material more quickly. Strategies include lots of note taking, rewriting notes, writing on index cards, or making your own written tests. These learners may excel in classes with essay exams.

Doing (D): This is also described as a kinesthetic learner. These learners learn by doing such as making models, diagramming information, and performing hands-on tasks. Kinesthetic learners may also enjoy reviewing material while walking or exercising. Activity is the key component to this learning type.

Reading (R): Learners with this learning preference will pick material up more quickly through reading. Study strategies include borrowing notes of other students to fill in information you may have missed. Highlighting and rereading is effective. Reading additional material on course content will also be helpful.

Listening (L): Students with the listening learning preference will benefit from study groups or studying with a partner. Listening to tapes, lectures, or review sessions may also be helpful. Sharing information and reading notes to others with the listening preference may be a good strategy.

Visualizing (V): Visual learners learn best by picturing or "seeing" information in their mind. They may benefit from closing their eyes and trying to recall or see a page of information. Effective study strategies may include using various color pens to write notes and taking notice of the shape, color, and size of the paper and highlights to assist with visual recall.

Adapted from Sladyk K. *OT Student Primer: A Guide to College Success*. Thorofare, NJ: SLACK Incorporated; 1997:39-41.

✓ Leave some space between concepts in case you wish to add material later.

✓ Use regular 8.5-by-11 inch paper. Smaller notebooks are easier to carry but not functional for taking good notes.

✓ Take time after class to summarize your notes. Summarize your notes in one page that covers the major concepts, specific points, and any "take home messages."

✓ Write good notes the first time. Recopying can be very time consuming. Rather than recopy,

Table 4-2

Effective Study Habits

Before Class

- Meet 30 min before class with a study group and discuss interesting course content.
- Try to relate the reading from class to observations in your clinical experiences.
- Find a study partner and quiz each other regularly.
- Use a calendar to mark classes and assignment due dates.
- Make "to-do" lists and prioritize your work.
- Talk to former students who have taken the class (learn the teacher's style).
- Ask for a syllabus before class begins. Buy books and read before the first class.
- Complete all assigned readings before class. Reread after class.
- Read the syllabus closely and check it often.
- Record the lecture, then listen to the tape after class. Stop the tape and ask yourself questions.
- Turn in all assignments on time. If you must miss a class meeting when an assignment is due, turn it in early.

During Class

- Arrive to class on time.
- Sit in the first or second row of lecture classes.
- Take notes on what you do not know, not what you do know.
- Ask questions.
- Relate material to other courses and/or your clinical experiences.
- If you are called upon and do not know the answer, politely say so.
- Keep side conversations during class to a minimum.
- Reading the newspaper or doing work for another class is disrespectful.
- Ask yourself key questions to help relate new information to past experiences, beliefs, or ideas. It is helpful to relate items to other athletic training classes (eg, information from evaluation class can be linked with information in your rehabilitation class).
- If you must miss a class, contact the instructor (most will request you email them) and explain why. Arrange, on your own, to have 2 or 3 other students take notes for you. It is your responsibility to figure out what you missed and need to hand in.

After Class

- Studying is more than reading; find ways to interact with the subject matter. Ask yourself questions.
- Imagine you were writing an exam. What points would you cover?
- Visit your instructor at least once or twice during office hours, introduce yourself (if he or she does not know you or you are unsure), and ask an intelligent question.
- Consider making flash cards (questions on front and answers on back) from your notes. Once you make them, carry them with you and study them between classes. Particularly if you have to memorize material (ie, origins and insertions of muscles, special tests for evaluation).
- Study in spare moments during the day, squeeze in chunks of new material.
- Schedule regular times in your personal calendar for study blocks. Two hours at a time if possible.
- Ask someone to proofread your work (every author needs an editor).
- Use highlighters and colored pens to make key points stand out.

Adapted from Pranger H. Learning as a college student. In: Sladyk K, ed. *OT Student Primer: A Guide to College Success*. Thorofare, NJ: SLACK Incorporated; 1997:37-47.

I Have Not Yet Begun to Procrastinate!

Is this your slogan? Do you always find time to do anything but what you are supposed to do? If left unchecked, procrastination can create significant stress for students and wreck havoc on their academic life. Wasted time cannot be recovered, and missed opportunities do not always come back around. If you think you are a procrastinator, maybe the following suggestions will keep you on task.

- Rational self-talk
  - Excuses will not hold up to rational inspection. You need to challenge the faulty logic behind each excuse.
  - Excuse: "I'm not in the mood to study."
  - Realistic thought: "Mood doesn't do my work, actions do."
  - Waiting for the right mood will not get anything done.
- Positive self-statements
  - Incorporate positive statements. "The sooner I get it done, the sooner I can play."
- Do not create a catastrophe
  - Do not jump to conclusions about outcomes. "I will fail" or "I'm no good at this." Negative predictions are not facts. Focus on the present and what positive steps you can take toward reaching your goals.
- Avoid perfectionism
  - Doing something imperfectly is better than not doing it at all. You can improve later with revisions.
- Design clear goals
  - Think about what needs to be done. Be specific. Set realistic goals for your project. If your goals are too big, they can overwhelm you and it will be easier to procrastinate.
- Set priorities
  - Write out what you need to get done in order of importance. This will allow you to set priorities. BE CAREFUL. Elaborate list making is a great way to procrastinate!
- Get organized
  - Have your materials ready before you begin.
- Use prompts and reminders
  - Notes stuck on the bathroom mirror, TV remote, and front door will remind you what needs to be done.
- Reward yourself
  - Self-reinforcement can help you develop your "do it now" attitude. Reward yourself with the completion of tasks. Do not overdo it! But the reward of a 30-minute walk for an ice cream cone after 2 hours of studying can be helpful on a sunny day when you would rather not be studying!
- Work in groups
  - Working with friends from the same class can help keep you all on task.

Adapted from University of Wisconsin-Madison. *Greater University Tutoring Service Study Skill Handbook*. Madison, WI: Author; 2008.

summarize your notes and interject some items from your reading to support concepts from class.

✓ Sit close to the front. There are fewer distractions and you will have an easier view of the board.

✓ Ask one or two classmates to share notes with you. This will allow you to see how others interpret the same information.

Improving your note-taking skills will enhance the learning experience. Good notes allow you to move beyond just writing down what was said and move toward truly interacting with the course content.

READING ASSIGNMENTS

Reading assignments for athletic training classes can be challenging. Chapters in athletic training texts often contain a significant amount of anatomical information and terminology. Developing an active reading plan will help you get the most out of your reading assignments. The biggest piece of advice for any student in college courses is to DO YOUR READING as it is outlined in your syllabus. Much like taking notes, you will need to develop an approach. Table 4-3 outlines a 3-step reading plan that includes planning your reading by asking questions, reading

---

Table 4-3

Three-Step Active Reading Strategy

I. Pre-Plan and Ask Questions

- Do not just dive in!
- Skim the pages by searching for main points.
  - Read the objectives at the beginning of the chapter.
  - Read the chapter summary.
- Scan the pages and read the highlighted definitions, formulas, or key facts.
- Ask yourself the following:
  - How does this information relate to previous topics?
  - What am I supposed to learn?
  - Why it this material important?
  - Formulate potential exam questions.

2. Read the Chapter Actively

- Use the headings to focus your reading.
- Think about your potential questions and think of new questions as well.
- Take a 5-minute break when you burn out or get sleepy.
- Read with the goal of learning not just finishing.

3. Review

- Reread the chapter summary.
- Evaluate for yourself if you met your goals.
- Try to relate your reading to something
  - Tie the material to your clinical experience.
  - Relate the material to previous lectures.
- Ask more questions!

Adapted from Pranger H. Learning as a college student. In: Sladyk K, ed. *OT Student Primer: A Guide to College Success.* Thorofare, NJ: SLACK Incorporated; 1997:37-47.

---

the chapter actively, and reviewing what you have read. Your reading assignments coupled with your class notes and insights from your professor will provide you with a knowledge base from which you can draw and connect to your larger athletic training program.

HEALTHY HABITS FOR THE ATHLETIC TRAINING STUDENT

TIME MANAGEMENT

Time management is a consistent theme put forth by any student who has been successful in college. Making a schedule, setting aside time to study, mak-ing lists, and prioritizing your tasks can all be found in Table 4-2. To get a more realistic view of what it takes to manage your time as an athletic training student, graduate students from a variety of athletic training postcertification programs were asked to describe key time management skills that they would share with new athletic training students. They provided the following recommendations:

- ✓ Account for every hour in a week. Schedule appropriate sleep, time in class, and time in your clinical setting. What is left is your time to study, socialize, etc. You may have more time than you realize.

- ✓ Be sure you understand the time commitments of your clinical experience.

- ✓ Blend your classroom assignments with the clinical setting. You can review and work with concepts in your clinical time; it is like studying without trying to study.

- ✓ Do not wait until you are in a hole before you ask for help.
- ✓ Invest in a day planner or calendar system.
- ✓ Keep a list of all the things you need to do and refer to it often.
- ✓ Keep a regular study schedule.
- ✓ Manage your time and communicate with ACIs, professors, and advisors often.
- ✓ Plan everything, including time for yourself.
- ✓ Read ahead. Use the syllabus as a planning device.
- ✓ Set aside time every day to study core athletic training concepts.
- ✓ Stay organized and review your schedule often.
- ✓ Take time to learn about your own learning style so you can study effectively.
- ✓ Use the small chunks of time between classes purposefully.
- ✓ Write EVERYTHING down.

STRESS MANAGEMENT AND HEALTHY HABITS

College can be a challenging time for students to maintain healthy habits. Good eating and sleeping habits are challenging for college-age students. Weight gain has been documented as a college health problem. A 2007 University of Minnesota study, which surveyed 10,000 students across 14 campuses in Minnesota, found that 39% of all students fell within the overweight or obese/extremely obese categories, and 70% of students gained a significant amount of weight between the start of college and the end of sophomore year (an average of 9 pounds). The report states that food choices, not volume, were the most common culprit.

Alcohol consumption and the resulting associated risk behaviors are well documented for this age group. Data from several national surveys indicate that about 4 in 5 college students drink and that about half of college student drinkers engage in heavy episodic consumption. The US Surgeon General and the US Department of Health and Human Services have identified binge drinking among college students as a major public health problem. Binge drinking is typically defined as consuming 5 or more drinks in a row for men and 4 or more drinks in a row for women.

Given the potential pitfalls, students must use great caution in selecting appropriate activities to manage the stress of their academic program and personal lives. Athletic training students as care providers in training need to look at the big picture and develop healthy habits themselves. The same graduate athletic training students who discussed time management in the preceding section have outlined these thoughts on stress management and healthy habits:

- ✓ Athletic training (like all health care) is about serving others. You have to take time out to help yourself.
- ✓ Avoid drama. Being a helpful friend does not mean you have to take on other people's stress. Keep yourself healthy first.
- ✓ Dealing with injuries can be stressful and as a student you need to expose yourself to some stressful situations. However, let your ACIs be very helpful in this area.
- ✓ Do not feel like you have to do everything on your own. Your ACIs and instructors understand and they will be helpful. Talk to people when you are feeling the pressure.
- ✓ Do not forget to have fun. Make sure that if there is something you like to do (hobby, sport, interest), do not give it up; use it to help relieve stress.
- ✓ Exercise.
- ✓ Find comfort in your peers since they are likely going through the same stress.
- ✓ Find something outside of athletic training that you enjoy.
- ✓ I found my clinical experience to be a stress reliever. I was able to learn without the structure of a classroom. I loved the setting and using information in a practical manner.
- ✓ Make sure to schedule social time to relax.
- ✓ Stress can either hurt you or help you. Learn to take things one step at a time and not get overwhelmed by everything at once. Use good time management and organization and help keep the stress low.
- ✓ Stress management is a little different for everybody. Find what works best for you because there are bound to be stressful situations in the field of athletic training.
- ✓ Work out, hang out with friends, give yourself some time to recharge or you will burn yourself out.

It is worth noting that exercise was one of the most frequently noted stress management tools for athletic training students. It only stands to reason that those interested in physical activity would mention this fact. Students mentioned many healthy habits, including joining an intramural team, taking an activity course, learning meditation and yoga, pursing a hobby, maintaining good nutrition, and getting enough sleep. It is no mystery that those who take care of others need to care for themselves as well.

Student to Student: Keys to Success in an Athletic Training Program

Graduate students from a variety of athletic training postcertification programs were asked to reflect on their recent entry-level program experience and provide "keys" to success for new athletic training students. They identified the following key items:

- Ability to relate to diverse groups of people
- Ability to think outside the box
- Communication skills
- Creativity
- Dedication
- Empathy
- Enthusiasm
- Flexibility
- Inquisitiveness
- Interpersonal skills
- Love of learning
- Loyalty
- Open mind
- Passion
- Pro-active learner
- Self-motivation
- Sense of humor
- Study skills
- Team player
- Time management skills
- Willingness to challenge yourself
- Work ethic

TAKING EXAMS: DEALING WITH TEST ANXIETY

Taking exams is inherently stressful for students. Athletic training programs will likely include a variety of testing techniques, including written exams and oral practical examinations. Test anxiety is conceptualized as a situation-specific personality trait that has 2 psychological components: worry and emotionality. Worry refers to the cognitive side of test anxiety, whereas emotionality refers largely to a person's awareness of bodily arousal and tension. Students who get nervous before and during examinations often experience an increased heart rate and progressive anxiety. Test anxiety is not inherently harmful if the accompanying nervous energy is properly directed. If properly directed, this energy may enhance performance.[5] However, when this anxiety produces a negative performance, steps must be taken to better handle testing situations. Studies indicate that poorly managed test anxiety can lead to decreases in both performance and motivation, thus creating a difficult environment for success.

Test anxiety is causing problems if your anxious state is resulting in poor performance. "Blanking" on answers, physical symptoms, inability to focus your eyes on the page, and self-doubt can indicate a test anxiety problem. Some students with test anxiety experience physical distress symptoms such as headaches, nausea, faintness, and changes in body temperature. Other students may experience emotional changes such as wanting to cry or laugh too much, feelings of anger, or helplessness.[4,5] Test anxiety must be managed during the examination time to allow students the best opportunity to correctly respond to the exam questions and not allow their thinking abilities to be compromised. Strategies for managing test anxiety are designed to direct your anxiousness toward a positive performance. Common strategies for test anxiety include mental preparation, physical preparation, and relaxation techniques. Table 4-4 presents strategies for alleviating test anxiety. Students who are experiencing test anxiety are encouraged to contact their campus counseling center for assistance.

COURSEWORK: COMMON ASSIGNMENTS FOR THE ATHLETIC TRAINING STUDENT

Athletic training is an exciting area of study that incorporates many other disciplines. The ability to bring together anatomy, physiology, biomechanics, and other subject areas and apply these concepts to real injury scenarios allows instructors to be very creative in how they ask students to demonstrate their knowledge. While a large portion of your athletic training program will involve traditional written exams combined with oral practical tests, there are a limitless number of written and group projects that you may encounter. Being prepared for these learning situations will allow you to maximize the experience. The assignments and projects listed next are a small sample of common practice. The following list is a representative sample identified by athletic training students as their favorites:

Table 4-4
Managing Test Anxiety

Mental Preparation

Before the Exam

- Be thoroughly prepared. A confident knowledge of course material is the first step in reducing test anxiety.
- For clinical skills and oral practical exams, be sure you have practiced and can explain how the clinical skills are utilized.
- Review material. Review should be spaced throughout the week. This aids memory development and retention.
- Do not cram. A final review is fine, but trying to cover 2 months of material in 2 hours is not an effective way to prepare for an exam. Begin your review process early to help reduce last minute anxiety.
- Arrive at the exam location early. Relax, and do not talk about the test with friends. Frantic reviews are often more confusing than helpful.

During the Exam

- Some initial tension is normal. Generally, when you receive the test, stop for a moment, take a few deep breaths and exhale slowly, relax, and then start reviewing directions and test items.
- In a timed test, make a schedule for answering questions. Allow more time for higher-point questions. Pace yourself to answer as many questions as possible.
- Do not spend too much time on any one question. If you do not know the answer, quickly move on. You can always come back if you have time. Higher scores will usually result from trying all items.
- If you get stumped on a question, move on to questions you can answer. This will get your mental process and concentration ready for more difficult questions.

Physical Preparation

Before the Exam

- Develop good study habits and techniques. Adequate food and rest are important parts of any study program, especially before an exam. When people are tired, they become frustrated easier and experience more anxiety.

During the Exam

- Find a place where you will have some privacy (ie, well-lighted and comfortable). Bring everything you will need (scratch paper, pencils, calculator, etc). Avoid locating yourself near doors or other high distraction areas.

Relaxation Techniques

When used with mental and physical preparation, relaxation before and during an exam can aid retention and improve test performance.

- Let your body relax. Put your arms at your side, close your eyes, and let your mind go blank.
- Beginning with your head, first tense the muscles in the forehead and scalp for about 10 seconds. Then let them relax completely. Think about the difference and concentrate on making those muscles relax more and more.
- After about 30 seconds, repeat the process with the muscles of your face and jaw, neck, shoulders, arms, chest, etc until you reach your toes.
- While continuing to relax, imagine those situations in which you feel most tense and anxious. If you become anxious, stop imagining and relax again. Repeat the process of relaxation and imagining until you feel no anxiety while imagining.
- Practice relaxing at times when you feel anxious (ie, while studying, reviewing, or actually taking the exam [if time permits]). This will reduce tension and help clear your mind for study and review.

Adapted from The Greater University Tutoring Service. Study Skills Handbook. Madison, WI: University of Wisconsin Board of Regents; 2008.

✓ Athletic training facility design

✓ Case studies

✓ Developing an athletic training student handbook that includes policy and procedures

✓ Evidence-based research projects

✓ Lab assignments from the modalities course (it allowed me to put my physiology information to use)

✓ Literature reviews

✓ Mock evaluations

✓ Planning and developing a budget for an athletic training program

✓ Practical examinations with classmates playing the part of the patient

✓ Working on an actual research project being done by one of the athletic training professors

✓ Working with an ACI developing rehabilitation plans and criteria for progression for an actual patient

 ## Find a Teacher (and a Librarian!)

There is an old Zen saying that you should find a teacher, then practice. Any good teacher who is a source of learning should be treated preciously. You do not want to overlook an opportunity to learn. In this spirit, I would encourage all students to seek out a source of learning that is often overlooked. Do not just find a teacher, find a librarian!

Librarians are the gateway to so many resources. Librarians can help with the following:

● Access appropriate bibliographic databases like PubMed (MEDLINE)

● Provide instruction on how to manage and organize resources

● Give guidance on how to use online tools like RSS readers and MyNCBI (National Library of Medicine) to personalize your information resources

● Instruct you on various evidence-based practice resources to answer clinical questions

An athletic training student who can master the above tasks will be well on his or her way to becoming a scholarly clinician.

Indeed. Find a librarian.

WRITING PAPERS

Athletic training is a profession that requires excellent communication skills. The ability to communicate verbally and in writing is essential for professional success. Students should determine very early in their academic program if they have difficulty with written assignments. A candid self-assessment will allow you to get appropriate assistance if needed. Colleges and universities have writing improvement programs that are available for students and staff to improve their written expression. These are not necessarily remedial programs. Such improvement programs often focus on organizational skills, proper structure and format, appropriate use of resources, and editing strategies. The items below are suggestions to assist with the process[4]:

✓ Have a focused topic. Topics that are too broad will make for a difficult assignment. If you are unsure of what the instructor is looking for, get clarification. A broad writing assignment about evaluating abdominal injuries may be more focused by examining common complications associated with a specific injury. Try to pose your topic as a question to be answered or a problem to be solved.

✓ Select appropriate resources. It is more likely your professor will desire information gleaned from professional journals like *Journal of Athletic Training, American Journal of Sports Medicine*, etc rather than information from lay publications. Be sure you have selected original sources rather than taking information as someone else has cited it. Be wary of Internet resources that do not have appropriate references or copyright dates. Some professors will not allow resources from the World Wide Web.

✓ Use a system to organize your information. It is common to take notes, highlight articles, or use note cards to keep track of the information you plan to use. Taking some extra time to stay organized at this step will assist you as you write your paper.

✓ Write an outline for your paper. Different types of papers have different sections that are common to them. All have an introduction, body, and conclusion. In scientific writing, the structure of a literature review differs from a basic science paper or case report. Be sure you understand exactly what the professor is asking you to write. Table 4-5 shows the common heading used for articles published in the *Journal of Athletic Training*.

✓ Write your introduction. The introduction will allow you to establish some background for your paper, explain the focus, and reveal the purpose of the paper.

✓ Write the body of the paper. Use your outline and build your paper around the points you wish to

Table 4-5

Common Components of Athletic Training Manuscripts

Original Research	Case Report	Literature Review

*Structured abstract
   Objective
   Design/setting
   Subjects
   Measurements
   Results
   Conclusions
   Key words
	Structured abstract
	   Objective
	   Background
	   Differential diagnosis
	   Treatment
	   Uniqueness
	   Conclusions
	   Key words
		Structured abstract
		   Objective
		   Data sources
		   Data synthesis
		   Conclusions/recommendations
		   Key words

		Introduction
		Body of paper
Introduction	Introduction	Subsections by topic
Methods	#Case report (body)	Conclusion
Results	Discussion/conclusions	References
Discussion	References	
%Clinical implications		
Conclusion		
References		

* The structured abstract should be no more than 250 words.

The body of the case report should discuss the personal data, chief concern, relevant medical history, results of physical examination, treatment, criteria for return to participation, and deviation from expected findings (what makes the case unique).

% Clinical implications are presented in original clinical research studies. Basic science studies do not typically discuss clinical implications by section. However, the clinical implications may be part of the discussion as it relates to existing literature.

Adapted from Authors guide. *Journal of Athletic Training*. Revised 2006. Available at www.nata.org/jat/authors/authors_guide.pdf. Accessed April 19, 2009.

Evidence-Based Practice

What Is Evidence-Based Practice?

If we had to choose the newest phrase that has become embedded into the lexicon of health care in the past decade, a very strong case can be made for "evidence-based practice (EBP)." Evidence-based medicine, EBP, evidence-guided practice, and best practices all refer to the integration of the best research evidence with clinical experience and patient values to make a clinical decision. EBP focuses on research dealing with the daily practice of patient care. EBP may help prove accepted practices or make way for new practices. It can focus on evaluation and assessment, diagnostic testing, treatment protocols, preventative programs, or any aspect that influences patient care. EBP forces practitioners and educators to ask themselves, "How do we know what we know? What is the best evidence to influence our treatment approaches?" The combination of research, clinician knowledge and experience, and what is important to the patient will influence the application of EBP. EBP in not a recipe or road map for patient care; rather it is higher-order thinking and evaluation of information. Athletic training can benefit from embracing EBP to help provide greater scientific support for our scope of practice.

Questions and Sources of Evidence

Multiple EBP sources are available for clinicians who have pertinent clinical questions. Scholarship is driven by questions. The idea of scholarship is not the sole domain of academics. Clinicians need to develop an approach to scholarly clinical practice. A scholarly clinical practice would embrace EBP, determine gaps in our knowledge through clinical encounters, develop questions that will serve as precursors to research, and seek to bridge the perceived gap between academics and clinical practitioners.

(continued)

Evidence-Based Practice (continued)

Research is driven by questions. Simple, clear, well-formulated questions are at the heart of all good studies. It is these questions that will drive us to a more scholarly practice. EBP often relies on systematic literature reviews and meta-analysis to address clinically relevant questions. Databases dedicated to EBP literature, such as the Cochrane library (www.cochrane.org), are readily accessible. While the Cochrane library is a subscription service, many public institutions and libraries have access. In addition, health sciences libraries on many university campuses have dedicated Web portals to EBP topics with links to online resources. These web portals allow clinicians an excellent starting point for a systematic search of available literature. Examples include the following:

- Bibliographic Databases
  - PubMed (MEDLINE) *www.ncbi.nlm.nih.gov/pubmed*
  - SPORT Discus (sports medicine/fitness) *www.sportdiscus.com*
  - CINAHL (nursing and allied health) *www.ebscohost.com/cinahl*
- General evidence-based resources
  - Cochrane Library *www.cochrane.org*
  - PEDro *www.pedro.fhs.usyd.edu.au*

Questions abound in athletic training. A paradigm shift toward EBP is needed to develop a more scholarly approach to clinical practice. Athletic training students must be conversant with EBP and familiar with the resources available to answer relevant clinical questions.

---

get across. Use your sources wisely but do not let them dictate your paper. Writing a paper is not always a step-by-step process. Be flexible as ideas change and information presents itself. Be flexible but stick to the purpose of the assignment. Remember to summarize published work rather than just repeating it. This is the "detail" section of the paper.

✓ Write your conclusion. The conclusion should be a more general summary that links back to the purpose. Provide a summary for the reader if the information is quite complex. Conclusions often provide a general statement on what is missing in the literature and it may call for additional research.

✓ Take time to revise. Have someone else read your paper for grammatical errors. Ask yourself if you had to read the paper aloud, would it flow nicely? Check the paper on several levels. Overall make sure the introduction is logical, and the body of the paper is of the appropriate depth. Be sure the conclusion is effective. Evaluate paragraphs individually. Do they have a logical sequence of topic sentences and summary sentences? Be sure to check your references.

✓ References. Choose a reference style (eg, Modern Language Association [MLS], American Psychological Association [APA], National Library of Medicine [NLM]) and use it for the entire paper.

✓ Do not be accused of plagiarism. It is inappropriate to represent work as your own when it has been quoted or paraphrased from another source. If you are uncertain, be sure to provide a citation.

FINANCIAL RESOURCES

The cost of attending college and completing a degree program is significant. Students must invest thousands of dollars toward higher education. Such a financial outlay requires that they are confident in their choice of academic programs. Do not waste your (or your parents') hard earned money on a program that does not excite you. Athletic training students will need strategies to pay for their education. A part-time job, work study programs, federal or state level financial aid, student loans, and scholarships are the most common financial resources available to students.

Part-time employment may prove difficult for the athletic training student. Athletic training programs require significant clinical time. However, many students work a set number of part-time hours during their program. Part-time jobs with a consistent schedule will allow students to plan their day to meet all of their personal and academic responsibilities. Jobs in the library, recreational sports, food services, housing, with professors, and countless others are common to the campus community. At some institutions, students can qualify for pay in conjunction with some of the service activities they may perform in the clinical setting. However, these for-pay services

The Journal of Athletic Training

One of the most important benefits of NATA membership for students is an on-line subscription to the *Journal of Athletic Training*. Since its initial publication in 1956, the *Journal of the National Athletic Trainers' Association* has undergone several changes to become the primary publication outlet for research in the field of athletic training and a valuable resource for anyone who works with physically active populations. The journal took a major step in 2007 by achieving indexing status in the National Library of Medicine's MEDLINE index. This placed the *Journal of Athletic Training* alongside the most respected journals published today.

The mission of the *Journal of Athletic Training* is to enhance communication among professionals interested in the quality of health care for the physically active through education and research in prevention, evaluation, management, and rehabilitation of injuries.

This peer-reviewed publication thrives due to the hard work of a volunteer editorial board and countless athletic trainers around the country who serve as reviewers for the *Journal of Athletic Training*. The process of peer review means that the articles are blind reviewed by practicing professionals prior to publication. This process helps uphold the highest standards and quality for publication. The journal is indexed in several locations, including MEDLINE (National Library of Medicine), PubMED Central, Focus on Sports Sciences and Medicine (ISI: Institute for Scientific Information), Research Alert (ISI: Institute for Scientific Information), Physical Education Index, SPORT Discus (SIRC: Sport Information Resource Centre, Canada), CINAHL (Cumulative Index to Nursing and Allied Health Literature), AMED (Allied and Alternative Medicine Database), and PsycINFO (American Psychological Association). Students familiar with the indexing of the journal will know which database to search when researching topics related to athletic training. To make that easier, *Journal of Athletic Training* articles are available through libraries that subscribe to PubMed Central search services. This allows articles to be viewed and printed from on-line sources. Through indexing and increased availability, manuscripts published in the *Journal of Athletic Training* will be cited frequently in other sports medicine-related research.

The journal will be an invaluable resource for students pursuing a degree in athletic training. Students are eligible to enter the annual student writing competition sponsored by the NATA. The winning manuscript is published in the *Journal of Athletic Training*. There is no greater tool to enhance your educational program and start you on the path of professional development than the habit of reading your professional journal.

The *Journal of Athletic Training* can be found on line at www.journalofathletictraining.org.

cannot be a compulsory requirement of their program.[6] These policies vary greatly for each program. Students should investigate the opportunities available on their individual campuses.

The financial aid office on your campus will have the most up-to-date information about the financial programs available to you. Federal financial aid programs are need based and require students to file paperwork to determine if they qualify for assistance. Students should contact their campus financial aid office to inquire about federal programs as well as programs specific to their state. Some scholarship programs will require students to be evaluated for financial need even though they may not qualify for any federal or state funds. The financial aid office on your campus may also have information regarding scholarships and other work programs to offset expenses. Student loans are another avenue for financing a student's education. Loans may be initiated from your financial institution or specific programs are offered through your campus financial aid office. Student loans are desirable based on their low interest rates and flexible repayment plans. However, educational

loans are serious financial obligations that must be repaid. It is your responsibility to understand and meet the terms and conditions of your loan agreement. Not all loans are alike; interest rates, repayment periods, and other allowances vary depending upon the loan program and the source of the loan. Students should not enter into a loan agreement without fully understanding the repayment obligations.

Athletic training students should explore every avenue available to see if they qualify for any scholarships. Scholarships may be earned through your major academic department, school, college, or university. Your parents or a guardian may be a member of a union or company that offers a scholarship. Scholarships may be offered from service clubs, banks, or businesses in your hometown. Students should be sure to investigate every possible source to be sure they have exhausted all avenues for funding. Your individual campus will have an office to direct you toward appropriate scholarships. In addition, you may wish to search the World Wide Web to investigate potential scholarships. The information you need is out there for free; there is no need to pay a fee or

Criteria for Eligibility for an NATA Undergraduate Scholarship

To be eligible for an NATA scholarship, the student shall:

- Be an NATA member.
- Be enrolled in an athletic training education program.
- Have an overall minimum cumulative undergraduate grade point average of 3.2 (based on a maximum of 4.0) from ALL institutions attended.
- Be at least a junior in college.
- Have performed with distinction as a member of the athletic training program. Note: Athletic training achievement is considered equally with academic achievement. Recipients of scholarships are expected to remain enrolled in an undergraduate program except if they are assigned to active military duty.
- Have conducted him- or herself on and off the field in a manner to bring credit to him- or herself, the institution, and the ideals of American higher education.
- Other examples of campus participation and leadership may also be considered.
- Once students are awarded a scholarship in one category, they are ineligible for another in that category.

Note: The above are general criteria for an undergraduate scholarship. Students should visit www.nata-foundation.org to review the specific scholarship application as well as review opportunities for graduate and doctoral scholarships.

Adapted from NATA-REF Scholarship Application. www.natafoundation.org/scholarship.html#eligible. Accessed July 25, 2008.

subscribe to a particular scholarship service. Once you are accepted into an athletic training program, you will then be able to investigate specific athletic training scholarships. Do not be discouraged if you do not earn a scholarship in your first year of college. Many scholarships are designed for students who have demonstrated excellent scholarship during their college experience. Keep trying!

There is more to that scholarship award than just money in your pocket. Any scholarship—no matter how big or how small—should make its way onto your resume. Students applying for graduate positions, professional schools, or employment should highlight their academic achievements. Do not be modest. If you have earned the achievement, then make sure you put it out there to be seen. A brief discussion of resumes is provided in Chapter 16.

ATHLETIC TRAINING SCHOLARSHIPS

Athletic training scholarships are offered at the state, district, and national levels. The opportunity to apply for scholarships is just one reason that students should join the NATA. The NATA-REF offers over 50 scholarships annually, each for $2000. To be eligible, students must have a minimum GPA of 3.2 on a 4.0 scale. Students must also be sponsored by a certified athletic trainer and be a member of the NATA. Several district and state scholarships follow criteria similar to the national scholarship program. Scholarships are offered for undergraduate, master's, and doctoral level students in athletic training.

Athletic training-specific scholarships may be offered by the athletic training program at your university, athletic department, or athletic conference. Students should check with the athletic training program director, head athletic trainer, or director of sports medicine about opportunities specific to his or her program.

PROFESSIONAL ORGANIZATIONS

The NATA's role in advancing the profession and serving the membership is well documented by both their mission and deed. Chapter 2 outlined the rich history of the organization. However, service to the certified membership is only one part of the organization's role. The NATA is dedicated to meeting the needs of student members as they pursue their athletic training education.

Students should view their membership as a resource that will provide them with tangible benefits. The opportunity to apply for scholarships as noted above is only one reason. The benefits to NATA membership that most impact students include the following:

✓ A subscription to the *NATA Journal* (a scientific, peer-reviewed journal)

✓ The monthly *NATA News*, a magazine provided only to members

✓ Employment services, including listings of jobs and graduate positions

✓ A discounted fee for the NATA-BOC examination

✓ Opportunities for scholarships

✓ Discounted registration fees for the National Symposium

Visit www.nata.org for the most up-to-date information about membership.

Membership in your district organization is included with your national dues. However, students should not discount the value of becoming a member in their state athletic training organization. Often the first opportunities to network with other professionals are at state meetings. Symposiums at the state level are more affordable than traveling to the national meetings. In addition, many state organizations have committees that call for student participation. It is never too early to network or get involved.

SUMMARY

The wise prospective athletic training student should learn as much as possible about the academic program he or she wishes to pursue. In addition, the best students often learn very early on how they like to study, how they like to interact with information, and if they have any underlying test anxieties. At some point in your college experience, it is common to have trouble with a specific subject or a specific assignment. Seeking out help is an indication that you are serious about your academic success and mature enough to address your problem. There are a variety of resources available to the athletic training student. Take advantage of your campus counseling and study services, take some time to learn about your learning style, watch for signs of test anxiety, and develop good study habits. The student who takes these factors into account will be well prepared for problems that may arise. Make good use of your resources—it is an investment that will pay off.

REFERENCES

1. Pranger H. Learning as a college student. In: Sladyk K, ed. *OT Student Primer: A Guide to College Success*. Thorofare, NJ: SLACK Incorporated; 1997:37-47.

2. Harrelson G, Leaver-Dunn D, Wright K. An assessment of learning styles among undergraduate athletic training students. *Journal of Athletic Training*. 1998;33:50-53.

3. Stradley SL, Buckley BD, Kaminski TW, Horodyski M, Fleming D, Janelle CM. A nationwide learning-style assessment of undergraduate athletic training students in CAAHEP-accredited athletic training programs. *Journal of Athletic Training*. 2002;37(4 Supplement:S141-S146.

4. The Greater University Tutoring Service. *Study Skills Handbook*. Madison, WI: University of Wisconsin Board of Regents; 2008.

5. Hancock DR. Effects of test anxiety and evaluative threat on students' achievement and motivation. *Journal of Educational Research*. 2001;94:284.

6. Commission on Accreditation of Athletic Training Education. *Standards for the Accreditation of Entry-Level Athletic Training Education Programs*. Available at http://caate.net/documents/standards.6.30.08.pdf. Accessed April 19, 2009.

WEB RESOURCES

National Athletic Trainers' Association
www.nata.org
This site offers links to NATA committees, publications, position stands, and all aspects of the professional organization. A special section reserved for members allows access to employment listings and other member benefits.

National Athletic Trainers' Association Research and Education Foundation
www.natafoundation.org
The NATA-REF site provides details on previous research funded by the foundation, details on upcoming calls for research proposals, information on education opportunities, and scholarship information for students.

Journal of Athletic Training
www.journalofathletictraining.org
This site provides valuable information for authors and subscribers to the *Journal of Athletic Training*. Resources include guide for authors, links to abstract supplements, editorials, and an index of titles from recent publications.

Greater University Tutoring Services (GUTS) UW-Madison
http://guts.studentorg.wisc.edu
This site from the UW-Madison is typical of study skills and counseling sites available through most university and college campuses. The site includes information about tutoring and an extensive section on study skills.

ℹ Career Spotlight: Educational Program Clinical Coordinator

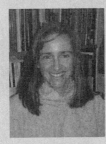

Shari Clark, MS, LAT

Assistant Faculty Associate

University of Wisconsin—Madison Athletic Training Education Program

My Position

I am the athletic training education program clinical coordinator and an instructor at the University of Wisconsin–Madison. My responsibilities include coordinating clinical field placements that occur in conjunction with core athletic training eduction program classes with specific instructors and ACIs (approved clinical instructors). This includes placement, site evaluation, clinical supervisor evaluation, and field visits. I also teach some of the core athletic training classes within our program.

Unique or Desired Qualifications

My undergraduate degree was in physical education with an emphasis in exercise physiology. I worked in cardiac rehabilitation and as a research assistant in exercise and aging. I came back to pursue athletic training and also received a master's degree in curriculum and instruction with an emphasis in health education. I have worked as a physician extender, high school athletic trainer, and also as an athletic trainer in a rehabilitation clinic.

Favorite Aspect of My Job

I love the interaction with the students in both the classroom as well as during their field experiences. I enjoy watching them take the information from class and apply it in their field experiences. They have an excitement for learning and passion for the profession that is very rewarding to be a part of. It has allowed my passion for athletic training to be turned into an opportunity to give back to the program that gave me so much.

Advice

Make the most of every opportunity given. You can learn something valuable from every situation you encounter. Stay positive, always question, look to learn more, and find ways to challenge yourself to be the best that you can be!

SECTION II

COMMON
INJURIES AND CONDITIONS

CHAPTER 5

UNDERSTANDING ATHLETIC INJURY
TERMINOLOGY AND CLASSIFICATION

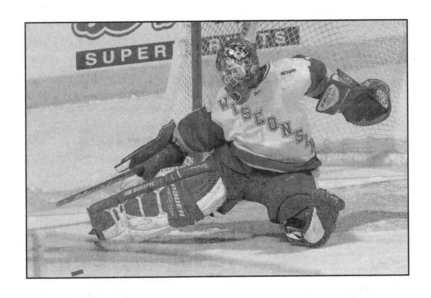

I am very envious of the students today and the preparation that they receive in athletic training education programs. My professional experiences with the NATA-BOC and the evolution of the certification exam have left me impressed with the quality of professional preparation athletic training students receive.

Brad Sherman, MEd, LAT
Director, University of Wisconsin Hospital Sports Medicine
(1981-2001)
Past President of the NATA-BOC

The development of a professional vocabulary and creating a framework to understand athletic injury are 2 early steps in an athletic training student's evolution as an emerging professional. The value of learning appropriate terminology cannot be understated. The athletic trainer's ability to communicate, both orally and in writing, with an array of medical professionals is a vital professional skill. To be an allied health professional means to be joined and aligned with other health professions. To do so, a common ground must exist so that we can communicate. This common ground includes the nomenclature we use to discuss injuries as well as the symbols and abbreviations we use to document medical records. Communication and documentation allow us to record progress, document findings, bill for services, and perform a host of other vital functions as an athletic trainer.

Understanding athletic injury begins with a basic understanding of anatomical structures: bone, muscle, tendon, ligament, cartilage, nerve, vascular tissue, and the specific organs that are subject to athletic injury. The proper function of any anatomical area is dictated by the integrity of the structures comprising that body part. Compromise the integrity of the structure and the desired function is lost or limited. For example, proper function of the knee is dictated by several structures. Muscles move the joint, ligaments provide stability, bones provide structure and support, nerves supply information and activate muscles, and cartilage helps provide protection and support to the joint. Injure any one of these tissues and the overall function will be influenced. Structure dictates function. To begin to learn about the aspects of athletic injury, it is essential to classify them properly.

This chapter will provide a starting point for understanding injury by presenting appropriate terminology and a system for the classification of athletic injuries. Upon completion of the chapter, the student will be able to:

- ✓ Define common terminology used in athletic training
- ✓ Identify common abbreviations and symbols used in documentation
- ✓ Utilize word parts and word roots to better understand medical terminology
- ✓ Explain the concept of injury mechanism
- ✓ Identify how specific tissues are injured
- ✓ Describe how injuries are classified and how the severity is graded
- ✓ Discuss how injuries are scientifically studied

DEVELOPING A PROFESSIONAL VOCABULARY

MEDICAL TERMINOLOGY: A WORD PART APPROACH

Myositis, osteoarthritis, and *avascular* are all examples of medical terms. You need to learn to break the words into specific parts in order to understand medical terms and use them appropriately. Most medical words are composed of specific word parts. The word parts are prefix, word root, and suffix. These parts may sometimes be connected by vowels to create the complete medical term. A prefix is the word part that appears before the word root, while the suffix appears after the word root.

The 3 examples above can be broken down using the word part approach. When the word *myositis* is broken into parts, we see that *myo* means muscle and *itis* means inflammation, so myositis = inflamma-

tion of the muscle. Osteoarthritis has all 3 parts. The prefix *osteo* meaning bone, the word part *arth* refers to a joint, and *itis* is inflammation, so osteoarthritis = inflammation of the bone in the joint. Avascular takes a common word and adds the prefix *a*, which means without, so avascular = without blood supply. Refer to Table 5-1 for a list of common medical prefixes, word parts, and suffixes.

These terms will become second nature with time and practice. Understanding the word part concepts and putting these words to use will allow you to communicate effectively with your instructors, clinical supervisors, and fellow students. Keep in mind that when you communicate with the athlete or the lay public, you may need to adjust your vocabulary accordingly.

ABBREVIATIONS, SYMBOLS, AND SOAP NOTES

The recording of medical information is an important job responsibility for any allied health professional. Common examples of documentation include evaluation of injuries, treatment plans, rehabilitation progress, physician visits, and discharge from care. These forms of documentation are a medical-legal responsibility of the professional athletic trainer. Proper documentation allows a patient's care to be recorded accurately and can protect the sports medicine team from claims of negligent care. Documentation allows the athletic training professional to keep appropriate paper work and have a record that will allow proper communication with physicians, other athletic trainers, and other health providers.

One of the most common documentation techniques is the SOAP note. SOAP stands for subjective, objective, assessment, and plan. It is an acronym that allows you to keep different types of information separate. Subjective information is usually what is told to you by the patient and includes the history and any information relating to his or her pain. Objective information can be observed or measured and includes findings from your physical examination of the patient. The assessment is your impression of the evaluation or sometimes your listing of the problems. The certified athletic trainer can help provide a diagnosis of the injury. This is best done in consultation with the physician. The plan is what you will do next, and it may be immediate care or part of a long-term rehabilitation effort.

Within the context of the SOAP format, you may have to write several notes pertaining to one injury situation. This can become a lengthy and tedious process. The use of common symbols and abbreviations

Table 5 -1

Common Word Parts

a	no, not, without	*gastro*	beginning	*orrhagia*	hemorrhage
ab	away from	*glyco*	sugar	*orrhaphy*	suture
ac	pertaining to	*gram*	record	*orrhea*	flow, discharge
ad	toward	*graph*	recording device	*orrhexis*	rupture
algia	pain	*hemo*	blood	*osis*	condition of
an	pertaining to	*hetero*	different	*ostomy*	new opening
ar	pertaining to	*homo*	same	*oto*	ear
arthro	joint	*hydro*	water	*otomy*	incision
auto	self	*hyper*	high	*ous*	pertaining to
brach	arm	*in*	not	*patho*	disease
cardio	heart	*inter*	between	*peri*	around
cephal	head	*intra*	within	*plasty*	surgical repair
chondro	cartilage	*ism*	condition of	*pnea*	breathing
colic	large intestines	*ist*	specialist	*pneumo*	lung, air
cranio	skull	*itis*	inflammation	*poly*	many
cyan	blue	*ive*	pertaining to	*post*	after
cyto	cell	*kinesio*	movement	*pre*	before
dento	teeth	*laryng*	larynx	*psych*	mind
derma	skin	*leuko*	white	*pyo*	pus
di	two	*lipo*	fat	*retro*	behind, backwards
dia	through	*litho*	stone	*rhino*	nose
dynia	pain	*logy*	study of	*sclero*	hardening
dys	bad, difficult	*macro*	large	*stasis*	stopping, controlling
eal	pertaining to	*mal*	bad	*sub*	under
ecto	out, without, away	*micro*	small	*supra*	above
extomy	excision	*mono*	single	*syn*	joined, fused
encephal	brain	*myel*	spinal cord	*syno*	synovial, joint capsular
endo	inside	*myo*	muscle	*tachy*	over
epi	above	*necro*	dead	*teno*	tendon
erythro	red	*nephro*	kidney	*thera*	therapy
eu	good	*neuro*	nerve, brain	*thermo*	heat
ex	out	*oid*	resembling	*trophy*	growth, nutrition
fibro	fiber	*oma*	tumor	*uni*	one

Adapted from Ginge K. *Writing Soap Notes*. Philadelphia: FA Davis; 1990

that are accepted by several allied health and medical specialties can make documentation and communication much easier. Table 5-2 outlines some common abbreviations and symbols used in documentation of medical records.

THE LANGUAGE OF INJURY

Discussing injuries with patients and lay people can lead to the use of terms that are not befitting of a student wishing to become an allied health professional. As an athletic training student, it is important to dismiss inappropriate injury terminology as soon as possible. From this point forward you will no longer accept terms like *tweaked, pulled, cranked,* and *dinged* when discussing an injury or injuries. Students who use terms properly will have an advantage when communicating with the CIs and allied health professionals they encounter in their clinical experiences. Athletic training students who understand and use proper terminology will present themselves in a professional light and be taken seriously as a student of their discipline. Improper use of terms can lead to confusion for patients and lead instructors and supervisors to doubt your knowledge of specific content.

A list of terms and definitions specific to athletic injuries that sometimes lead to confusion and are frequently misused (examples can be found during the sports segment of the evening news or by reading the sports section of the newspaper) can be found next. This list can serve as a starting point for

---

Table 5-2

Examples of Abbreviations and Symbols Used for Documentation

Abbreviations

AAROM	active assisted range of motion
AROM	active range of motion
BP	blood pressure
CC	chief concern
c/o	complains of
D/C	discontinue, discharge
DX	diagnosis
FWB	full weight bearing
FX	fracture
HR	heart rate
Hx	history
LBP	low back pain
LE	lower extremity
NWB	non-weight bearing
O:	objective
P.H. or PHx	previous history
PROM	passive range of motion
PT	physical therapy
PWB	partial weight bearing
q	every
qd	every day
qid	four times a day
ROM	range of motion
RROM	resisted range of motion
Rx	treatment, prescription, therapy
S:	subjective
SOAP	subjective, objective, assessment, plan
SP	status post
Sx	symptoms
tid	three times daily
UE	upper extremity
WNL	within normal limits

Symbols

(L)	left
(R)	right
↑	increase
↓	decrease
@	at
♀	male
♂	female
#	pound
=	equals
+	plus, positive
-	negative, minus
~	approximate
Δ	change
1°	primary, 1st degree
2°	secondary, 2nd degree
X	number of times

Examples

Patient CC LBP x six weeks = patient's chief concern is low back pain for 6 weeks.

AROM (L) Knee = 0° to 110° = Active range of motion in the left knee is 0° to 110°

Adapted from Ginge K. *Writing Soap Notes*. Philadelphia: FA Davis; 1990

---

understanding the language of injury and developing good habits for the proper use of terminology.

SPRAIN VERSUS STRAIN

A sprain is an injury to a joint and most often involves injury to the ligament(s) and to the joint capsule. A strain is an injury to muscular tissue or the muscle tendon complex.

Examples of proper use:
- ✓ The player sustained a third-degree sprain of the medical collateral ligament of the right knee.
- ✓ The sprinter sustained a second-degree muscle tendon strain to the left hamstring.

ACUTE VERSUS CHRONIC

An acute injury is a recent injury with a rapid onset. An acute injury may also refer to an injury in the early stages of inflammation. A chronic injury is defined by its slow onset and long duration. Acute injuries are often followed by a chronic phase. However, chronic injuries need not be preceded by an acute phase.

Examples of proper use:
- ✓ The acute injury was treated with ice and compression.
- ✓ Joe was diagnosed with chronic tendonitis of his right rotator cuff tendon.

DISLOCATION VERSUS SUBLUXATION

A dislocation (also called a luxation) is the complete disarticulation of a joint. A subluxation is a partial or incomplete dislocation followed by an immediate and spontaneous relocation.

Examples of proper use:

✓ Abduction and external rotation of the shoulder is a common position for a dislocation injury.

✓ Repeated subluxation of the glenohumeral joint left Roger with significant laxity in his shoulder.

SIGN, SYMPTOM, AND SYNDROME

These terms are often confused. A sign is something that the athletic trainer can observe or measure, while a symptom is something the patient describes to you. For example, I observe my patient has a pale appearance (a sign), and she describes that she has no appetite (a symptom). A syndrome is a collection of signs and symptoms.

Examples of proper use:

✓ Redness and swelling are signs of an inflammatory response.

✓ Nausea and loss of appetite are symptoms of the influenza.

✓ A concussion is a syndrome characterized by several signs and symptoms (loss of memory, dizziness, nausea, etc).

-OSIS, -ITIS, AND -ALGIA

These 3 suffixes commonly reference an athletic injury. Their similarity can lead to some confusion for the student. Remember that -osis means a condition of, -algia is the generic reference for pain, and -itis is the most common of the 3 and means inflammation.

Examples of proper use:

✓ Following a third-degree sprain of the anterior cruciate ligament, it is common to have blood contained within the knee joint. This condition is known as a hemiarthrosis.

✓ The physician was concerned about Joan's metatarsalgia, or pain in the metatarsals of the foot, so she ordered a radiograph (x-ray).

✓ Jim had played too much tennis on vacation and developed some tendonitis in his right shoulder.

EDEMA, EFFUSION, AND ECCHYMOSIS

Swelling is a common finding when you evaluate an athletic injury. The type and location of that swelling dictates what it is called. Edema is swelling as a result of the collection of fluid in connective tissue. An effusion is a collection of fluid contained within a joint space or joint capsule. Ecchymosis refers to the discoloration that often accompanies edema. Bruising is a form of ecchymosis.

Examples of proper use:

✓ The edema surrounding Bill's ankle made it difficult for him to wear his shoe.

✓ The physician explained that the effusion in April's knee joint may be a sign of a more serious ligament injury.

✓ A few days following his third-degree hamstring strain, Drew had a large patch of ecchymosis along his posterior thigh.

CONCENTRIC VERSUS ECCENTRIC

A concentric muscle contraction occurs when a muscle shortens and there is movement at the joint. Concentric contractions are sometimes called positive contractions. If I flex my bicep muscle to drink a glass of water, I must perform a concentric contraction of the bicep muscle. An eccentric muscle contraction is when a muscle lengthens against resistance. Eccentric contractions may also be referred to as negative contractions. Eccentric contractions have a greater association with muscle injury and delayed onset muscle soreness (DOMS). When you walk downhill, it is natural for your quadriceps muscles to lengthen against the resistance provided by your body weight and the incline; this is an example of an eccentric contraction.

Examples of proper use:

✓ The repeated bending of the knee during the exercise session produced a concentric contraction for the hamstring muscle group.

✓ The athletic trainer informed Jim that he needed to perform eccentric (lengthening) contractions as part of his rehabilitation program.

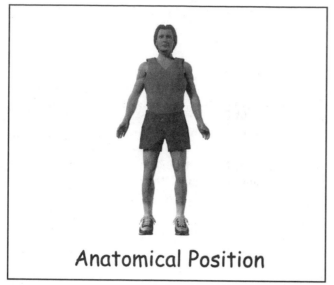

Anatomical Position

Figure 5-1. A diagram of anatomical position. This position serves as a starting or reference point when studying movements of specific joints.

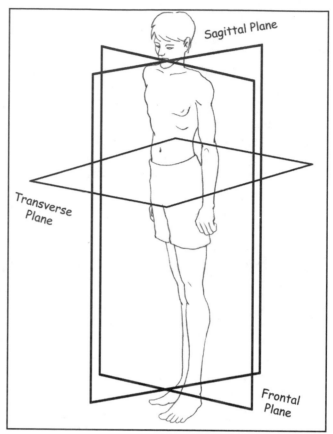

Figure 5-2. The sagittal, transverse, and frontal planes.

THE LANGUAGE OF MOVEMENT AND BODY POSITION

The athletic training student who masters the language of movement and body position will have a solid foundation for understanding injury and better utilizing his or her knowledge of anatomy. An athletic trainer must have points of reference when evaluating injuries and describing how injuries occur. Any discussion of movement and body position should begin with knowing the anatomical reference position. Figure 5-1 illustrates the anatomical position. To stand in anatomical position is to stand erect with your feet shoulder width apart and your arms hanging relaxed at your sides with the palms facing forward. This in not a normal standing position; however, it is the body position used as the reference point for discussing anatomical movements.

The terms provided below describe the relationship of specific body parts to other parts of the body or objects external to the body. The following are common terms with which students should be familiar:

- ✓ Superior (cranial): Closer to, or toward the head
- ✓ Inferior (caudal): Farther away from, or toward the feet
- ✓ Anterior (ventral): Toward the front of the body
- ✓ Posterior (dorsal): Toward the back of the body
- ✓ Medial: Toward the midline of the body
- ✓ Lateral: Moving away from the midline of the body

- ✓ Proximal: Closer to the trunk (eg, the elbow is proximal to the wrist)
- ✓ Distal: Away from the trunk (eg, the foot is distal to the knee)
- ✓ Superficial: Toward the surface
- ✓ Deep: Inside the body, away from the surface

The body is divided into 3 cardinal planes that bisect it in 3 dimensions. The cardinal planes are reference points that can be thought of as imaginary flat surfaces. The 3 planes are sagittal, frontal, and transverse. These planes are represented in Figure 5-2. The sagittal plane divides the body into halves (straight down the middle of your nose into right and left halves), forward and backwards movements take place in the sagittal plane. The frontal plane divides the body into anterior and posterior halves (this would be like dividing your body to represent the front and back), lateral movements away from and toward the midline take place in the frontal plane. Lastly, the transverse plane separates the body into top and bottom halves, movements that occur parallel to the ground take place in the transverse plane. Table 5-3 shows some examples of movement in these 3 planes.

Table 5-3

Joint Movement Terminology

Primary Movements	Cardinal Plane	Example
Flexion/extension	Sagittal	The shoulder, elbow, wrist, hip, knee, and ankle all move in the sagittal plane
Abduction/adduction	Frontal	Frontal plane movements also include lateral bending of the trunk, depression and elevation of the scapula, and lateral movements of the wrist
Rotation	Transverse	Rotational movements of the arm and leg take place in the transverse plane Eversion and inversion of the foot are also considered rotational movements
Horizontal abduction/adduction	Transverse	Movement of the arm or leg in the transverse plane away from or toward the midline.

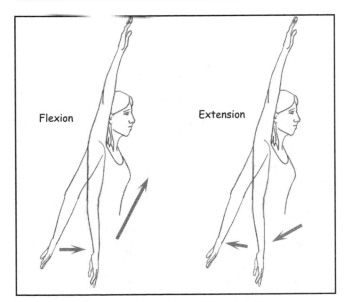

Figure 5-3. Flexion and extension of the shoulder.

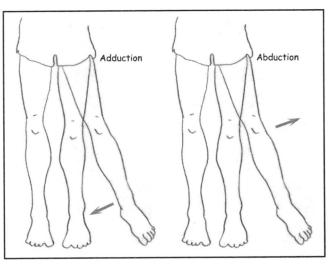

Figure 5-4. Abduction and adduction of the hip.

Understanding movements as they relate to the planes of the body and each specific joint is a logical starting point for the athletic training student. The movements represented below are a logical starting point for the prospective athletic training student:

✓ Flexion/extension
✓ Abduction/adduction
✓ Internal rotation/external rotation
✓ Pronation/supination
✓ Inversion/eversion

Figures 5-3 thru 5-7 provide examples of the movements listed above.

INJURY CLASSIFICATION

ACUTE AND CHRONIC INJURY

Injuries can be classified based on several characteristics:

✓ Did the injury occur rapidly or did it appear gradually?
✓ Is the injury life threatening or of lesser severity?
✓ Did the injury cause the patient to miss any of his or her normal physical activities?

The answers to these questions help shed light on how athletic injuries are classified. The simple

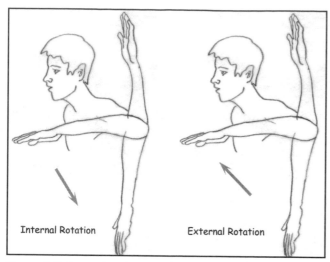

Figure 5-5. Internal and external rotation of the shoulder.

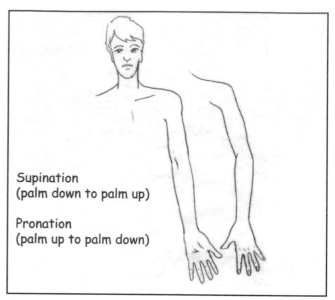

Figure 5-6. Pronation and supination of the forearm.

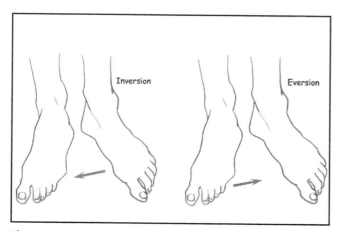

Figure 5-7. Inversion and eversion of the ankle.

definition of an injury is an act that causes damage or hurt. In the sports medicine setting, an athletic injury is defined as a medical condition resulting from athletic activity that causes a limitation or restriction on participation. An athletic injury may also be defined as an injury that requires the patient to seek medical treatment.[1]

Injuries can be classified as acute or chronic. An acute injury has a rapid onset. When we see an athlete fall in the course of a practice or competition, it is likely a result of an acute injury. It is immediate. Landing on an opponent's foot and sustaining a fracture is an acute injury. A chronic injury is an injury that progresses over time and has a slow onset. Developing a case of tendonitis in the posterior tibialis tendon during several weeks of distance running is an example of a chronic injury. Onset time is not the only way to determine an acute versus chronic injury; physiologic factors must also be considered.

The body responds to injury by activating an inflammatory process. This process is a series of physical, chemical, and vascular events. Swelling, pain, and redness are associated with the acute stages of the inflammatory process. Healing injuries will progress from acute inflammation to stages of repair and remodeling. The athletic trainer must be able to determine when an injury is in the acute stage based on the signs and symptoms of inflammation, not just the time elapsed since an injury occurred. Knowing the stage of injury healing is essential to proper management and will assist in selecting the proper course of treatment. Chronic injuries may be referred to physiologically as subacute. These injuries require a different course of treatment compared to those still classified as being in the acute inflammatory process.

Mechanism of Injury

How an injury occurs is called the mechanism of injury (MOI). Compression, shear, and tension are mechanical forces that can contribute to injury. Compression occurs when tissues absorb force, shear occurs when tissues are pulled in opposite directions in relation to one another (eg, perpendicular along an axis), and tension occurs when tissues are pulled in opposite directions (such as a stretching or elongating motion). Plant and cut on a pass route and the rotation may cause a shear force to specific ligaments in your knee. Stretch muscle or tendon beyond their limits and the tension force may cause a strain. Missing the baseball and getting hit in the leg is an example of compressing the tissue, which can lead to a hematoma or possibly a fracture. Understanding the MOI is essential information in the injury evaluation process and is helpful to the athletic trainer as he or she makes an appropriate referral or treatment plan for the patient.

The Cardinal Signs
of Inflammation

The inflammatory process is a natural and needed response to injury. However, how an athletic trainer treats or manages an injury is dependent upon what stage of the inflammatory process is present. The recognition of temperature, color, and pain as indicators of injury can be traced back to the Roman and Greek origins of medicine. Allied health and medical professionals rely upon recognition of the signs of inflammation to determine appropriate referral and treatment strategies. The cardinal signs of inflammation often indicate an acute injury or the presence of infection. The indicators of inflammation are pain, heat, swelling, redness, and loss of function.

Indicator	Cause
Pain	Increased chemical activity and direct tissue damage.
Heat	Increased metabolic activity.
Swelling	Chemical and vascular changes allow fluid to leak into cellular spaces.
Redness	Increased blood flow and increased metabolic activity.
Loss of function	Inability to perform desired activities due to tissue damage, swelling, and pain.

INJURY SURVEILLANCE

Injury surveillance is an essential tool in determining the scope of athletic injuries under a variety of conditions. Injury surveillance studies gather data to better understand the rate, type, and severity of injuries under specific conditions for a given sport or activity. Such studies can yield valuable information that can assist with rule modifications, safety precautions, examination of equipment and participation conditions, and appropriate staffing decisions. Injury surveillance requires careful consideration of the data collection methods (who and how) and an agreement of the terms of the data collection—specifically how an injury is defined. Injuries may be defined by the outcome of the injury itself. The common definition of an athletic injury used for injury studies has a component of restriction or loss of participation from an activity. This is referred to as a time-loss injury. Time-loss data are key components for injury surveillance

studies. This type of research is known as injury epidemiology. Injury epidemiology is the study of injury trends for the purpose of discovering their root causes and preventing them in the future. Many of these studies rely heavily upon the participation of athletic trainers to document and record the number of participates in practices and games as well as the types and severity of injuries that occur. Table 5-4 presents an example of injury surveillance data on injury rates for intercollegiate student-athletes participating in men's and women's basketball.

The most severe injury is the catastrophic injury. A catastrophic injury is defined as any severe spinal, spinal cord, or cerebral injury. There are 3 categories of outcomes associated with a catastrophic injury: fatal, nonfatal with permanent disability, and serious with no permanent disability. The National Center for Catastrophic Sports Injury Research at the University of North Carolina–Chapel Hill has tracked catastrophic injuries since 1982. Fatalities are further classified as being either direct or indirect. A direct fatality is one that results from trauma sustained during participation in a sport or activity. An indirect fatality is caused by systemic failure as a result of exertion while participating in a sport or activity or by a complication secondary to a nonfatal injury.

Football is associated with the greatest number of catastrophic injuries. There were a total of 10 high school direct catastrophic injuries for the 2005 football season; the lowest number since The National Center for Catastrophic Sports Injury Research began collecting data. College football was associated with 1 direct catastrophic injury in 2005, which is also the lowest number since the Center was started in 1982.[2] In addition to the direct fatalities in 2005, there were also 10 indirect fatalities. Eight of the indirect fatalities were at the high school level and 2 were at the college level. The causes of the high school indirect deaths were heat stroke (1), lightning (1), heart related (3), and unknown (3). The college indirect deaths were attributed to heat stroke and viral meningitis.

In addition to the fatalities, there were 6 permanent disability injuries in 2005. Three were cervical spine injuries and 3 were brain injuries. This number is a decrease of 6 when compared to the previous year's data. Five of the injuries were at the high school level and one at the college level. Serious football injuries with no permanent disability accounted for 3 injuries in 2005—all at the high school level. High school athletes were associated with 1 cervical spine fracture and 2 brain injuries with full recovery.[2]

Catastrophic injuries have been examined by gender as well. Data collected from 1982 thru 2000 showed a total of 78 direct and 48 indirect catastrophic injuries to high school and college female athletes.[3] These data include injuries from cheerleading, which

Table 5-4

Injury Data for NCAA Division I Men's and Women's Basketball

NCAA Division I	♂ Basketball	♀ Basketball
Team seasons	20	20
Exposures	39,354	36,358
Injuries	1440	1630
Nontime loss	1135	1366
Time loss	305	264
Injury rate/1000 exposures	36.6	44.9
Nontime loss	28.8	37.6
Time loss	7.8	7.3
Incidence density ratio	3.7	5.2

Terms

Injury and time loss: When an injury or illness evaluation identifies the complaint to be sufficient to require the player to be restricted from participation, it is reported as a time-loss incident. Any injury or illness that is not sufficient to be initialized as a time-loss incident and that causes the athletic trainer to conduct an evaluation of the player's complaint is reported as a non–time-loss incident.

Incidence density ratio (IDR): Nontime loss injury rates divided by time-loss injury rates produced an IDR. This ratio allows the investigators to make judgments concerning the magnitude of difference between the conditions under consideration. An IDR of 1.0 would represent no difference between the 2 conditions.

Adapted from Powell JW, Dompier TP. Analysis of injury rates and treatment patterns for time-loss and non–time-loss injuries among collegiate student-athletes. *Journal of Athletic Training*. 2004;39(1):56-70.

 # Grades and Degrees

Various criteria may be used to classify the severity of a sprain or strain injury. A physician will diagnose an injury to a joint or muscle and classify it by the grade or degree of the injury. This classification is used to indicate severity. A 1st degree or Grade I injury is the least severe, while a 3rd degree or Grade III is the most severe.

Sprains

Injuries to ligaments are sprains. Injuries to ligaments are classified by the amount of damage to the tissue and the resultant instability.

- Grade I (1st degree) sprain causes some stretching or slight tearing of ligamentous fibers with no instability to the joint. If your patient experiences a Grade I sprain, he or she may experience some pain and swelling. Functional ability may or may not be limited. Discoloration (ecchymosis) is most often absent. While most people with mild sprains usually do not need an x-ray, it is always advisable if there is any bony tenderness, the patient is an adolescent, or the injury does not improve.

- Grade II (2nd degree) sprain causes partial tearing of the ligament. The patient will have some laxity and pain with joint testing. A grade II sprain will present with ecchymosis, moderate pain, and swelling. In the ankle or knee, a patient with a grade II sprain will experience loss of function and will have difficulty bearing weight. An x-ray should be obtained to determine if a fracture is present. MRI may also be needed to further assist the physician with diagnosing the severity of injury and the specific tissues involved.

- Grade III (3rd degree) sprain is a complete tear or rupture of the ligament. Initial pain may be severe; however, it is not unusual for patients with Grade III injuries to have little pain after the nerve fibers have been disrupted. Swelling and ecchymosis are usually severe, and the patient will have significant instability at the joint. An x-ray or MRI will be needed to determine the specific tissues involved and the severity of the injury. Grade III sprains may lead to instabilities that require surgical repair.   (continued)

Grades and Degrees (continued)

Strains

Strains, which are injuries to muscle tissue, are classified by the amount of damage to the muscle fibers and the resulting dysfunction.[1]

- Grade I (1st degree) muscle strains result in some tearing of muscle fibers. There may be tenderness to the touch and pain with active muscle movement. Grade I strains usually do not cause limitations in the ROM.
- Grade II (2nd degree) muscle strain injuries will be painful with active contraction of the muscle and a greater number of fibers will be disrupted. A small defect may be palpable in the muscle. Some swelling and discoloration may occur. ROM will likely be decreased and painful.
- Grade III (3rd degree) muscle strain injuries result in a complete rupture of muscle-tendon tissue. This often takes place at the junction of the muscle and tendon tissues or sometimes in the tendon itself. Patients with Grade III injuries will have significant loss of function and may present with unusual defects in the muscle due to the contractile nature of the muscle fibers. Pain may be great with the initial injury but subside quickly if the rupture is complete and the nerve fibers disrupted. Grade III muscle-tendon ruptures may require surgical repair.

Reference

1. National Institute of Arthritis and Musculoskeletal Skin Diseases. Sprains and strains. Available at www.niams.nih.gov/hi/topics/strain_sprain/strain_sprain.htm. Accessed May 5, 2008.

---

represents the highest number of direct injuries in both the interscholastic and intercollegiate levels. Catastrophic injuries to female athletes have increased largely due to increased participation and the evolution of cheerleading to a gymnastic-like activity.[1]

Understanding the data associated with the epidemiology of all sports injuries (catastrophic and otherwise) allows athletic trainers to make informed decisions regarding proper medical coverage for practices and events. The decrease in catastrophic football injuries noted above illustrates the importance of data collection and being sure that the information is passed on to those responsible for conducting football programs. It is unlikely that all athletic injuries, unfortunately even catastrophic events, can be eliminated, but reliable data collection and analysis prevention programs, rule changes, and improvements in medical coverage may help reduce their incidence.

Moving Beyond Surveillance

Injury surveillance has proven an important tool in defining the scope of the injury problem. However, injury surveillance alone only provides one piece of the puzzle. What should be done with this information? The issue of injury from sport and recreation has significant economic implications. Roughly 7.3 million young people participate in high school-sanctioned athletics in the United States.[4] The rate of injury among this group is substantial; these injuries lead to emergency room visits, hospitalizations, sur-

geries, and lost school/work days. These factors have real economic costs and place strain on the health care system.[5] 2003 data from the Injury Cost Model of the US Consumer Product Safety Commission (CITE) revealed that the injuries in the top 5 female and male high school sports cost an estimated $588 million in direct expenses and $6.6 billion in indirect expenses. Finding ways to prevent injury, even those not considered life threatening, can have significant economic impact. The next step beyond injury surveillance is prevention. Surveillance can establish the problem, but further studies must be undertaken to address root causes that can then lead to appropriate prevention models.[6]

McGuine[6] performed a systematic review of the quality of 29 studies that identified either injury risk factors or injury prevention. The objective was to identify the available research regarding risk factors and prevention of injuries in high school athletes. This review concluded that the risk factors for injury in several sports such as soccer, American football, and basketball have been documented. However, other sports are less well represented in the current literature. The risk factors for injuries to the ankle, head, and knee have been identified to a limited degree. Upper extremity injury risk factors are less well known. There is a need for high-quality prospective studies to further identify injury risk factors and injury prevention strategies for high school athletes. Table 5-5 presents examples of high-quality risk factor and injury prevention studies.

Table 5-5

Examples of High Quality Injury Risk Factor Studies

Risk Factor Studies of Specific Sports

Sports	Study (Lead Author, Year)	Subjects	Variables Studied	Sample-Size Estimation	Analysis	Data Reported	Results	Quality Rank
Baseball, basketball, soccer, and softball	Powell, 2000	75,000 varsity athletes from multiple schools for 3 years	Sex, location, and type of injury Session and severity	Not provided	Chi-square	Injury rates, relative risk, 95% CI	Males at greater overall risk of injury Baseball/softball RR = 1.27 (1.15 to 1.39) Soccer RR = 1.14 (1.07 to 1.22) Females at greater risk of knee injury Basketball RR = 1.44 (1.20 to 1.71) Soccer RR = 1.46 (1.24 to 1.71)	High
Cheerleading	Schulz, 2004	1675 female competitive cheerleaders from 44 squads for 3 years	Injury history, body mass index, grade level, coaches' education and training	Not provided	Poisson regression	Injury rates, relative risk, 95% CI	Increased risk of injury with injury history RR = 2.2 (1.1 to 4.7) Higher levels of coach education, qualification, and training associated with lower risk of injury RR = 0.5 (0.3 to 0.9)	High

Risk-Factor Studies for Specific Injuries

Injury	Study (Lead Author, Year)	Subjects	Variables Studied	Sample-Size Estimation	Analysis	Data Reported	Results	Quality Rank
Ankle sprains	Beynnon, 2005	416 female and 247 male soccer, basketball, and lacrosse players (4 years)	Sex, sport, level of competition	Yes	Cox proportional hazards regression Wald statistic	Injury rates, relative risk, 95% CI	No difference in the rate of injury based on sport and sex	High
Concussions (second)	Zemper, 2003	7197 male football players for 2 years	Self-reported previous history of concussion	Not provided	Chi-square	Injury rates, relative risk, 95% CI	Previous concussion increased risk of second concussion RR = 5.8 (4.8 to 6.8)	High

Relative risk (RR) is the risk of an event (in this case injury) relative to exposure. RR is a ratio of the probability of the event occurring in the exposed group versus the control (nonexposed) group.

Adapted from McGuine TA. Sports injuries in high school athletes: a review of injury-risk and injury prevention research. *Clin J Sport Med.* 2006;16:6.

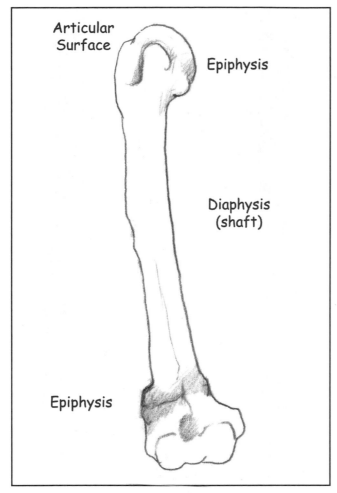

Figure 5-8. Anatomy of a typical long bone.

SPECIFIC INJURY CLASSIFICATIONS

The definition of injury by type (acute or chronic) only gives us information in very general terms. To learn more about specific injuries and how they are classified, we need to examine the type of tissues involved. This section discusses the general types of injuries specific to the involved tissues. Specific athletic injuries are discussed in greater detail in Chapters 6 to 9.

INJURIES TO BONE

A fracture is a disruption in the continuity of bone. Fractures are described as being either open or closed depending upon the integrity of the skin. An open fracture is one that disrupts the skin, while a closed fracture does not. An open fracture is sometimes referred to as a compound fracture; however, this term can be confusing and has fallen out of favor. Understanding fractures, how they are classified, and

how they heal will require some basic knowledge of bones in general.

The bony tissue that makes up our skeletal system is often thought of like the frame of a house—it provides support and protection. However, unlike the rigid materials that frame a home, bony tissue is constantly changing thanks to the activity of specific cells. The working cells of bony tissue are the osteoblast and osteoclast. An osteoblast is a bone cell responsible for the production of new bone, while osteoclasts allow absorption and removal of bone cells. The activities of these cells provide a living and constantly changing tissue. When a fracture has been immobilized, osteoblasts produce extra bone at the site of the fracture to allow for protection and healing. This extra bone is called a callus. The presence or absence of the bony callus on x-ray (radiograph) assists the physician in his or her evaluation of the amount of healing that has taken place. Once immobilization is no longer needed, the bone will remodel based on the stresses placed upon it and the process of osteoclast absorption and osteoblast production. The combination of normal stress plus this cellular activity allows the bone to adjust to the demands placed upon it. This bone's ability to change based on the stress placed upon it is known as Wolff's law.

Long bones are the bones found in our extremities as part of the appendicular skeleton. Knowing the various parts of the long bones is essential for the athletic trainer who must be able to evaluate potential injuries to this tissue. The structure of long bones includes the diaphysis, a distal and proximal epiphysis, articular surface, and the periosteum (Figure 5-8). The diaphysis is the shaft of the bone. The epiphysis is the end of the bone and the area of the bone where growth takes place. In a skeletally immature patient, this region is called the growth plate. The growth plate, also known as the epiphyseal plate or physis, is the area of growing tissue near the ends of the long bones in children and adolescents. Each long bone has at least 2 growth plates, one at each end. The growth plate determines the future length and shape of the mature bone. When growth is complete (sometime during adolescence), the growth plates close and are replaced by solid bone. Because the growth plates are the weakest areas of the growing skeleton—even weaker than the nearby ligaments and tendons that connect bones to other bones and muscles—they are vulnerable to injury. Injuries to the growth plate are called epiphyseal or physeal injuries. Injuries to adolescent athletes must be treated with care to ensure that the growth plate is not compromised. Often what appears to be a ligamentous injury in an adolescent may prove to be an epiphyseal injury.

The membrane that covers the bone (except at the articular surface) is called the periosteum. Tendons

Figure 5-9. Types of fractures. (A) Spiral. (B) Greenstick. (C) Buckle (torus). (D) Transverse. (E) Comminuted.

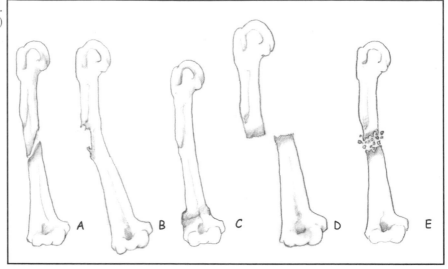

that connect muscle to bone attach at the periosteum. This membrane is also highly vascular and provides nutrition to the bone. The articular surface is the end of the bone that articulates with other bones to help form a joint. This surface is covered with articular cartilage, which protects the bone during movement. Unlike other tissues, articular cartilage does not heal or regenerate. Injuries to this tissue can have long-lasting effects.

Fractures to bone can result from a variety of injury mechanisms. The mechanism of injury will often dictate the type or classification of fracture. Acute fractures may be classified based upon the extent of the damage or deformity to the cortex of the bone. Fractures that do not disrupt the cortex include the following:

✓ Buckle (torus) fracture: This is a fracture that disrupts but does not break the cortex. These fractures appear wrinkled or buckled.

✓ Greenstick fracture: A greenstick fracture is one that breaks one side of the cortex of the bone, and results in the opposite side being bent or deformed.

The following fractures all can be classified as complete fractures because the cortex of the bone is disrupted:

✓ Spiral fracture: A fracture caused by a twisting force, resulting in a spiral-shaped fracture line.

✓ Oblique fracture: A fracture in which the fracture line is angled in relation to the long axis of the bone.

✓ Transverse fracture: Produces fracture lines that are at a right angle to the long axis of the bone.

✓ Comminuted fracture: A fracture is classified as comminuted if it results in 3 or more fragments.

Figure 5-9 presents examples of these fractures.

Fractures that involve the epiphyseal plate or physis deserve special mention. Growth plate injuries can occur in growing children and adolescents. In these skeletally immature patients, a serious injury to a joint can easily damage a growth plate rather than the ligaments that stabilize the joint. Trauma that would cause a sprain in an adult might cause a growth plate fracture in a child. Growth plate fractures occur twice as often in boys as in girls, partly because girls reach skeletal maturity at an earlier age than boys. As a result, their bones finish growing sooner, and their growth plates are replaced by stronger, solid bone. Thirty-three percent of all growth plate injuries occur in competitive sports such as football, basketball, or gymnastics, while about 20% of growth plate fractures occur as a result of recreational activities such as biking, sledding, skiing, or skateboarding.[7]

Epiphyseal injuries are classified using the Salter-Harris classification (Figure 5-10), which divides most growth plate fractures into the following 5 categories based on the type of damage[1]:

1. Type I—Fracture through the growth plate: The epiphysis is completely separated from the end of the bone or the metaphysis through the deep layer of the growth plate. The growth plate remains attached to the epiphysis.

2. Type II—Fracture through the growth plate and metaphysis: This is the most common type of growth plate fracture. It runs through the growth plate and the metaphysis, but the epiphysis is not involved in the injury.

3. Type III—Fracture through growth plate and epiphysis: This fracture occurs only rarely, usually at the lower end of the tibia, which is one of the long bones of the lower leg. It happens when a fracture runs completely through the epiphysis and separates part of the epiphysis and growth

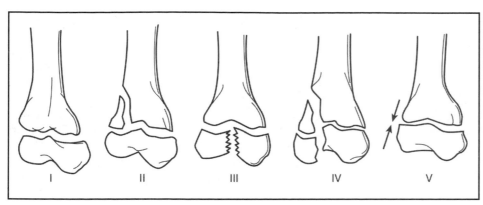

Figure 5-10. The Salter-Harris classification divides growth plate fractures into 5 categories based on the type of damage.

plate from the metaphysis. Surgery is sometimes necessary to restore the joint surface to normal.

4. Type IV—Fracture through growth plate, metaphysis, and epiphysis: This fracture runs through the epiphysis, across the growth plate, and into the metaphysis. Surgery is frequently needed to restore the joint surface to normal and to perfectly align the growth plate.

5. Type V—Compression fracture through the growth plate: This uncommon injury occurs when the end of the bone is crushed and the growth plate is compressed. It is most likely to occur at the knee or ankle. Prognosis is poor, since premature stunting of growth is almost inevitable.

A newer classification, called the Peterson classification, adds a Type VI fracture, in which a portion of the epiphysis, growth plate, and metaphysis is missing.[7] This usually occurs with open wounds or compound fractures and often involves lawnmowers, farm machinery, snow equipment, or gunshot wounds. All Type VI fractures require surgery (as well as many multiple corrective or reconstructive surgeries). Bone growth is almost always stunted with such severe trauma. With good fortune, the athletic trainer will never see this type of injury.

Bones are living, constantly changing structures. Normal healthy bone responds to physical stress and demands with a cycle of bone loss (breakdown) followed by bone formation (production). If the amount of bone loss exceeds production, the result is a stress fracture. Weight-bearing bones (lower extremity) and bones susceptible to repetitive stress are the most common sites of stress fractures. Stress fractures often develop when there is a change in the volume of physical activity, the intensity of physical activity, a change in footwear, or a change in playing surfaces. Correcting biomechanical deficiencies and making appropriate adjustments to activity are key treatment considerations.

Some common stress fracture locations include the tibia (lower leg), metatarsals (foot), femoral neck (thigh), and tarsal navicular (mid foot). Stress fractures are not exclusive to the lower extremity. Pain in the spine may result from a stress reaction to the vertebrae, and some sport activities can lead to stress reactions in locations other than the lower extremity. Tennis (nondominant ulna) and rowing (ribs) are examples of such sport activities. Persistent pain with impact activities, pain that does not resolve with rest, and pain at night are all common signs of a possible stress fracture. The location of the stress fracture is commonly point tender to touch, while soft tissue injuries are often more diffuse. Stress fractures present a challenge to the athletic trainer in developing a rehabilitation program that will allow a gradual return to activity to prevent a recurrence.

INJURIES TO MUSCLE AND TENDON

An injury causing tearing to the fibers of a muscle is called a strain. Studies estimate that injuries to muscles represent between 10% to 30% of all athletic-related injuries. A report of injury patterns in 10 selected high school sports (5 boys and 5 girls) revealed 23.2% of the reported injuries were strains.[7] Strain injuries are graded from first thru third degree based on the amount of damage to the tissue. Muscle strain injuries are caused by over stretching of the muscle or an overload to the tissue caused when the muscle must absorb forces while under tension. Muscle is a unique tissue that has the ability to both contract and be stretched. It is elastic and can adapt over time. Sitting for an extended period of time and having tightness in your hamstrings when you get up is an example of how rapidly muscles can adapt. Maintaining flexibility and properly warming up the muscle tissue prior to activity are keys to preventing injury.

Any discussion of muscle injury must also include injuries to tendons. Tendons attach muscle to bone, and the location where muscle and tendon come

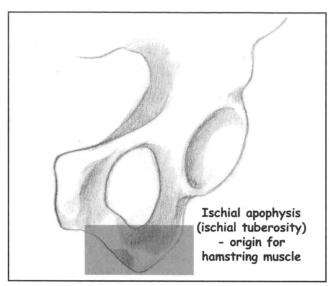

Ischial apophysis
(ischial tuberosity)
- origin for
hamstring muscle

Figure 5-11. An apophysis may be a site of inflammation (apophysitis) or a location for an avulsion fracture. Apophyseal avulsions should be evaluated and ruled out in skeletally immature patients.

together is called the muscle-tendon junction. The muscle-tendon junction is a common site of a strain injury. The anatomical connection between muscle and tendon is vast. Tendons are strong connective tissues composed of collagen. They differ from muscle tissue in that they do not have a contractile element. Tendons do adapt with stresses and can be warmed to assist in this process. Connective noncontractile tissue penetrates the muscle extensively. It is not uncommon to see muscle strain injury also referred to as muscle-tendon strain injury in deference to this anatomical arrangement.

Injuries to the tendon itself may be either acute or chronic. The most common chronic injury is tendonitis. Tendonitis is an inflammation of the tendon caused by repetitive stress (overuse), changes in intensity or volume of an activity, or biomechanical alterations in movements. For example, a runner who has tightness in the posterior muscles of the lower leg may develop an alteration in his or her running gait, leading to Achilles tendonitis. In addition, "too much too soon" is the perfect recipe for tendonitis. Individuals just starting a conditioning program or those returning to a sport following rehabilitation must take extra care to gradually increase activity to avoid these overuse injuries. Acute tendon ruptures are less common than overuse injuries, but they can occur in physically active populations. A rupture of the Achilles tendon is not uncommon, particularly among middle-aged recreational participants.

The location on a bone where a muscle originates or inserts (via tendon) often will adapt due to the force exerted by the muscle or muscle group. This area of bone is called an apophysis. Apophysitis is inflammation where the tendon arises from the bone at this location. It is possible to avulse or rupture the apophysis completely away from the larger bone. These injuries are mentioned alongside muscle-tendon injuries because they are often associated with mechanisms of injury common with muscle strains. Often, an apophyseal injury will be misidentified as a third-degree muscle strain. If the athletic trainer suspects a rupture to an apophysis (Figure 5-11), a radiograph and referral to the physician are essential.

A contusion is another soft tissue injury that most often affects muscle tissue. A contusion is a closed injury caused by a direct blow that compresses the underlying tissues. Contusions are usually point tender and display edema and ecchymosis. While often a minor injury, an improperly managed contusion can lead to a myositis ossificans. Myositis ossificans is a condition that develops when there is continued bleeding in a muscle following a contusion. Calcification within the muscle can result over time. This calcification is an abnormal bone growth that can result in pain and dysfunction of the affected muscle group. The quadriceps is the most common location for such an injury. The formation of calcification in a location where it does not belong is called an ectopic calcification. An ectopic calcification can also occur in tendons and is called calcific tendonitis.

A final chronic connective tissue injury to be aware of is fascitis, which is inflammation of connective fascia. Although not a true injury to the muscle tendon unit itself, it is often caused by tightness or restrictions in a muscle group that lead to pain and inflammation in a specific group of fascia. This condition is common to the plantar aspect of the foot (plantar fascitis).

INJURIES TO JOINTS

Injuries to joints represent some of the most common conditions the athletic trainer will encounter. A joint or articulation is the point where 2 bones join. Joints are classified based on their ability to move. A freely moveable joint is called a diarthrotic joint; commonly called a synovial joint. Synovial joints are supported by a joint capsule or ligaments. The capsule is lined with a synovial membrane that produced fluid, and the articular surfaces (ends of the bones) are covered with an articular cartilage. Articular cartilage is called hyaline cartilage. Synovial joints may also have a fibrocartilaginous disk or meniscus that separates the articular surfaces while providing stability and shock absorption to the joint. The knee is an example of a synovial joint that contains a meniscus (Figure 5-12). The ankle is also a synovial joint; however, it does not contain a meniscus.

Structure Governs Function

The maxim "structure governs function" is commonly used in the area of sports medicine. It is often attributed to Dr. Andrew Taylor Still, the founder of osteopathic medicine. It is appropriate to think about as we begin to "understand injury." This chapter discusses how specific tissues can be injured. The integrity of the tissue (the structure) is partly responsible for its ultimate function. If the ligament is sprained, its structure may not allow for full function.

Understanding that "structure governs function" allows practitioners to think of function beyond just the affected joint. Function can apply to the "whole" person. Athletic trainers provide care to people, not just injuries. It is important to always remember that function extends beyond just the ankle or knee. An athletic training student that develops a philosophy that looks at the whole person and recognizes the relationships between function and structure is well on his or her way to success.

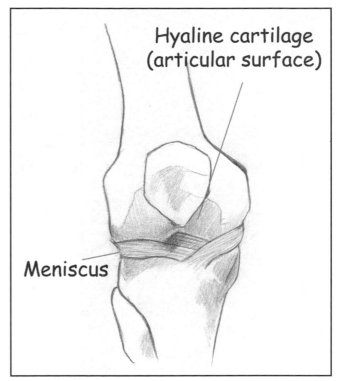

Figure 5-12. The knee is a synovial joint that includes a fibrocartilage meniscus.

Acute injuries can occur to synovial joints when forces cause the ligaments or capsule to extend beyond their limits. An injury to a ligament or the capsular tissue of a joint is called a sprain. Like muscle strains, a sprain is graded in degrees of severity (first to third). Sprains to the ankle are the most common sprains with which the athletic trainer will deal. The National Institutes of Health report that ankle sprains are the most common injury in the United States. Approximately 1 million ankle injuries occur each year, and 85% of them are sprains.[8] The knee and the shoulder are also common areas for sprain injuries.

If an articulation is forced beyond its anatomical limits of motion, it may either sublux or dislocate (luxation). A subluxation is a partial separation of 2 articular surfaces, while a dislocation is the complete separation of the articular surfaces from one another (Figure 5-13). In athletics, dislocations to the fingers are the most common, followed by dislocations at the shoulder (glenohumeral joint).[7] When an articulation dislocates for the first time, the athletic trainer must have the joint evaluated for a possible fracture. A fracture that involves the articular cartilage is called an osteochondral fracture. These types of fractures have significant ramifications for the long-term health of the articulation and must be treated with care. It is not uncommon for subsequent instabilities to take place in a joint that has been subluxed or dislocated. Untrained personnel should never attempt to reduce a joint that has been dislocated. Proper evaluation, referral, and rehabilitation are essential for patients with joint instabilities.

Chronic injuries are most often caused by repeated trauma, overuse, changes in workload or volume, and biomechanical insufficiencies. These mechanisms of injury apply to chronic injuries to synovial joints as well. One category of chronic injury is osteochondrosis, or degenerative changes to the ossification centers of bones. Osteochondritis dissecans (OCD) is an inflammatory condition that includes a loose body or fragment in a joint. These loose bodies are sometimes referred to as joint mice. A patient with OCD may have chronic pain and inflammation and lose the ability to move the joint freely. Patients with degenerative or inflammatory changes to the articular surfaces are said to have osteoarthritis. An inflammation of the synovial capsule that surrounds the joint is called synovitis. Patients with chronic pain and unexplained swelling should be referred to the physician for evaluation and management.

Chronic soft tissue inflammation can also occur in the bursa. Bursa are fluid-filled sacs or potential spaces that are found in areas of increased friction at synovial joints, between tendons and bone, at locations of bony prominence, and near tendons and ligaments. The suffix *-itis* indicates that bursitis is an inflammation of the bursa. Bursitis is caused by repetitive trauma, overuse, and biomechanical insufficiencies. In severe chronic cases, the bursa may develop calcific deposits or degenerate.

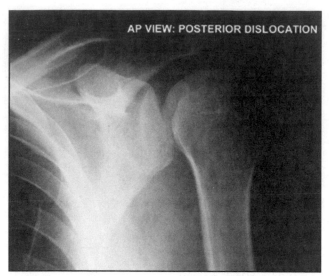

Figure 5-13. Radiograph of a posterior glenohumeral dislocation. (Courtesy of Dr. Ken Schreibman, University of Wisconsin–Madison School of Medicine and Public Health.)

NEUROVASCULAR INJURIES

Normal musculoskeletal function relies on input from sensory nerves to our central nervous system and output by motor nerves to the periphery. This constant flow of information controls our ability to perceive pain, have motor reactions, maintain smooth motor movements, and have an awareness of our surroundings. Within the context of athletic injuries, nerve injuries are most often secondary injuries associated with another primary injury. Fractures or dislocations may cause compression to nerves when bones are forced into improper positions. Nerves may be stretched or compressed by direct changes in body position or direct blows. Nerve injuries can present as mild changes in sensation or by weakness in specific muscle groups. Burning pain, radiating pain, and numbness are often associated with nerve injuries. Neuritis is inflammation of a particular nerve and is often associated with a nerve entrapment. A nerve is said to be entrapped when it is compressed between bone or soft tissue. A group of nerves that leaves the spinal cord in a specific region is known as a plexus. A stretch injury that results in paresthesia (numbness/changes in sensation) and weakness is called a neuropraxia. A stretch or compression injury to the brachial plexus of the upper extremity is a common athletic-related nerve injury.

Compartment syndromes are injuries to vascular and nerve tissues that are caused by increases in pressure in the extremities. The anatomical arrangement of bones and soft tissues in the extremities take the shape of compartments. It is difficult for pressure caused by swelling to dissipate in these compartments. Acute compartment syndromes are the result of swelling and pressure secondary to a traumatic event. These syndromes are characterized by increasing pain, loss of muscle function due to compression of nerves, and compromise of blood flow due to compression of vascular tissues. If left unattended, an acute compartment syndrome may lead to tissue death. The anterior/lateral portion of the lower leg is the most common location for a compartment syndrome; however, it can also occur in the thigh and forearm. A subacute compartment syndrome can sometimes present following prolonged exercise.

SUMMARY

Medical terminology provides a common ground for the athletic trainer to communicate with other allied health professionals and team physicians. The athletic training student who develops a working vocabulary and understands common word parts will be better equipped to complete class readings, interpret journal articles, and communicate in an effective, professional manner. Taking the time to develop these skills early can pay great rewards in the future.

Understanding injury begins with knowing the types of injuries that can occur and how each specific tissue is affected. Learning how tissues respond to acute and chronic conditions allows the athletic trainer to make appropriate referral and management decisions. Knowing the various types of injury, what tissues are affected, and how injuries are classified is a common starting point for all athletic training students.

REFERENCES

1. National Institute of Arthritis and Musculoskeletal Skin Diseases. Sprains and Strains .Available at www.niams.nih.gov/hi/topics/strain_sprain/strain_sprain.htm. Accessed May 5, 2008.
2. Mueller FO, Cantu RC. Annual Survey of Catastrophic Football Injuries 1977—2000. Chapel Hill, NC: National Center for Catastrophic Sport Injury; 2001.
3. Mueller FO, Cantu RC. 24th Annual Report: Fall 1982—Spring 2006. Chapel Hill, NC: National Center for Catastrophic Sport Injury; 2007.
4. National Federation of State High School Associations 2006-2007 athletes participation summary. Available at www.nfhs.org. Accessed August 12, 2008.
5. US Consumer Product Safety Commission, Directorate of Economic Analysis. Injury costs for high school athletes in baseball, basketball, football, soccer, softball, track and wrestling. Obtained through a data request January 2006. In: McGuine, TA. Sports injuries in high school athletes: a review of injury-risk and injury prevention research. *Clin J Sport Med.* 2006;16:6.

Beyond the Mona Lisa

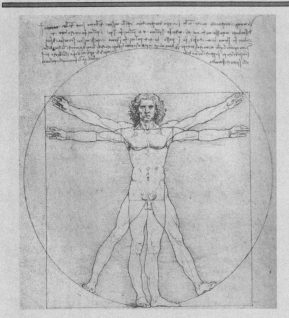

Maybe you should thank Leonardo da Vinci next time you are studying anatomy. What comes to mind when you hear da Vinci? The Mona Lisa? A popular novel? The Renaissance? Well, in addition to being a painter, sculptor, inventor, and engineer, he was also the best-informed anatomist of his day. He completed some 30 human dissections in addition to the countless animals he studied. He left behind over 800 anatomical drawings.

He also understood that pictures were the best medium for recording what he learned. The anatomical information in his day described the body in words. To this Leonardo said, "With what words [can you] describe the whole arrangement... more detail you write concerning it, the more you will confuse the mind of the hearer."

So Leonardo cut and drew. He created a pictorial vocabulary for all to see. He invented cutaway sections. He made his own crude x-rays by laying semitransparent tissue over underlying organs and bones. Leonardo the artist brought the dead back to life and gave them new life even as Leonardo the surgeon cut them into pieces.

His anatomical discoveries were many:

- He was the first to identify the sinus cavities.
- He was first to identify the heart as a muscle.
- He was the first to see that the heart was four chambered.
- He showed us that every muscle had another muscle working in opposition to it.
- He anticipated the existence of microscopic capillaries 150 years before they were identified.
- He used casting to determine the shape of internal cavities.

Leonardo was driven by his art and the sense of beauty that he found in the bodies he dissected. He also trumpeted the coming of a new age of empirical science when he warns us that, "If you wish to demonstrate in words... do not meddle with things appertaining to the eyes by making them enter through the ears, for you will be far surpassed by the painter."

Do yourself a favor and search online or go to the library to get a look at Leonardo's original anatomical drawings. When you are studying the drawings in this text or viewing the interactive anatomical images on the companion Web site, take a minute to think about the old master who decided that the picture would be worth more than a thousand words. Leonardo da Vinci—anatomist and much more than the creator of Mona Lisa's smile.

Adapted with permission from Leinhard JH. Engines of Our Ingenuity. Episode #637: Leonardo, Anatomist. [transcript]. Available at www.uh.edu/engines/epi637.htm. Accessed April 10, 2007.

6. McGuine TA. Sports injuries in high school athletes: a review of injury-risk and injury prevention research. *Clin J Sport Med.* 2006;16:6.
7. Peterson L, Renstrom P. *Sports Injuries: Their Prevention and Treatment.* 3rd ed. Champaign, IL: Human Kinetics; 2001.
8. National Institute of Arthritis and Musculoskeletal Skin Diseases. Growth Plate Injuries. Available at http://www.niams.nih.gov/Health_Info/Growth_Plate_Injuries . Accessed June 7, 2008.

WEB RESOURCES

Medical Terminology Web
http://ec.hku.hk/mt

A Web site produced by the English Centre and designed primarily for students majoring in dentistry, medicine, and nursing, the pages show a selected list of the frequently found terms that students may encounter. The purpose of this Web site is to help students recognize technical terms and assist them in building a professional vocabulary.

National Institute of Health
www.nih.gov

Extensive government site maintained by the National Institutes of Health and all of the centers affiliated with it. Search capabilities allow visitors to access a wide range of information.

American Orthopedic Society for Sports Medicine
www.aossm.org

The AOSSM is a national organization of orthopaedic surgeons specializing in sports medicine, including national and international sports medicine leaders.

National Center for Catastrophic Injury Research
www.unc.edu/depts/nccsi

The National Center for Catastrophic Injury Research collects and disseminates death and permanent disability sports injury data that involve brain and/or spinal cord injuries. The research is funded by a grant from the NCAA, the American Football Coaches Association, and the National Federation of State High School Associations. This research has been conducted at the University of North Carolina at Chapel Hill since 1965.

ⓘ Career Spotlight: Athletic Training Program Director

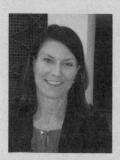

Dawn Hammerschmidt, MEd, ATC

Assistant Professor/Curriculum Coordinator

Athletic Training Education Program

Minnesota State University Moorhead

My Position

I am currently the curriculum coordinator for the athletic training education program at MSUM. My position requires oversight of all aspects of the athletic training major. This includes curricular decisions, clinical requirements, program assessment, teaching, advising, recruiting, retention, university committees, student club advising, and occasional clinical coverage/supervision.

Unique or Desired Qualifications

To obtain a position in higher education (professor), one must secure the appropriate education and professional experience. Most universities require at a minimum a master's degree while securing tenure usually requires a terminal degree (PhD, EdD).

Favorite Aspect of My Job

Without question, the opportunity to be around students who are eager and motivated to pursue a degree in athletic training.

Advice

Find something that you are passionate about—if you are passionate about your career, life is a whole lot simpler! Basically, you have to really like what you do in order to thrive and survive in the "real world."

CHAPTER 6

COMMON INJURIES TO THE LOWER EXTREMITY

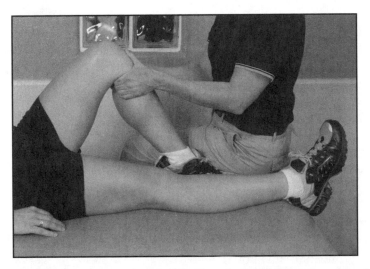

A good athletic trainer needs to be a hard worker, I think you have to enjoy helping people, and I think it takes someone who has some interest or passion about the activities our patients are involved in. You need to enjoy the environment you are in.

Scott Barker, MS, ATC
Head Athletic Trainer
California State University, Chico

INJURIES TO THE LOWER EXTREMITY

Students always laugh when I compare the limbs of a human to those of a dog (or any other 4-legged creature). However, it is not funny at all. Comparative anatomy is a rigorous subject at many universities and one that gives great insight into our own function. Humans walk on 2 feet. To hear the evolutionists tell it, at some point 4 million years ago, primitive man took those first shaky steps with knuckles up off the dirt and stood up. Why? To see over the tall grass and look for food, to reach and grasp? Maybe they knew someday there would be baseball and thought, "Who can pitch bent over like this?" Well, the latter is a stretch. It does not matter how it happened—the facts are in. We walk upright and because of that our discussion of the structure and function of the lower extremity often comes back to our evolutionary past. The strength of the hip joint, position of the specific muscles, and the wide, or limited, ROM at specific joints all come back to the fact that we walk upright. We support our weight, run, jump, land, and use our lower extremity in countless ways during physical activity. The ability of the bones, muscles, and joints of the lower extremity to generate force, absorb the impact of running and walking, and adjust to the forces placed upon them during activity will dictate whether we see injuries in these structures. Next time you see someone kick a soccer ball, thank our early ancestors. After all, they stood up and got it all started.

97

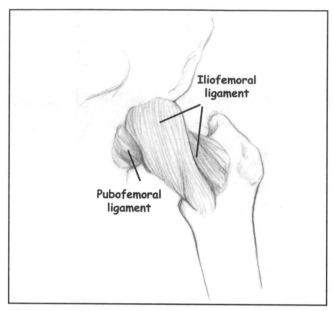

Figure 6-1. Anterior view of the hip, capsule, and ligaments.

Upon completion of this chapter, the student will be able to:

✓ Understand the anatomy of the lower extremity, including specific articulations at the hip, knee, ankle, and foot

✓ Recognize common injuries and conditions to the lower extremity

✓ Recognize common mechanisms of lower extremity injury

✓ Appreciate the athletic trainer's role in assessment and referral

 Treatment and Rehabilitation

Chapter 13 provides an overview of the initial care and management of acute athletic injuries, and some general concepts of rehabilitation are presented in Chapter 14. In the course of discussing common injuries in Chapters 6 to 9, only initial care issues are discussed. A comprehensive discussion of long-term management, rehabilitation, and reconditioning are outside the scope of this introductory text. Athletic training students in an accredited education program will receive instruction and clinical experience in each of these important educational competency and professional domain areas.

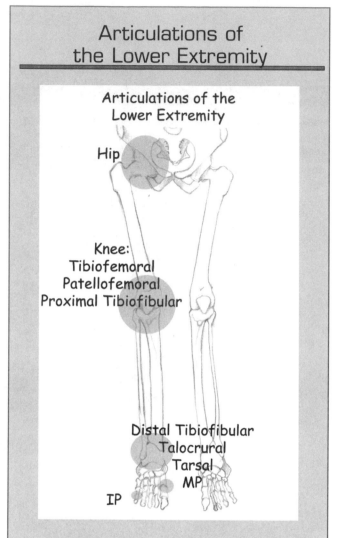

The articulations of the lower extremity include the hip, knee (tibiofemoral), patellofemoral, proximal and distal tibiofibular, ankle, (talo-crural), subtalar (talocalcaneal), foot (tarsal-metatarsal and metatarsal-phalange), and the interphalangeal joints of the toes.

Complete muscle and skeletal illustrations for the lower extremity are provided in Appendix D.

LOWER EXTREMITY ANATOMY

HIP

The femur articulates with the pelvis to form the hip joint. The round head of the femur acts as a "ball" that fits in the acetabulum of the pelvis or "socket." The hip joint is surrounded by a strong group of ligaments, including the ligamentum teres, transverse acetabular, iliofemoral, pubofemoral, and inguinal (Figure 6-1). A strong capsule and large muscle

Table 6-1

Major Muscles, Primary Actions, and Innervations at the Hip

Muscle	Action	Innervation
Gluteus maximus	Extension/adduction	Inferior gluteal
Gluteus medius and minimus	Abduction/internal rotation	Superior gluteal
Tensor fascia latae	Adduction/flexion/internal rotation	Superior gluteal
Iliacus	Flexion	Femoral
Psoas major	Flexion	Femoral and lumbar
Rectus femoris	Flexion	Femoral
Sartorius	Flexion/external rotation	Femoral
Pectineus	Adduction/flexion	Femoral

Adductors
  Longus
  Brevis
  Magnus
	Adduction/flexion	Obturator

Gracilis	Adduction	Obturator

Deep rotators of the hip
  Piriformis
  Obturator internus
  Obturator externus
  Quadratus femoris
	Lateral rotators	Second sacral
		Branch from sacral plexus
		Obturator
		Branch from sacral plexus

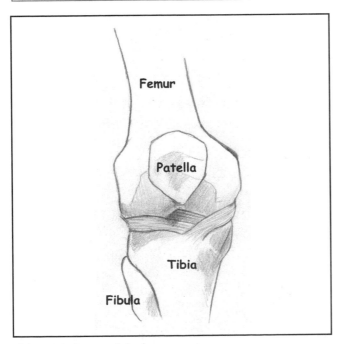

Figure 6-2. Bones of the knee.

groups on all sides support the joint. These muscles include the hip flexors, hip extensors, abductors, and adductors. The muscles that act on the hip joint and their actions are presented in Table 6-1. The muscles of the hip allow for the movements of flexion, exten-sion, abduction, adduction, internal rotation, and external rotation. The hip is a very stable articulation that does not have the excessive mobility found in the shoulder.

KNEE

The knee is the largest joint in the body and repre-sents 2 specific articulations: the tibiofemoral articu-lation and the patellofemoral articulation (PF). The bones that make up the knee joint include the patella, femur, tibia, and fibula (Figure 6-2). The femur and tibia are strong bones that support the knee joint and bear weight. The fibula is the smaller of the 2 bones of the lower leg and only bears a small percentage of weight. The patella is encased in a large tendon and slides back and forth in the groove of the distal femur. The motions possible at the knee joint include flexion and extension. A small amount of tibial rotation can also take place at the knee joint. The knee is somewhat unstable based on its shape and unique arrangement. The large femur sits atop the flat tibia; the rounded end of the femur can roll and slide back and forth on the tibia. The shape of the tibia is improved by the presence of 2 fibrous cartilages. They are known as the medial and lateral menisci (Figure 6-3) and help reduce joint shock and stress.

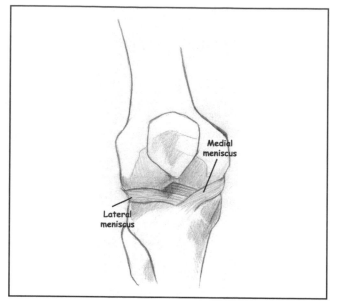

Figure 6-3. The menisci are a common site of injury at the knee joint.

Figure 6-4. Four main ligaments of the knee.

Table 6-2
Major Muscles, Primary Actions, and Innervations at the Knee

Muscle	Action	Innervation
Hamstrings		
Biceps femoris	Flexion/external rotation	Sciatic
Semimembranosus	Flexion/internal rotation	Tibial
Semitendinosus	Flexion/internal rotation	Tibial
Popliteus	Flexion/internal rotation	Tibial
Gastrocnemius (Calf)	Flexion	Tibial
Quadriceps		
Rectus femoris	Extension	Femoral
Vastus intermedius	Extension	Femoral
Vastus lateralis	Extension	Femoral
Vastus medialis obliques	Extension	Femoral

The 4 primary ligaments of the knee are the anterior cruciate (ACL), posterior cruciate (PCL), medial collateral (MCL), and lateral collateral (LCL) (Figure 6-4). The cruciate ligaments arise from the femur and attach to the middle of the tibial plateau. The ligaments are named based on their insertion (anterior and posterior) onto the tibia. These ligaments control the anterior and posterior slide of the femur on the tibia. They form an "X" pattern in which the ligaments cross in the middle of the knee. The MCL helps stabilize the inside of the knee joint. This ligament connects the femur and the tibia. The MCL is a broad ligament that has both a deep and superficial layer. The deep layer has an anatomical connection to the medi-cal meniscus while the superficial layer is consistent with the joint capsule. The LCL supports the lateral side of the knee and attaches the femur and the fibula. Unlike the MCL, it does not attach to the meniscus. The LCL is thicker and more distinct than its medial counterpart. The shape of the bones, the presence of the menisci, and the ligaments all contribute to static stability. However, this is not enough. The knee relies heavily on muscles to provide dynamic support.

The muscles that act on the knee joint are presented in Table 6-2. The primary movers of the knee joint are the large muscle groups of the thigh and lower leg. The thigh muscles include the quadriceps on the anterior aspect, and the hamstrings on the posterior aspect

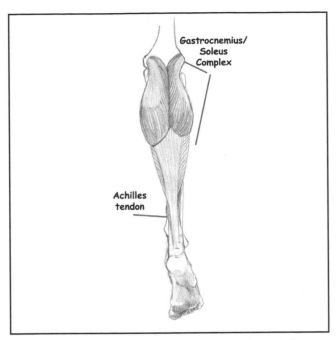

Figure 6-5. Gastrocnemius/soleus complex. The Achilles tendon is a common site of chronic injury.

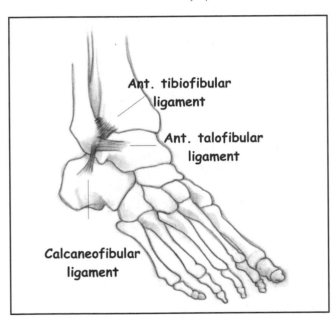

Figure 6-7. Ligaments of the ankle, lateral view.

of the knee. These muscle groups help extend and flex the knee, respectively. The gastrocnemius/soleus complex, or calf muscles, also help support the knee and assist in knee flexion (Figure 6-5). Other muscles that act on this joint include the popliteus, gracilis, tensor fascia latae, plantaris, and sartorius. It is only through strong muscles surrounding the knee joint that the inherent instability is overcome. As we will see, this is often not enough to prevent injury.

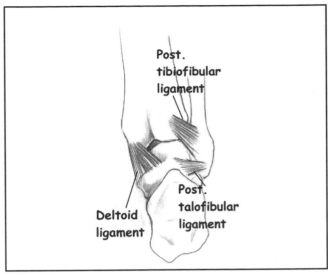

Figure 6-6. Ligaments of the ankle, posterior view.

ANKLE/FOOT

The foot is attached to the lower leg at the talocrural (ankle) joint. The tibia, fibula, and talus make up the ankle joint. The true ankle joint allows movement in plantar flexion (pointing of the toes) and dorsiflexion (pulling the foot up). However, the ankle is most often injured when the ankle rolls inward or outward. These motions are called inversion and eversion, respectively. The subtalar joint (talus and calcaneus) allows for these movements. The ankle joint is easily identified by the medial and lateral malleoli on each side of the ankle. These bony prominences are the distal ends of the fibula (lateral) and tibia (medial). The talus has a rectangular shape that is wider at the front. When the ankle is pulled into dorsiflexion, the talus fits snugly between the tibia and fibula. This stable arrangement combined with the ligamentous structures provides for a strong joint when in this position. However, when the foot is plantarflexed, the joint is not as stable. The longer lateral fibula, weaker lateral ligaments, and the loose position of the joint make rolling (inverting) your ankle very easy in this position.

Ligaments that provide support to the ankle joint are found on all sides of the articulation. The medial side of the ankle is much more stable in comparison to the lateral aspect. The deltoid ligament is a broad triangular-shaped ligament that supports the medial ankle. The lateral ligaments include the anterior talofibular, calcaneofibular, and posterior talofibular. The structure of the ankle is dependent upon the close proximity of the fibula and tibia to give shape to the joint. The anterior and posterior tibiofibular ligaments help hold the ends of the tibia and fibula together (Figures 6-6 and 6-7).

Table 6-3

Major Muscles, Primary Actions, and Innervations at the Lower Leg/Ankle

Muscle	Action	Innervation
Anterior tibialis	Dorsiflexion/inversion	Deep peroneal
Posterior tibialis	Plantar flexion/inversion	Tibial
Extensor hallicus longus	Extension (great toe)/dorsiflexion	Deep peroneal
Extensor digitorum longus	Extension of toes/dorsiflexion/eversion	Deep peroneal
Gastrocnemius (calf)	Plantar flexion	Tibial
Soleus	Plantar flexion	Tibial
Peroneus longus	Eversion/plantar flexion	Superficial peroneal
Peroneus brevis	Eversion/plantar flexion	Superficial peroneal
Flexor digitorum longus	Flexion of toes/plantar flexion/inversion	Tibial
Flexor hallicus longus	Flexion of great toe/plantar flexion/inversion	Tibial

The muscles that act on the ankle joint and help support the foot originate in the lower leg and cross the ankle joint. The largest muscle group is the gastrocnemius/soleus complex, which crosses the ankle joint and inserts via the strong Achilles tendon. This tendon is a common site of overuse injury, and this strong muscle group helps plantarflex the foot. On the lateral side of the ankle, the peroneal muscle group helps support the ankle and prevents inversion injuries. The peroneal tendons split below the lateral malleolus and insert in different locations. The peroneus longus supports the arch of the foot while the peroneus brevis inserts into the base of the fifth metatarsal. This insertion point is of particular interest to the athletic trainer and a common site for injury. The tibialis posterior, flexor digitorum, and flexor hallicus all cross the medial side of the ankle. These muscles can work to invert/plantarflex the foot as well as flex the digits and great toe. The large tibialis anterior crosses the front of the ankle and acts to dorsiflex the foot. The extensor digitorum longus and extensor hallicus also cross the front of the foot and as their names imply act to extend the digits and great toe. All of these muscle groups provide dynamic support to the ankle. Table 6-3 outlines the muscles of the lower leg and their primary movements.

Each foot has 26 bones (7 tarsal bones, 5 metatarsals, and 14 phalanges) and 38 individual articulations (Figure 6-8). The foot consists of 2 distinct arches: the longitudinal and the transverse. The longitudinal arch runs in an anterior/posterior direction and can be divided into lateral (outer) and medial (inner) regions. The transverse arch runs medial to lateral and is best visualized at the metatarsal heads. The anatomy of the foot is such that it can withstand impact forces over twice the body weight. The bones of the foot are supported by an extensive network of ligaments in the mid foot region. In addition, muscles/tendons originate on the lower leg, cross the ankle, and insert at the foot to support the bones of the foot. The tendons that extend the foot and phalanges are quite superficial on the dorsal surface of the foot and can sometimes be the site of inflammation or irritation. On the plantar surface (bottom), thick layers of skin and a broad band of fascia extend from the calcaneus (heel) to the front of the foot to provide protection.

INJURIES TO THE HIP AND THIGH

FRACTURES AND INJURIES TO BONE

Traumatic fractures to the femur or pelvis are not particularly common in sports; however, they can occur if there is a significant force. A vaulting injury in track and field, falls with equestrienne sports, or high-velocity direct blows would be the most likely mechanisms for a traumatic fracture to the femur or pelvis. An athlete with this type of injury would present with significant amounts of pain and have a logical mechanism for fracture. Proper stabilization and immediate transport to a medical facility or evaluation is essential. An open fracture to the femur is a medical emergency and should be treated as such. There are other bony injuries to the hip that the athletic trainer must be able to recognize.

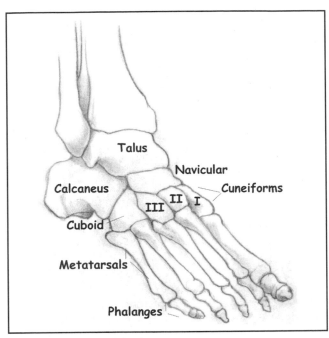

Figure 6-8. Bones of the foot.

While commonly thought of as an injury to the lower leg or foot, stress fractures can occur in the hip region to the pelvis or the femoral neck. Stress frac-

tures constitute 10% to 20% of all injuries presented to sports medicine clinics and 7% to 10% of those affect the femurs, pubic rami, iliac crests, and sacroiliac (SI) joints.[1] This injury is a result of repetitive trauma due to overuse. Femoral neck stress fractures may occur on the tension (superior) or compression (inferior) surface of the bone. The location of this stress fracture has significant implications. Tension surface femoral neck stress fractures often affect older runners and are at risk for nonunion or malunion (poor healing) and possibly avascular necrosis (loss of blood supply and bone death). Compression side stress fractures occur in younger runners and generally do well with protected activity and gradual return to activity.[1] These fractures are more common in female distance runners who may have nutritional deficiencies and menstrual irregularities (see Chapter 12). An athlete with a stress fracture will have generalized pain in the hip region, night pain, or pain with ambulation. Given the risk for poor outcome, physicians who suspect a femoral stress fracture will likely order computed tomography (CT) and/or MRI diagnostic tests to assist with diagnosis. The athletic trainer must consider the possibility of a stress fracture in patients who fit the above profile and have unresolved pain in this area. Rest, nonimpact training, and referral to a physician are the proper courses of action.

 ## Stress Fractures in the Female Athlete

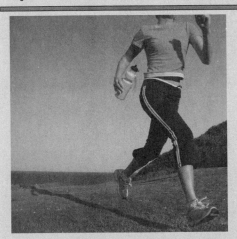

Female athletes may be at risk for stress fractures as a result of biomechanical, endocrinological, and nutritional factors.

A recent topic of increased interest in the sports medicine world has been the amount of stress fractures that seem to be occurring in the competitive female athlete.

The definition of a stress fracture is a partial to complete fracture of bone due to its inability to withstand repeated nonviolent stresses. When a bone is stressed in this manner, the bone responds by trying to adapt its form and function to meet the external stresses placed upon it. A stress fracture occurs when the rate of healing is unable to keep up with the rate of breakdown that is being caused by the repetitive stress placed upon it.

Athletes with a stress fracture commonly complain of very specific point tenderness directly on a bone that gets worse while running and improves with rest. They are most susceptible at the beginning of a sport season due to the rapid increase in physical activity that is required of them at this time. Stress fractures are treated with rest from impact activities for about 6 to 8 weeks or whenever pain-free running is possible.

Causes of Stress Fractures

The 3 main causes of stress fractures are biomechanical problems, endocrinological problems, and dietary problems. We are all familiar with the biomechanical causes of stress fractures such as running on hard surfaces; improper footwear; and malformation problems such as forefoot hyperpronation, rearfoot valgus, and cavus (high arch) and planus (flat arch) deformity of the feet. These problems cause stress fractures in both the male and female athlete. The key to the rise in stress fractures in females is

(continued)

Stress Fractures in the Female Athlete (continued)

proving to be secondary to the endocrinological and dietary problems that commonly occur in the female athlete.

Biomechanics Issues

It is essential that female as well as male athletes wear the proper athletic shoes for their sport and their level of training. In general, it is a good idea to replace your training shoes each sport season or every 6 months. Even if the shoe does not look worn, a large portion of the shoes' ability to support your foot and absorb shock is diminished as the material in the shoes breaks down.

In addition to simply getting new shoes, it is essential that those athletes who have a planus deformity purchase shoes that support the arch very well. If an athlete with these foot types has ongoing problems with medial lower leg and knee pain or a history of stress fractures, it would be wise for him or her to consult with a sports medicine physician or a podiatrist about obtaining either custom or noncustom arch supports/orthotics. This intervention can drastically change the discomfort associated with training in these individuals as well as prevent future stress fractures.

When biomechanical issues are determined to be a likely cause for a stress fracture, proper flexibility and strengthening exercises for the lower leg and ankle are just as important as proper footwear. A gradual progression into training is also much more important for individuals with biomechanical problems.

Endocrinological Issues

There is considerable evidence to support endocrinological disorders as a predisposing factor for stress fractures. One pertinent study performed by Barrow and Saha[1] evaluated 240 female distance runners. They noted that women with very irregular menses (0 to 5 per year) had an incidence of stress fractures of 49%. Those with irregular menses (6 to 9 per year) had a 39% occurrence, while those with regular menses had an occurrence of 29%. Another study by Lloyd and Triantafyllou[2] reviewed 207 female athletes and found that those individuals with absent or irregular menses had an incidence of 24% while those with regular menses had a 9% incidence of stress fractures. A recent study by Bennell et al[3] showed that restrictive dietary patterns and eating disorders are also a causative factor in the occurrence of stress fractures.

The reason stress fractures occur more frequently in amenorrheic females is due to a decrease in the rate of estrogen production. This causes a decreased absorption of minerals in bone, which decreases the bone mineral density and thus causes a decreased ability of the bone to withstand the repeated microtrauma induced by competitive athletics. Likewise, poor nutritional habits hinder the ability of bone to repair and maintain itself because the components needed in the healing process are not present in sufficient quantity. In both cases, stress fractures are often the inevitable result in a female that is training very competitively.

These athletes are commonly helped by estrogen replacement therapy designed to normalize and/or restore normal estrogen levels and also by dietary counseling. Coaches, athletic trainers, and parents usually become aware of these problems first and should encourage their athletes to see a sports medicine physician for monitoring, counseling, and treatment as deemed necessary.

Note: This information is part of the UW Health Sports Link Sports Updates Information Series and is reprinted with permission of UW Health, Madison, WI.

References

1. Barrow GW, Saha S. Menstrual irregularity and stress fractures in collegiate female distance runners. *Am J Sports Med.* 1988;16(3):209-216.
2. Lloyd T, Triantafyllou SJ. Women athletes with menstrual irregularity have increased musculoskeletal injuries. *Med Sci Sports Exerc.* 1986;18(4):374-379.
3. Bennell KL, Malcolm SA, Thomas SA, et al. Risk factors for stress fractures in female track and field athletes: a retrospective analysis. *Clin J Sport Med.* 1995;5(4):229-235.

Adolescents are susceptible to a specific group of injuries to bony structures at the hip. Avulsion fractures can occur when the strong muscles that act to flex the trunk or hip pull away from their bony origin or insertion (see Considerations for the Skeletally Immature Patient on p. 105). These injuries commonly take place at the anterior superior iliac spine (ASIS) where the rectus femoris muscle originates, the lesser trochanter of the femur where the iliopsoas inserts, and the ischial tuberosity, which is the origin of the hamstring muscle group. Younger athletes are prone to these injuries due to their skeletal immaturity. Their growth plates have not fully closed and the strong forceful muscle actions can cause the avulsion. Athletes with a suspected avulsion injury will have pain, may report hearing a sound associated with the avulsion (pop or snap), and will have decreased function of the involved muscle. Protection, rest, ice, compression, and elevation (PRICE) followed by a referral to the physician is the appropriate care for this injury.

There are 2 injuries to the hip commonly found in children and adolescents that the athletic trainer must be aware of, and those are the slipped capital femoral epiphysis and Legg-Calvé-Perthes disease. A slipped capital femoral epiphysis is a disruption of the growth site of the femoral head. The cause is unknown and can present in either acute or chronic fashion.[2] Pain may be present in the general hip region and can refer to the knee. In later stages, the patient may have a limp and difficulty with motion at the hip joint. Severe cases may require surgical repair while less severe cases will respond to rest and nonweight bearing.[3] Legg-Calvé-Perthes disease is a condition that results in deterioration of the articular surface of the femur at the hip joint. The femoral head can take on a flattened appearance. The mechanism that causes the vascular changes is not clearly understood.[2] A young person with this condition may have pain in the groin or knee and walk with a limp. The signs and symptoms most often appear over time. If the condition is caught early, treatment to reduce weight bearing can help improve the blood flow and allow the femoral head to regain its shape. Both conditions if untreated can cause secondary hip problems later in life.

A chronic condition that occurs at the bony ends of the pubic bones in the pelvis is called osteitis pubis. This inflammation at the pubic symphysis can be caused by muscle imbalances and repetitive stress. This condition is common to ice hockey players, soccer players, and runners. Active women who have had children are susceptible to osteitis pubis due to subtle movement at the pubic symphysis. Signs and symptoms include general pain in the groin region and will be point tender directly over the pubic symphysis. Radiographs (x-rays) may show changes to the bone ends at the location of discomfort. Rest, careful strengthening, and anti-inflammatory medications are common methods of follow-up care.

The diagnosis of a sports hernia as a common cause of persistent groin pain has been increasingly recognized in the absence of other pathological findings.[2] Sports hernia syndrome is thought to be caused by a congenital weakness of the muscles of the abdominal wall at the inguinal channel. Unlike a traditional hernia, there is no evidence of a bulge of tissue, although

 ## Considerations for the Skeletally Immature Patient

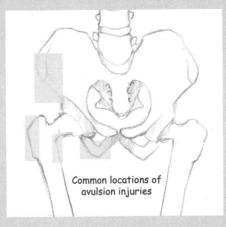

Common locations of avulsion injuries

In adolescents, the strength of muscles and tendons may be greater than the areas of growing bone when they originate or insert. When the bone is pulled away at this location, the resulting injury is an avulsion fracture. Avulsion fractures are commonly found in the growth centers of flat bones—like those found in the pelvis. These fractures often occur due to the rapid and forceful loads these large muscles can generate. Any skeletally immature patient (child or adolescent) with tenderness to the bone in these areas should be fully evaluated by a physician and a radiograph obtained. These injuries must be distinguished from musculotendinous injuries to best determine a course of action.

Common sites for an avulsion injury at the hip and pelvis include the following:

- Origin of the tensor fascia latae and sartorius muscles
- Origin of the rectus femoris muscle
- Origin of the hamstring muscles: biceps femoris, semitendinosus, and semimembranosus
- Insertion of the iliopsoas muscle
- Insertion of the gluteus medius muscle
- Growth zone of the iliac crest attachment site for the abdominal oblique, transverse abdominal, and the gluteus medius muscles

Bibliography

Peterson L, Renstrom P. *Sports Injuries: Their Prevention and Treatment.* 3rd ed. Champaign, IL: Human Kinetics; 2001.

it is speculated that these athletes are more susceptible to hernia later in life. Symptoms include pain that is vague and deep in the groin. The pain is often worse on one side, but it may radiate laterally and across the midline down the inside of the thigh into the adductor region. Pain is sometimes felt in the scrotum and testicles. Physical exam can reveal increased pain over the pubic tubercle on the painful side. Athletes report stabbing pain and discomfort with running, stopping, and quick changes of direction. Sports hernias are treated through surgical repair and reinforcement of the muscular wall. Reported results indicated that 87% of athletes can return to full activity in 2 months and the remaining 13% show improvement.[2]

Soft Tissue Injuries

Sprains and Dislocations

The hip joint is well supported. A deep articulation, strong ligaments, large muscle groups on all sides, and a substantial capsule contribute to its stability. Therefore, it is rarely subject to a true sprain injury. However, sprains to the hip joint can occur. A sprain of the hip can occur with a forceful twisting motion, impact, or a blow to the hip with the foot firmly planted.[2] Spain injuries are difficult to grade (1st thru 3rd degree); however, sprain injuries to the hip will be painful with all motions, particularly rotation and patients may require assistance (crutches) with ambulation. Initial care should include PRICE and a physician referral for an x-ray.

Although an uncommon event in sports, the hip can be dislocated. When this happens, it will require a significant force. The MOI is a force transmitted through the femur with the hip flexed followed by a posterior dislocation. The patient will be lying on his or her back with the injured leg internally rotated and flexed.[4] Dislocations of the hip should be considered a medical emergency. The dislocated hip presents with an obvious deformity and substantial pain. It is important to monitor the athlete's circulation in the lower extremity and to check for signs of shock.

Muscle-Tendon Injuries

The muscles that surround the hip allow for the movements of hip flexion, extension, abduction, adduction, and internal and external rotation. During physical activity, each of these large muscle groups must generate and absorb large amounts of force. When muscle fibers are stretched or are incapable of properly absorbing force during activity, they may be subject to strain-type injuries. Muscle strain injuries regularly occur in these muscles. Muscle strains are graded from 1st (least severe) to 3rd degree (most severe). Initial treatment of muscle strains should adhere to the PRICE concept. Athletic trainers must be aware of the possibility of avulsion fractures associated with severe muscle injury and evaluate and refer accordingly.

 ## Injury Spotlight: Hip Dislocation

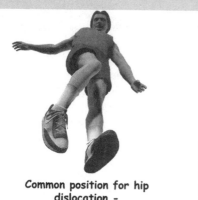

Common position for hip dislocation - adduction/internal rotation

Mechanism of Injury

The hip is in a flexed position and a force is applied through the long axis of the femur. The hip will most often dislocate in the posterior direction.

Affected Structures

Disruption of the joint capsule and ligamentous structures. Hip dislocations require great force, therefore the patient may have concurrent musculoskeletal injuries. Complications include possible damage to the acetabulum and potential loss of circulation to the femoral head. The health of the femoral head has implications for long-term health and function of the lower extremity.

Signs and Symptoms

Pain; swelling; gross deformity; palpable defect; affected extremity will often be flexed, rotated, and angled toward the opposite limb.

Initial Care

This injury requires activation of an emergency plan and transportation of the athlete to a medical facility. The extreme pain requires the athletic trainer to monitor for shock, circulation, and sensation to the lower extremity.

Bibliography

Peterson L, Renstrom P. *Sports Injuries: Their Prevention and Treatment.* 3rd ed. Champaign, IL: Human Kinetics; 2001.

The thigh is made up of 2 prominent muscle groups: the quadriceps (anterior) and the hamstrings (posterior). The primary role of these groups is to extend and flex the knee joint while working together to provide

Injury Spotlight: Snapping Hip

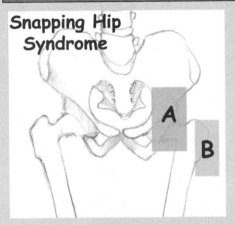

Snapping Hip Syndrome

Description

Snapping hip syndrome is a benign condition that is characterized by a painful and/or audible snap. The sound or sensation often occurs when the limb moves from a flexed, abducted, and externally rotated position to extension and internal rotation. The snapping hip can be described as external snapping or internal snapping.

Mechanism of Injury

Snapping hip is an overuse injury that is often more of a nuisance than debilitating. Runners, gymnasts, track and field hurdlers, and dancers may experience snapping hip. The cause is often tightness of specific structures and/or muscular imbalances at the hip.

Affected Structures

External snapping hip is associated with the movement of the iliotibial band (tensor fascia latae) or gluteus maximus tendon over the greater trochanter of the femur. Internal snapping is less common but can be more pronounced than external snapping and is usually caused by the iliopsoas tendon passing over the anterior hip capsule, lesser trochanter of the femur, femoral head, or iliopectineal eminence. However, other causes of internal snapping may need to be ruled out. Internal snapping may also be caused by the biceps femoris passing over the ischial tuberosity, the iliofemoral ligaments moving over the femoral head, iliopsoas bursitis, acetabular labral tears, hip subluxation, or intra-articular loose bodies.[1]

Signs and Symptoms

External snapping hip symptoms are associated sounds/sensations or discomfort on the lateral aspect of the hip. Moving the hip from flexion to extension may reproduce the external snap. Internal hip snapping is associated with anterior hip pain or snapping sensations. Internal snapping may be reproduced during the snapping hip maneuver (ie, movement of the flexed, abducted, and externally rotated hip to an extended and internally rotated position). Performance in runners is not always impaired with snapping hip syndrome.

Radiographs, MRI, or CT exams may help determine if intra-articular abnormalities are the cause of internal hip snapping. In the most extreme cases, arthroscopy of the hip may be indicated.

Initial Care

Treatment of snapping hip syndrome involves adjusting activities, analgesic care, stretching of the appropriate musculature, and muscular strengthening of the hip to address imbalances. Stretching will focus on hip abduction and external rotation. A full postural evaluation that examines any other possible biomechanical abnormalities is essential.

Reference

1. Paluska SA. An overview of hip injuries in running. *Sports Med.* 2005;35(11):991-1014.

Bibliography

Peterson L, Renstrom P. *Sports Injuries: Their Prevention and Treatment.* 3rd ed. Champaign, IL: Human Kinetics; 2001.

dynamic stability to the knee, particularly when the foot is in contact with the ground. The hamstrings act as secondary stabilizers to the important ACL. During the course of flexion, extension, and powerful acceleration and deceleration activities, these muscles may be subject to muscle strain injury. The nature of these injuries is often sport specific. Certainly, strains to the hamstring group are common in sports that require strong bursts of powerful lower extremity movements such as track and field sprinting, football, and soccer. Muscle injuries are classified (from less to more severe) as 1st thru 3rd degree. These injuries often present with pain, stiffness in the muscle group, discomfort with activity, and weakness. Initial care involves PRICE with full rehabilitation requiring a focus on regaining strength and flexibility.

Contusions to the quadriceps muscle group are common and hold the potential for complications if they are not treated properly. A contusion in the quadriceps muscle will bleed and cause a hematoma. If left untreated, the pooling of this blood can cause the formation of a myositis ossificans. Myositis ossificans is a calcium-rich, bone-like formation in the muscle. Attempts to continue to participate or "run it off" following a contusion can increase the risk for myositis ossificans. In addition, too vigorous treatment following a contusion (ie, massage over the contusion or use of heat during the acute inflammation phase) is another risk for calcification.[3] Contusions to the quadriceps should be treated with PRICE with ice and compression applied in a slightly stretched position (knee bent). If a myositis ossificans takes place, it can be seen on radiograph. Once identified, the treatment is based on the limitation (if any) caused by the ossification. Some cases may require surgical removal.

Other Soft Tissue Injuries

One of the most common acute soft tissue injuries to the hip is a contusion called a hip pointer. A hip pointer is a contusion to the top of the iliac crest. The direct blow is the MOI for the hip pointer. Muscles that help control the trunk insert at this location, and a blow to this region can cause significant pain and loss of function for the patient. Initial care involves PRICE with physician referral if needed. The iliac crest can be protected with additional padding; however, the movements of the trunk easily aggravate the condition and return to activity must be gradual.

Bursitis of the greater trochanteric bursa is a common chronic injury that can cause pain in the hip region. The greater trochanter is a bony projection off of the proximal femur. The tensor fascia latae covers the greater trochanter and travels distally to the tibia. This structure (a muscle that becomes a band of tendon) muscle is also called the iliotibial band. If this muscle is tight, the pressure increases over the top of the greater trochanter, causing irritation of the bursa. The role of the bursa is to decrease friction between structures. When the bursa is irritated, the natural response is to become inflamed. Greater trochanteric bursitis can be improved with therapeutic treatment and flexibility of the tensor fasciae latae.

INJURIES TO THE KNEE

FRACTURES AND INJURIES TO BONE

While acute traumatic fractures to the femur and tibia at the knee joint are not common, they may occur with a significant force. Of particular concern is any fracture that extends through the epiphyseal plate (growth plate) of an adolescent or any fracture that compromises the articular surface. A fracture that extends from the bone into the articular surface

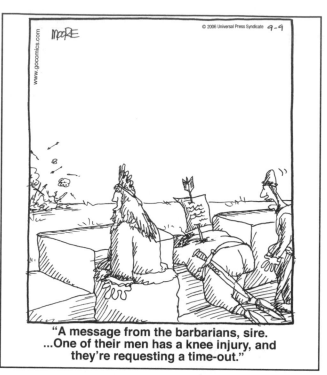

"A message from the barbarians, sire. ...One of their men has a knee injury, and they're requesting a time-out."

is an osteochondral fracture. Fractures to the femur, tibia, or fibula can take place with mechanisms commonly associated with sprain injuries. The athletic trainer must take careful precaution to evaluate an athlete's level of pain, locations of point tenderness, or any potential deformities when evaluating an acute knee injury. If any of the above are present, the athlete should have the limb immobilized and be transported for radiographs and a complete evaluation.

The patella is subject to fracture due to its exposed anterior position and its attachment to the very strong quadriceps and patellar tendons. Patellar fractures occur as a result of a direct blow or with a very forceful contraction of the quadriceps with the lower extremity in an immovable position. The direct blow could occur from a fall on a hard surface, hit from a helmet, direct blow from a bat, or a host of possible situations. Initial care of a suspected fracture should follow the PRICE procedures and referral for radiographs and a full evaluation.

OCD is a localized separation of a fragment of bone and articular cartilage from the normal bone. This injury is seen following trauma or repetitive injury. Loose bodies float in the joint and are called joint mice. Seventy-five percent of all cases of OCD take place in the medial femoral condyle.[2] Most cases of OCD in young patients are sport related. In most cases, loose bodies that interfere with normal joint function will need to be surgically removed.

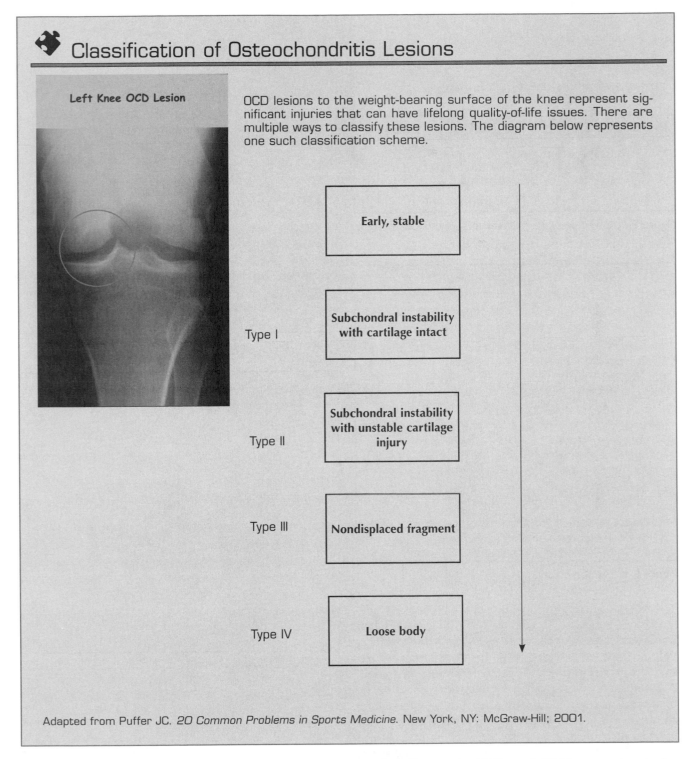

Classification of Osteochondritis Lesions

Left Knee OCD Lesion

OCD lesions to the weight-bearing surface of the knee represent significant injuries that can have lifelong quality-of-life issues. There are multiple ways to classify these lesions. The diagram below represents one such classification scheme.

	Early, stable
Type I	**Subchondral instability with cartilage intact**
Type II	**Subchondral instability with unstable cartilage injury**
Type III	**Nondisplaced fragment**
Type IV	**Loose body**

Adapted from Puffer JC. *20 Common Problems in Sports Medicine*. New York, NY: McGraw-Hill; 2001.

SOFT TISSUE INJURIES

Sprains and Dislocations

Ligament injuries to the knee are common in sport and physical activity. The 4 primary ligaments of the knee are the MCL, LCL, ACL, and PCL. The collateral ligaments (MCL and LCL) primarily provide support to varus and valgus forces (Figure 6-9) while the cruciate ligaments (ACL and PCL) prevent anterior and posterior translation of the tibia on the femur. Ligament sprain injuries can occur as isolated events (a sprain to one ligament) or in combination (injuries to more than one ligament). When forces are placed upon the ligaments that exceed their tensile strength, they will stretch or rupture. The type of force—single plane, rotational, or in combination—determines the ligament injury (isolated or in combination).[3]

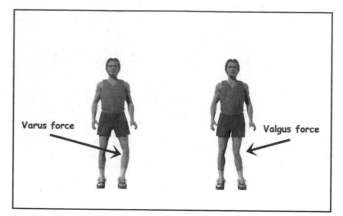

Figure 6-9. Common forces that cause injury to the collateral ligaments of the knee.

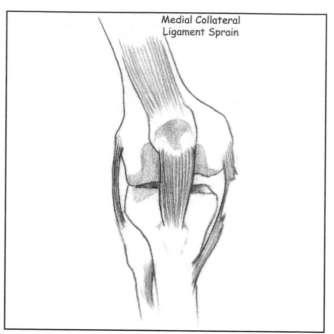

Figure 6-10. Sprain to the MCL.

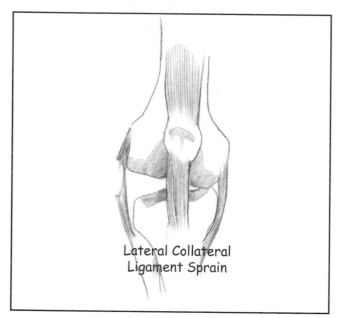

Figure 6-11. Sprain to the LCL.

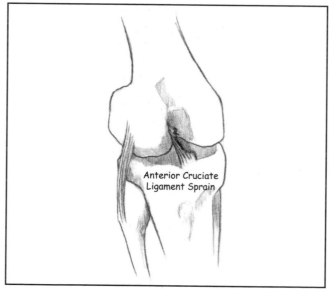

Figure 6-12. Sprain to the ACL.

Sprains to the MCL (Figure 6-10) take place when the lateral aspect of the knee is hit and the resulting valgus force causes the MCL to stretch or rupture. Like all sprain injuries, the degree of injury is graded. A 1st-degree MCL sprain will have few fibers of the ligament torn while a 3rd-degree injury represents a complete rupture of the tissue. The MCL can also be injured in combination with the ACL. Initial care of this injury involves PRICE and referral to a physician for complete evaluation followed by a rehabilitation program. Surgery is not recommended for isolated MCL injuries.[5] The MOI for the LCL injury is effectively the opposite of the MCL. The knee receives a blow to the medial aspect, resulting in a varus force that causes the LCL to stretch or rupture (Figure 6-11). Sprain injuries to the LCL are not as common as injuries to the MCL. The initial care for theses injuries is essentially the same.

The cruciate ligaments seem to receive the most attention of the 4 major knee ligaments, in particular the ACL (Figure 6-12). It is hard to pick up a sports page or national magazine without reading about an athlete who has had an ACL injury. The sports medicine community has made great strides in the ability to identify, surgically reconstruct, and functionally rehabilitate the ACL injury to allow for safe return to competition. While many questions about this injury have been answered, many still need to be addressed. In particular, why do women have a higher incidence of ACL injuries than men? The incidence of ACL

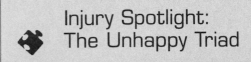

Injury Spotlight: The Unhappy Triad

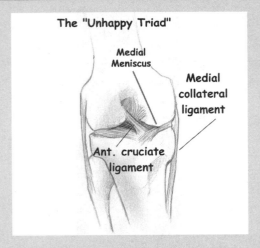

The "Unhappy Triad"

Medial Meniscus

Medial collateral ligament

Ant. cruciate ligament

Mechanism of Injury

A blow to the lateral aspect of the knee with the foot fixed with concurrent femoral internal rotation and external rotation of the fixed tibia.

Affected Structures

ACL, MCL, and medial meniscus. Also known as O'Donoghue's triad. Research suggests that complete ruptures of the ACL and MCL are less associated with concomitant meniscal tears than when the ligaments receive 2nd-degree sprain injuries.

Signs and Symptoms

Pain, joint effusion, tenderness at MCL and along joint line, loss of function. Patient may not be able to ambulate without support depending upon the severity of the sprain injuries.

Initial Care

PRICE with referral for an orthopedic evaluation and diagnostic testing.

Bibliography

Shelbourne KD, Nitz P. The O'Donoghue triad revisited: combined knee injuries involving anterior cruciate and medial collateral ligament tears. *Am J Sports Med.* 1991;19:474-477.

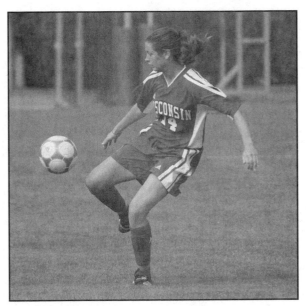

Figure 6-13. Female soccer players are more likely to injure their ACL than their male counterparts. (Courtesy of University of Wisconsin–Madison Athletic Communications.)

injuries among women basketball players is twice that for men, and female soccer players are 4 times more likely to suffer an ACL tear than their male counterparts (Figure 6-13).[6] Several theories have been put forth to explain this trend (anatomical, hormonal, and neuromuscular issues), yet none at this date are conclusive.

The ACL is usually injured when an athlete is decelerating, plants the foot, externally rotates the femur, and has the knee in a valgus position (Figure 6-14).[3] This is the classic "noncontact" ACL injury. A forced hyperextension of the knee (from a blow) is also a possible MOI for this ligament. Patients who have torn the ACL often report hearing a pop, will have an episode of instability (knee buckles out from under them), and cannot continue with activity. An athlete with a complete ACL sprain will produce a swollen joint (effusion), have difficulty with motion, and need assistance with ambulation. If left untreated, most patients without an ACL ligament cannot continue with physical activity. The knee has repeated episodes of instability (buckling). Repeated instability can lead to damage to the articular surfaces and possible meniscal injuries, each of which can affect the long-term health of the knee joint. Surgery is recommended for patients who are active.

The PCL is often injured when the tibia is forced backwards. This occurs when the knee is flexed and a force is transmitted through the anterior portion of the tibia (Figure 6-15). A patient with a PCL tear may report feeling a pop in the knee and have some swelling in the popliteal fossa (back of the knee); however, this injury does not produce the instability associated with the ACL sprain. An athlete who has a logical mechanism for a PCL injury will need to have a thorough examination to see if there is laxity when moving the tibia backwards. While initial treatment will follow the PRICE approach, long-term treatment

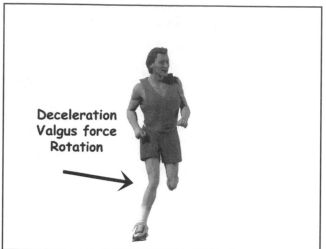

Figure 6-14. MOI for the ACL.

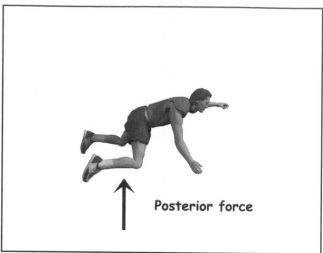

Figure 6-15. MOI for the PCL.

varies. Nonoperative treatment of PCL injuries is commonplace and many high-level athletes can function without the PCL. The benefits of surgical repair or reconstruction of the PCL and the need to study the long-term effects of participation without a PCL is currently receiving attention.[5]

Dislocations of the knee are medical emergencies that should be considered limb threatening. Dislocations of the tibiofemoral articulation are uncommon; however, they can occur in sport. The MOI involves excessive rotational forces combined with either valgus or varus positioning. These injuries involve multiple ligament damage and often happen in the posterior/lateral direction. The location of the popliteal artery in the back of the knee makes it easily compromised. In addition to potential vascular compromise, the peroneal nerve can also be injured in a dislocation, causing possible disability at the ankle. Initial care involves activation of an emergency plan, immobilization, identification of a distal pulse, and immediate transport.

Other Soft Tissue Injuries

A variety of soft tissue injuries can take place in and about the knee joint. Injuries to the medial and lateral meniscus can happen when the foot is planted in a weight-bearing position and then rotated. The menisci are crescent-shaped fibrocartilage disks that absorb shock to the knee and help give the joint its shape. The classic MOI for a meniscus tear is a plant-and-cut–type movement. When the knee is in full extension or flexion, the menisci are compressed between the joint surfaces of the tibia and the femur. These positions can put the menisci at greater risk. Tears to the meniscus may be identified acutely or a small tear to the meniscus can present as a chronic injury. Signs and symptoms include effusion (swell-

ing in the joint), clicking or snapping, pain going up or down stairs, and joint line pain. Patients with these signs and symptoms must be referred for an orthopedic examination and an MRI. Injuries to the medial meniscus are more common than the lateral meniscus due to its anatomical attachment to the MCL. The medial meniscus tear makes up one third of the "unhappy triad."

Jumper's knee or patellar tendonitis is an overuse chronic condition that is seen frequently in jumping sports (eg, volleyball, basketball). The patellar tendon serves to insert the large quadriceps tendon into the tibia. The patella is embedded in this tendon and slides through the groove of the femur. An individual with weakness in the quads who cannot absorb the forces of jumping and landing is at risk for patellar tendonitis. This injury is also seen in individuals with tightness and poor flexibility at the quadriceps and hip flexor muscle groups. Changes in mechanics of movement due to inflexibility or weakness are common causes of overuse injuries like jumper's knee. Initial care includes modification of activities, treatment for discomfort (ice or heat), and rehabilitation to improve strength and flexibility.

In adolescents, anterior knee pain and discomfort of the patellar tendon may be due to Osgood-Schlatter disease or Sinding-Larsen–Johansson disease. "Disease" is a bit of a misnomer really because both diseases are orthopedic conditions that cause anterior knee pain and are common in growing patients. Osgood-Schlatter's is an apophysitis that results in excess bone formation and an increase in size of the tibial tuberosity due to increased tension at the insertion of the patellar tendon. Sinding-Larsen–Johansson disease is sometimes called a traction tendonitis. While Osgood-Schlatter occurs at the tibial tubercle, Sinding-Larsen–Johansson is a painful inflammation at the inferior pole of the patella. Radiographs of both of these conditions may show a fragment or the presence of an ossicle. Treatment includes PRICE, modification of activities, and careful strengthening of the surrounding musculature. Discomfort from this condition usually subsides as the athlete moves closer to skeletal maturity. While the pain will decrease with age, the resultant "bump" will remain. In some instances, surgical removal of the painful ossicle is necessary.

The prepatellar bursa sits on the anterior aspect of the patella. This bursa, when not inflamed, is quite thin and not noticeable. However, if the knee is contused on a hard surface, the bursa can become inflamed and cause significant swelling. This is an acute or traumatic bursitis. Bursitis of the prepatellar bursa is also known as turf knee due to its common occurrence on hard artificial surfaces. This condition may be referred to by layperson's as water on the knee. Inflammation of the prepatellar bursa should not be confused with an effusion within the knee joint. This swelling is external and comes from the bursa itself. Initial care involves using compression to decrease swelling and ice for comfort. These injuries can recur, thus proper padding and protection are essential as the athlete returns to activity. Chronic bursitis can also be found in and around the knee joint. Two common chronic injuries include suprapatellar bursitis and pes anserine bursitis. Bursitis, like most overuse injuries, is caused by repetition, changes in workout volume or intensity, or mechanical changes due to weakness and inflexibility. Care of these chronic injuries requires rest and addressing the underlying cause of the injury (weakness, flexibility, etc).

Neurovascular Injuries

Neurovascular injuries to the knee are not common, and if they do occur, they are often associated with trauma such as fractures or complete knee dislocations. It is worth noting that the peroneal nerve resides in a very superficial location and is easily susceptible to trauma. The nerve can be easily contused or irritated secondary to tape or an ill-fitting knee brace or sleeve. The nerve is easily compressed along the head of the fibula. Pressure on this nerve can cause weakness in dorsiflexion of the ankle (drop foot). Contusions should be treated with care as not to cause greater pressure on the nerve. Return of normal strength and sensation varies a great deal.

INJURIES TO THE PATELLOFEMORAL ARTICULATION

The PF is a distinct joint that sits above the knee (tibiofemoral articulation). The patella is a wedge-shaped bone that sits in the groove created at the distal end of the femur. The patella is a sesamoid bone, meaning it is encased in a tendon (the patellar tendon). The strong quadriceps muscles serve to stabilize the patella as it passes through the groove during flexion and extension of the knee. These muscles act as dynamic stabilizers to the patella. If the knee is in extension, the patella is quite mobile. As the knee goes into flexion, the patella sits deeper into the femoral groove. The patella is also held into the groove by the lateral and medial retinaculum. These structures provide static stabilization to the PF joint.

The majority of PF joint problems stem from the patella not moving properly through the femoral groove. The tendency is for the patella to be pulled laterally and compress against the lateral femoral condyle. In severe cases, it can even dislocate. Several problems can arise if there are changes to the structures that provide dynamic or static stability to the patella. Problems with the PF joint can be exaggerated by other structural problems such as pronated (flat) feet, weak muscles, tight static structures, and a large quadriceps (Q) angle. Q angle is the angle of pull of the quadriceps muscle group and is identified using the ASIS, mid point of the patella, and tibial tubercle as a guide (Figure 6-16).

Common injuries and conditions to the PF joint include patellofemoral stress syndrome (PFSS), subluxation of the patella, and dislocation of the patella. PFSS is a catch-all term for retropatellar (behind the patella) and peripatellar (on the patella) pain resulting from physical and biomechanical changes in the patellofemoral joint. These changes may include overuse, overload, biomechanical problems, and muscular dysfunction.[7] Subluxation occurs when the patella is pulled laterally during a quadriceps contraction on an extended knee and partially moves from the femoral groove.[1] Repeated subluxations will result in damage to the articular surfaces and cause pain. Progressive instability of the patella may lead to a full dislocation.

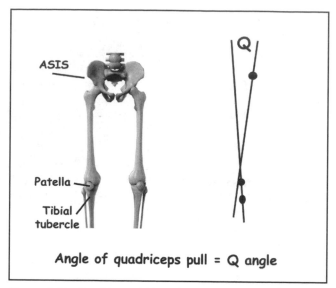

Figure 6-16. Quadriceps (Q) angle.

A dislocation occurs when the patella moves laterally and comes to rest outside the femoral groove. A dislocated patella will cause significant soft tissue disruption on the medial aspect of the knee.

Treatment of patellofemoral problems can prove to be challenging for the athletic trainer. Treatment includes PRICE for acute inflammation followed by a rehabilitation program that addresses muscular weakness, tightness of static structures, and biomechanical insufficiencies.

INJURIES TO THE LOWER LEG

There are some specific injuries to the lower leg that the athletic trainer must be able to identify and properly refer. These include muscle strains, chronic tendonitis, stress fractures, and compartment syndromes. The muscles of the lower leg cross the ankle joint and provide movement at the ankle, foot, and toes. These muscles and their associated tendons also provide support for the arches of the foot. Lower leg muscles tend to have long tendons that cross the ankle and insert in various locations on the foot. These muscles and tendons are subject to muscle strain injury. The nature of these injuries is often sport specific. The gastrocnemius (calf) muscle, anterior tibialis, peroneals, and posterior tibialis are commonly strained in the lower leg. Like all muscle injuries, these strains are classified as 1st thru 3rd degree. These injuries often present with pain, stiffness in the muscle group, discomfort with activity, and weakness. Initial care involves PRICE with full rehabilitation requiring a focus on regaining strength and flexibility.

Tendonitis occurs in many of the tendons of the muscles identified previously. Like all overuse tendonitis problems, changes in intensity and frequency of activity are common causes of these injuries. Biomechanical alterations due to foot position (pronation), muscle weakness, or lack of flexibility (common in the gastrocnemius) are contributing factors to tendonitis. Initial care includes modification of activities, treatment for discomfort (ice or heat), and rehabilitation to improve strength and flexibility.

Tendon ruptures can occur in the lower leg. A rupture of the large Achilles tendon is one of the more common complete tendon ruptures in sport and physical activity. The injury rate increases with age, making this a more common injury among middle-aged recreational athletes when compared with their younger counterparts. The ratio of men to women who sustain this injury is 6:1 with the average age being 35 to 40 years.[2] Sudden forceful plantar flexion movements can cause these injuries, which are common in court sport athletes. Signs and symptoms include a painful sensation in the tendon that may be accompanied by an audible pop. The classic sensation is one of being kicked in the calf. The tendon will have a palpable defect and the patient will be unable to ambulate without a limp. Initial care includes PRICE, including the use of crutches for ambulation. First-aid providers should avoid initially placing the athlete's foot in a walking boot or orthopedic appliance, which may force the ankle past a neutral position. If this happens, a partially torn tendon may be placed on stretch and further damage the tissue. Prompt referral to a physician is essential. Surgical repair of the tendon is required for the complete rupture. Surgical repair has shown good results for return to activity. Seventy-five percent of top level professionals and 90% of recreational tennis players who ruptured the tendon and had subsequent repair returned to their desired level of tennis.

Stress fractures can occur to the lower leg and are common in repetitive impact sport activities. Running is the most common sport activity that can lead to a stress reaction in the bones of the lower leg. Stress fractures can be found in both the tibia and the fibula. Skeletal differences, variations in gait, poor running conditions, hard surfaces, prior injury, and poor training techniques are common causes of stress fractures. Signs and symptoms include pain with activity that does not change when the athlete has warmed up. The pain may increase upon completion, be uncomfortable at night, and will be located in a specific spot (point tender). An athlete who has signs and symptoms of a stress fracture should be referred to the physician for further evaluation. Impact loading activities should be stopped in favor of cross-training nonimpact activities.

Injury Spotlight: Medial Tibial Stress Syndrome

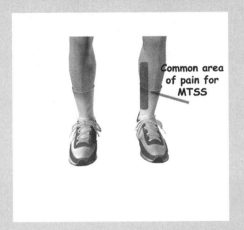

Common area of pain for MTSS

Mechanism of Injury

Medial tibial stress syndrome is also referred to as "shin splints." This chronic condition has many possible causes, including overuse, changes in footwear, changes in playing surfaces, and pronation of the rearfoot. Often a "catch-all" diagnosis, treatment will be more effective if a specific cause of pain is identified.

Affected Structures

The medial tibia, periosteum, medial soft tissue structures (ie, posterior tibialis tendon), and anterior structures (extensor muscles and tendons) may be involved.

Signs and Symptoms

Diffuse pain and tenderness along the medial tibial margin. Swelling may be present. The pain is most pronounced over the distal third of the tibia. Pain will ease with rest and return with activity.

Initial Care

Ice, rest, and identifying the underlying cause of the discomfort are keys to treatment. Proper referral and diagnosis to rule out a stress fracture are appropriate. Gradual return to activity upon reduction of symptoms will help prevent recurrence. It is of particular importance to evaluate and correct any biomechanical insufficiencies.

Bibliography

Peterson L, Renstrom P. *Sports Injuries: Their Prevention and Treatment*. 3rd ed. Champaign, IL: Human Kinetics; 2001.

Compartment syndromes are injuries that involve an increased pressure that is localized to a specific compartment of the lower leg. The leg is divided into compartments that are walled off by tight fascia, the tibia and fibula, and the interosseous membrane. Following an acute injury like a contusion, the swelling from a hematoma cannot disperse due to the tight nature of the compartments in the lower leg. The anterior compartment can be affected by such an injury. Compartment syndromes cause compression of neurovascular structures and if left unattended, can lead to tissue death (necrosis). An acute compartment syndrome secondary to trauma should be considered a medical emergency. Signs and symptoms include pain, tightness and swelling of the tissue, shiny appearance to the skin, reduced circulation to the foot, decreased sensation to the foot, and absence or weakness in dorsiflexion of the ankle. Initial care should include ice and elevation; however, compression should NOT be used in this situation. The athlete should be referred immediately for further evaluation and testing of the intercompartmental pressures.

Compartment syndromes can also be chronic or caused by exertional activities. Chronic compartment syndromes will present signs and symptoms during physical activities or at the end of specific physical activities. These may occur to the anterior or deep posterior compartment of the lower leg. If they are persistent and do not respond to conservative therapy, surgical intervention may be needed. The surgery involves releasing the fascia around the compartment to relieve symptoms.

INJURIES TO THE ANKLE AND FOOT

FRACTURES AND INJURIES TO BONE

The ankle and foot may be fractured from injury mechanisms similar to those found with ankle sprains. The same MOI that may produce a sprain to the lateral ankle ligaments can also cause a fracture to the medial malleolus (distal tibia). Likewise, an eversion mechanism can cause a sprain to the medial ligaments or a possible fracture to the lateral malleolus (distal fibula) (Figures 6-17 and 6-18). Avulsion fractures in the ankle take place when a piece of bone is pulled off with the ligament. Avulsion fractures can also occur at the insertion location of a tendon such as peroneal tendon insertion at the base of the 5th metatarsal. The distal fibula and tibia may also be fractured when inversion or

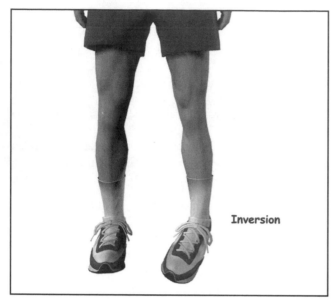

Figure 6-17. Inversion of the ankle, common MOI for lateral ligament injury.

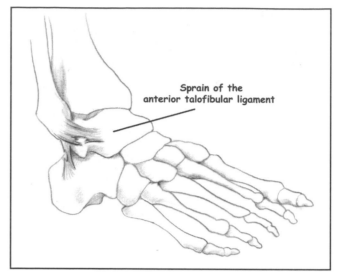

Sprain of the
anterior talofibular ligament

Figure 6-18. Injury to the anterior talofibular ligament.

eversion mechanisms of injury are combined with rotation. In addition, spiral fractures to the fibula are a common injury with the inversion and rotation MOI. For the above reasons, all second- and third-degree ankle sprains, or any ankle sprain with persistent pain should have a radiograph.

There are some fractures that are specific to the foot. A Jones fracture is a fracture at the proximal third of the 5th metatarsal of the foot. Sir Robert Jones identified the Jones fracture in the early 1900s. In fact, Jones sustained this very injury while dancing! The peroneus brevis tendon inserts into the base of the 5th metatarsal. Inversion stress of the ankle puts the base of the 5th metatarsal at risk for either a Jones fracture (proximal third) or a true avulsion of the tendon. Jones fractures can occur secondary to an underlying stress fracture. Signs and symptoms include pain, point tenderness, and the patient may report a "popping" sensation. The base of the 5th metatarsal has poor blood supply and may have an extended healing period. Surgery to repair the bone using a screw to fix the fracture is a common course of action for active patients.

Stress fractures to the foot are frequent injuries among athletes who participate in impact loading activities. The tarsal navicular and metatarsals are locations that are subjected to stress fractures. A stress fracture to the metatarsals, most often the 2nd metatarsal, is called march fractures. Poor or ill fitting footwear, skeletal differences, variations in gait, hard surfaces, prior injury, and poor training techniques are common causes of stress fractures. Signs and symptoms include pain with activity that does not change when warmed up. The pain may increase upon completion, be uncomfortable at night, and will be located in a specific spot (point tender). An athlete who has signs and symptoms of a stress fracture should be referred to the physician for further evaluation.

Traumatic or repeated injuries to the ankle can make the joint susceptible to osteochondral lesions. If the talar dome is compressed against the joint surface of the tibia, a compression fracture to the chondral surface can occur. Repetitive trauma to the joint surface can result in OCD lesions much like those discussed in the knee. If fragments of the bone and articular cartilage come loose, the ankle may have loose bodies that compromise normal function.

SOFT TISSUE INJURIES

 ### Jones and Lisfranc: Who?

Anyone with a fantasy football team knows that if you become too familiar with Jones or Lisfranc, chances are your guy is done for the year. While the injuries that bear their name may be bad news for coaches and fans (not to mention the poor guy with the actual injury), the story behind the names is remarkable indeed.

Sir Robert Jones (1857 to 1933)

A fracture to the proximal aspect of the 5th metatarsal is known as a Jones fracture. Robert Jones identified this fracture by personal experience. He fractured his 5th metatarsal while dancing. That story alone is amusing enough until you scratch the surface a bit and find that Sir Robert Jones is regarded as one of the finest surgeons of his time and a humanitarian in all aspects of his life. At the young age of 31, Jones became the Surgeon Superintendent in charge of the health, surgical work, and hospitals required for the 20,000 laborers and their families along the route of the Manchester ship canal during its 8-year construction. His surgical skills developed rapidly in this setting. During World War I, Jones placed his services at the disposal of his country and succeeded in obtaining a wide acceptance of his methods in the field and in the hospitals of Britain. Through his effort, greater emphasis was placed on saving limbs and restoring injuries as much as possible. Later in his career, he became a crusader for health issues that impact children such as improved housing and better milk supplies.

Jones wrote many books and articles and is widely recognized as one of the great orthopedic surgeons of the last century. Robert Jones was knighted, made a Major General, and recognized by countless European institutions and governments. Harvard, Yale, McGill, and Smith all conferred degrees upon him and he received the Medal of Distinguished Service from the United States government.

Jacques Lisfranc (1790 to 1847)

Jacques Lisfranc did gain some favor and recognition as a surgeon after obtaining his medical degree in 1813. Today, Lisfranc has an injury named after him that he never saw (see injury highlight on p. 120). As a field surgeon in Napoleon's army, Jacques Lisfranc served on the Russian front. He made a name for himself through an amputation technique to treat the common occurrence of gangrene from frostbite. To save time (he did many surgeries a day) and to avoid having to cut through bone, Lisfranc cut through a series of joints in the mid foot. This route became known as the Lisfranc joint. The joint describes the boundary between the rigid mid foot and the weight-bearing forefoot.

He left the army in 1814, and from then on chiefly concerned himself with the improvement of surgical methods. In 1826, he got his own department at L' Hospital de la Pitié in Paris and soon commenced teaching clinical medicine. Despite his recognition as a teacher and surgeon, he was not a popular person. His bellicose manners made any close friendships between him and his colleagues impossible.

Their names are forever attached to injuries, and because so will be repeated into the next centuries and beyond. More often than not, those names will be repeated with little thought to who they were. Yet, with each name there is a story. Jones, the beloved surgeon and humanitarian, was so much more than a foot injury. Lisfranc, the troubled former field surgeon, struggled to be close to his colleagues (maybe he had seen too much on Napoleon's battlefield). Perhaps there is a lesson to be learned from this history. Every injury belongs to a real person; some wonderful and some not so wonderful. However, as athletic trainers we treat people who happen to have injuries—not just the injuries themselves. It is not "my ACL patient" but rather "my patient who has an ACL injury." There is a difference. Take the time to learn the whole story.

Bibliography

Schriebman K. Famous Feet. Athletic Training Lecture Series. UW-Madison October 2006.
Who Named It? Dictionary of medical eponyms. Available at www.whonamedit.com. Accessed March 5, 2008.

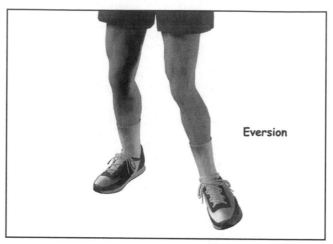

Figure 6-19. Eversion of the ankle, common MOI for medical ligament injury.

Injury Spotlight: High Ankle Sprain (Syndesmotic Sprain)

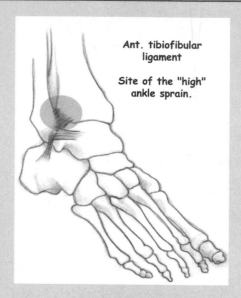

Ant. tibiofibular ligament

Site of the "high" ankle sprain.

Mechanism of Injury

Forced external rotation and forced dorsiflexion of the ankle. This injury is commonly seen in football athletes. It is estimated that 10% of all ankle injuries include a tear of the distal syndesmosis.

Affected Structures

The distal syndesmosis, anterior tibiofibular ligament. These injuries are often associated with medial side eversion stress injuries to the ankle (deltoid ligament). True isolated syndesmotic injuries without associated medial ligament stress or fracture are rare.

Signs and Symptoms

Pain, swelling, point tenderness at the anterior aspect of the ankle between the tibia and fibula. Athlete may be unable to bear weight. External rotation of the ankle will be painful (often done by the athletic trainer to test for this injury).

Initial Care

PRICE with an emphasis on controlling pain and swelling. Assistance with ambulation is essential (walking boot or crutches). The patient should be referred for radiographs and a complete orthopedic assessment. High ankle sprains require a longer recovery time when compared to other common ankle injuries.

Bibliography

Peterson L, Renstrom P. *Sports Injuries: Their Prevention and Treatment.* 3rd ed. Champaign, IL: Human Kinetics; 2001.

Sprain Injuries to the Ankle and Foot

The ankle sprain is the most common injury that occurs in sport and physical activity. During 2000, an estimated 1.2 million physician visits were the result of ankle sprain injuries, while an additional 675,000 physician visits were ankle fractures.[8] The costs associated with treating ankle injuries are significant. In 1999, the US Consumer Products Safety Commission estimated that the costs of treating ankle injuries in soccer and basketball players age 14 to 19 were approximately 1.56 billion dollars.[9] Ankle sprains are often identified by the mechanism that caused the injury (ie, an inversion sprain) or the degree of injury (ie, a 2nd-degree eversion sprain).

Inversion sprains can often take place in combination with plantar flexion. This MOI is common and can take place when someone lands on his or her foot, steps off a curb, or steps in a hole (see Figure 6-17). An inversion/plantar flexion mechanism will usually cause damage to the anterior talofibular ligament (Figure 6-19). A true inversion mechanism can cause damage to one or more of the 3 lateral ankle ligaments (anterior talofibular ligament, calcaneofibular ligament, and the posterior talofibular ligament). Eversion mechanisms are less common and usually result when someone lands on the lateral aspect of the ankle. Eversion injuries stretch or rupture the triangular deltoid ligament located on the medial aspect of the ankle (see Figure 6-18). As with all injuries to ligamentous tissue, sprains to the ankle are graded on a scale from 1st to 3rd degree. A 1st-degree sprain will have few fibers of the ligament torn while a 3rd-degree injury represents a complete rupture and will present with marked laxity of the joint.

An injury to the ligaments that hold the distal tibia and fibula together is called a high ankle sprain. This injury involves a rotational component that forces the talus to rotate and spread the tibia, causing damage to the tib-fib ligament. Plantar flexion and forced external rotation are common mechanisms for this injury.[2] A high ankle sprain is also called a syndesmotic sprain. The syndesmosis is the area between the tibia and fibula and is made up of the anterior and posterior tibiofibular ligaments and the interosseous membrane. These injuries should be evaluated with care since they are often associated with fractures.

High ankle sprains frequently take a longer period of time to recover when compared to other common ankle injuries.

Ankle sprains will present with a logical MOI, swelling, pain, and limitations in function based on the degree of injury. Initial care for the patient with an ankle sprain should include adherence to the PRICE protocol with an emphasis on ambulation without pain or limp. If the patient is unable to ambulate without a painful gait, a walking boot or crutches is recommended. As noted in our discussion of fractures, an x-ray is warranted to rule out fracture.

This Little Piggy Went To ...

Well, one little piggy got none (hopefully none of the conditions below). Injuries and conditions to the toes often come on slowly and do not receive attention until they are problematic. Recognizing these conditions and how they may contribute to other foot conditions is essential for the athletic trainer.

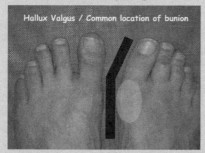

Hallux Valgus / Common location of bunion

Hallux valgus—If the angle of the great toe extends more than 10 degrees away from the midline of the body, it is known as a hallux valgus. Bony growth and a bursa formation can occur on the medial aspect of the base of the great toe (bunion). Proper footwear with enough toe box room is essential. Surgical removal of the painful bunion may be indicated.

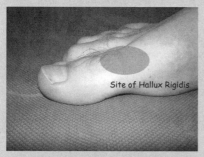

Site of Hallux Rigidis

Hallux rigidus—If the great toe has a history of repeated minor injury, small bone spurs may form on the top of the metatarsal phalangeal joint. Early osteoarthritis may also develop. The result is a limitation in movement specifically in dorsiflexion. Surgical intervention is sometimes needed to remove the spurs and restore motion.

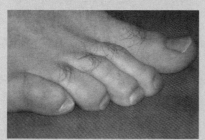

Hammer toes—A hammer toe is a flexion contracture that creates an inability to extend the toe at the proximal interphalangeal joint (PIP). Hammer toes may be caused by problems with the arch or by wearing shoes that are too small. Callus may form over the top of the PIP joint and on the end of the toes. Proper shoe fit is essential.

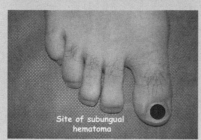

Site of subungual hematoma

Subungual hematoma—A blow to the toe or repeated pressure on the nail can create bruising under the nail. This bruising is common in runners and soccer players who wear shoes that are too small. This can also happen with a contusion.

Injury Spotlight: Lisfranc Injury

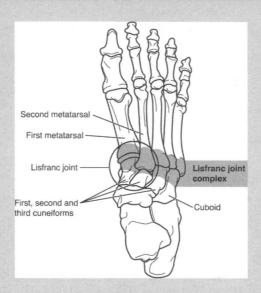

Mechanism of Injury

The Lisfranc injury may occur from a direct crushing MOI to the mid foot region. However, the more common mechanism is a longitudinal compression with the foot in plantar flexion. Imagine the foot trapped by the dorsum of the toes and falling backward, or the ballet dancer who falls off the toes, allowing his or her full body weight to fall on the dorsum of the foot. Often in football (the American variety), a player will be kneeling with the foot dorsiflexed and someone will land on the heel. The result is a large force crossing the ligaments and capsule of the tarsometatarsal joints.

Affected Structures

The Lisfranc joint is the joint between the 5 metatarsal bones and the midtarsal bones—the 3 cuneiforms and the cuboid bone. The second metatarsal bone is the key to stability of the Lisfranc joint because the Lisfranc ligament extends from the second metatarsal to the medial (first) cuneiform. While injury to this ligament is uncommon, it must be identified and treated with care or a resulting deformity (widening of the space between the proximal 1st and 2nd metatarsals) and chronic pain may be possible.

Signs and Symptoms

A patient with a Lisfranc injury may have swelling, point tenderness between the first and second metatarsal bases, asymmetry in the amount of space between the first and second toes, ecchymosis (discoloration) around the plantar aspect of the joint, pain with compression (squeezing) of the mid foot, pain with abduction and adduction of the toes, pain with abduction of the forefoot with the heel stabilized, and pain with weight bearing. Prompt referral to an orthopedist for complete assessment is required. Full diagnosis is reached though radiographic evaluation. A CT scan may be needed to make a final diagnosis. Any "mid foot" sprain with persistent pain that does not respond to treatment should be re-evaluated to rule out the Lisfranc injury.

Initial Care

Initial care for this injury requires immobilization with a walking boot and symptomatic care (ice, compression, and elevation). Long-term treatment of this injury may be conservative with immobilization. In general, stable, minimally displaced Lisfranc sprains are treated with immobilization until weight bearing is pain free (typically between 4 to 10 weeks). However, in unstable injuries, closed reduction or surgical fixation is often required to provide full anatomical restitution. Recovery from such a procedure and serious injury may take 9 to 12 months before sport activities can be resumed.

Bibliography

Ho VB, Hawkes NC, Fleming DJ. Radiology corner: subtle Lisfranc injury: low injury mid foot sprain. *Military Medicine.* 2007;172:xii-xiii.

Peterson L, Renstrom P. *Sports Injuries: Their Prevention and Treatment.* 3rd ed. Champaign, IL: Human Kinetics; 2001.

Other Soft Tissue Injuries

As noted previously, inversion ankle sprains are particularly common. An inversion sprain may result in an increased thickening of the synovium along the anterolateral aspect of the ankle joint (between the fibula and talus). This inflammation of the joint lining can cause the tissue to thicken, making it susceptible to entrapment in the joint. This condition is known as anterolateral ankle impingement. As the talus fits snugly into the ankle joint in full dorsiflexion, this condition causes pain for the patient. This condition is commonly seen in patients with chronic ankle instability. A snapping or locking sensation can sometimes occur. In addition, pain is experienced with pushing off of the ankle. Treatment includes using a heel wedge, stretching the tissue, and improving stability. In some instances, arthroscopic surgery can remove the resulting thickened lesion to alleviate pain.

Plantar fasciitis is an inflammation of the broad band of fascia that extends from the calcaneus to the front of the foot. The plantar fascia is located on the bottom or plantar surface of the foot. Activities that involve raising the heel off of the ground, running hills, and court sports that involve repetitive jumping are associated with inflammation of the plantar fascia. In addition, tightness in the gastrocnemius and soleus muscles can cause increased tension on the plantar fascia through the calcaneus. Overuse, rapid changes in intensity and frequency of workouts, and biomechanical alterations (ie, pronation) are also underlying factors. Signs and symptoms include pain in the heel that is worse in the morning. Care of plantar fasciitis includes treatments to decrease pain (heat and ice), therapeutic exercise to improve flexibility, and soft tissue massage to improve the mobility of the tissue. Like all overuse conditions, underlying biomechanical issues such as proper shoe support and addressing pronation of the rear foot must be addressed. The plantar fascia can also rupture acutely. An acute injury mechanism, pain, swelling, and limited function are all signs of a plantar fascia tear. Initial care will include PRICE. Acute injuries to the plantar fascia may be preceded by chronic plantar fasciitis.

Inflammation of the metatarsal phalangeal joint of the great toe can result from a sprain-type mechanism or repetitive trauma due to hyperextension. The layperson's name for this injury is turf toe. Turf toe got its name because of the common occurrence of this injury to athletes who participate on the hard surface of artificial turf. Despite its name, it is also common to court sport athletes or anyone who exercises or competes on hard surfaces. Shoes with a stiff forefoot will limit the hyperextension and help prevent or provide relief from turf toe. Signs and symptoms of turf toe include pain, swelling, point tenderness at the base of the great toe, and pain with active hyperextension. Treatment includes ice, support, and limitations in activity until symptoms subside. Taping support and appropriate footwear may be helpful in the long-term elimination of symptoms.

Neurovascular Injuries

In the distal portion of the foot, nerves that sit between the metatarsals and metatarsal heads are referred to as interdigital nerves. These nerves can become irritated due to pressure from repeated extension of the toes or from compression due to poorly fitting footwear. Localized swelling of the nerve between the metatarsal heads is called a neuroma. Inflammation of the nerve can cause pain and numbness at the site of the neuroma and also in the toe next to it. Commonly found between the 2nd and 3rd metatarsal heads, this condition is called Morton's neuroma. Signs and symptoms include pain, numbness, point tenderness between the metatarsal heads, and increased pain with squeezing of the metatarsal heads. Treatment involves improving the fit of the shoes, decreasing the inflammation (a physician may prescribe anti-inflammatory medication), and use of a pad to help relieve pressure in the area. Recurrent neuromas may require surgery for removal.

The area behind the medial malleolus below the retinaculum and the bones below lies the tarsal tunnel. The tendons of the posterior tibialis, flexor hallicus, and flexor digitorum run through the tarsal tunnel. Alongside these tendons you find the tibial nerve and the tibial artery and vein. Inflammation in this area that causes numbness and tingling along the medial and plantar aspects of the foot is a common finding for tarsal tunnel syndrome. Tarsal tunnel syndrome is also painful to a tapping over the region (called a Tinel's sign). Persistent tarsal tunnel inflammation may lead to weakness and atrophy. A normal course of care involves reducing the inflammation to relieve pressure on the tibial nerve.

SUMMARY

The injuries presented in this chapter represent an overview of common conditions the athletic trainer may see in the lower extremity. The injuries outlined above represent only a fraction of the possible injuries with which the athletic trainer must be familiar. The athletic trainer's ability to evaluate; provide initial care; and properly refer, treat, and rehabilitate a wide variety of injuries and conditions is rooted in his or her educational preparation and dedication to learning well beyond his or her certification. Students pursuing a degree in athletic training must be committed to establishing a strong academic foundation from which they can build their allied health career.

REFERENCES

1. Paluska SA. An overview of hip injuries in running. *Sports Med.* 2005;35(11):991-1014.
2. Peterson L, Renstrom P. *Sports Injuries: Their Prevention and Treatment.* 3rd ed. Champaign, IL: Human Kinetics; 2001.
3. Arnheim DD, Prentice WE. *Principles of Athletic Training.* 10th ed. New York: McGraw-Hill Higher Education; 2000.
4. Shultz SJ, Houglum PA, Perrin DH. Assessment of athletic injuries. In: Perrin D, ed. *Athletic Training Education Series.* Champaign, IL: Human Kinetics; 2000.
5. Sullivan AJ, Anderson SJ. *Care of the Young Athlete.* Oklahoma City, OK: American Academy of Orthopaedic Surgeons & American Academy of Pediatrics; 2000.
6. AOSSM. The Injured ACL: American Orthopedic Society for Sports Medicine; 1997. Available at www.aossm.org/ Publications/Stips/ACL.htm. Accessed January 27, 2002.
7. Juhn MS. Patellofemoral pain syndrome: a review and guidelines for treatment. *Am Fam Physician.* 1999;60:2012-222.
8. American Academy of Orthopedic Surgeons. Sprained ankle may not be minor injury. Available at www.aaos.org/wordhtml/ 2001news. Accessed February 28, 2002.
9. US Consumer Products Safety Commission Directorate of Economic Analysis. Injury Costs for Youth Soccer and Basketball. FOI Request Tim McGuine MS ATC; March 14, 2001.

WEB RESOURCES

American Academy of Orthopaedic Surgeons
http://orthoinfo.aaos.org
The American Academy of Orthopedic Surgeons (AAOS) supports this site that includes general injury information by body part, patient education materials, and information about locating an orthopaedic surgeon. The site also maintains links to sports medicine-related topics.

American Orthopedic Society for Sports Medicine
www.aossm.org
The AOSSM is a national organization of orthopaedic surgeons specializing in sports medicine, including national and international sports medicine leaders.

American Academy of Pediatrics
www.aap.org
The Web site for the AAP provides information regarding many aspects of providing care for children and adolescents. Professional publications sections allow for searches of current position statements and reports.

Acute Care for Ankle Sprains

Ankle sprains can be frustrating for both athletes and coaches. The following information is helpful in treating ankle injuries and getting athletes back in the game.

What Should Happen When a Player Injures an Ankle?

An effective method of dealing with ankle injuries includes a prompt and accurate diagnosis with an aggressive rehabilitation and injury prevention strategy. In the event of an ankle injury, evaluate the athlete on the field to rule out any obvious fracture. If you suspect a fracture, do not have the player put weight on the injured ankle and refer the player to a physician for diagnosis. If the athlete is able to tolerate weight bearing, ice, elevate, and compress the ankle. For high school athletes, the athletic trainer should talk to the player's parents and discuss referring the player to his or her physician for diagnosis of the injury. If the athlete is taken to an emergency room or urgent care clinic, impress on the parents that they follow up with their regular physician as well. When in doubt, refer any player you suspect of having a serious injury to his or her family physician.

The next step begins after the diagnosis of the ankle sprain. The goals of your treatment plan should be to decrease pain, increase functional ability, regain sport-specific skills, and prevent further injuries from occurring.

Crutches: As Long As You Have To, As Little As Possible

The athlete should use crutches when unable to bear weight without pain. However, rarely does a player need crutches to eliminate all weight bearing. Eliminating all weight bearing does not promote rapid healing. In addition, the strength, flexibility, and proprioception of the entire leg diminish within days of nonweight bearing.

A better method allows the athlete to begin weight bearing "as tolerated." This means that the level of pain indicates the extent crutches are used. Have the injured player concentrate on using crutches to assist with walking, trying to put the foot in the same functional position used in walking normally, and using the crutches to minimize the weight on the foot. As the player feels better, he or she simply allows an increasing amount of weight on the foot. Whenever possible, use an ankle boot to protect the ankle. Ankle boots put the foot in the necessary position while minimizing pain when walking. Many athletes are able to discard their crutches when they wear ankle boots. As soon as the player is able to walk without any pain, discontinue the boot and the crutches.

Ice Is Nice

The old standard of using PRICE is still effective in limiting the amount of pain an athlete feels following an injury. Ice should be used as long as there is swelling in the ankle, even if this means continuing this treatment for a week or more. Numerous studies have shown that the most effective and safe way to cool an injured body part is to apply bags of ice directly to the injury and compress the entire area with an elastic wrap. Place bags of ice on each side of the ankle and hold them in place with a 4- or 6-inch elastic wrap. Elevating the ankle while icing can further enhance the elimination of ankle swelling. Have the player ice, compress, and elevate the ankle for 20 minutes every 2 to 3 hours. When not icing, have the athlete wear an elastic wrap with a foam horseshoe around the lateral malleolus of the ankle to provide compression. Elevation whenever possible allows gravity to assist in removing the swelling.

Motion, Strength, and Endurance

ROM of ankle injuries will improve as swelling decreases. Gentle stretching, use of a slant board, and active movement can all assist in regaining motion. Following an ankle injury, and even a short period of immobilization, strength of the surrounding musculature will be lost. When the swelling has decreased and the athlete can tolerate movement, a strengthening program should be initiated. The athlete should work on all planes of movement using some form of resistance. Manual resistance from the athletic trainer, therapy bands, and surgical tubing are common exercise methods. In addition to regaining strength, the athletic trainer must initiate a program that addresses muscular endurance as well.

Active Rest Is the Best

When dealing with an ankle sprain, use "active rest." Keep the athlete from engaging in activities that cause pain in the ankle and encourage all other activities that do not cause pain. These activities include maintaining current levels of strength, flexibility, proprioception, and cardiac function as well as some limited sport-specific skills. The athletic trainer must be able to design and implement a return-to-play program for individual players. Some ideas for active rest are outlined next.   (continued)

Acute Care for Ankle Sprains (continued)

A player with a severe ankle sprain should be able to ride a stationary bike or swim to maintain cardiac function. Strength training for both the upper and, in some cases, lower body should also be carried out daily. Opposite limb balance exercises can help maintain appropriate levels of proprioception as well. As the player progresses and pain in the ankle diminishes, he or she could start running in chest-deep water in a swimming pool. Further progression could find the athlete running in waist or even thigh-deep water as weight bearing tolerance increases.

Progression to full-unassisted weight bearing is a sign that the athlete is probably ready to start a limited number of sport-specific activities that do not cause pain. For example, a football player can often participate in drills with limited stress on the ankle. As the player progresses, start more football-specific drills and activities. Lineman can work on exploding out from their stance, while receivers can work on cutting drills.

Ankle Bracing Versus Taping

Ankle taping used to be a standard practice following any ankle injury. However, brace technology has progressed significantly in the last several years and offers a safe, cost-effective alternative to ankle taping. Semirigid orthoses combine hard plastic with a liner and can be used both as a light ankle immobilizer and a brace when the athlete initially returns to sports. A lace-up brace does not offer the same level of support as the semirigid orthosis but is less costly and easier to fit in an athletic shoe. Lace-up braces offer the same if not more support than ankle taping while costing significantly less money over the course of an athletic season.

Ankle taping can be an effective means of ankle support if a skilled professional such as a certified athletic trainer does it. Ankle taping offers the advantage of being "custom fit" for each athlete and, if applied well, will limit excess ankle motion while maintaining normal ankle motion necessary to take part in various athletic activities. The high cost of ankle taping ($2.50 to $3 per application) should be considered when recommending the athlete choose this form of ankle support.

Return to Play

Generally, players can return to action as soon as they have regained their strength, balance, and ROM and can do all of their sport activities without any pain. To test this, have the player perform a series of running and functional activities tailored to his or her sport. With a little imagination, you can come up with your own set of criteria and tests for different positions. If the player limps or is unable to go full speed during the test, he or she is not ready to play. Repeat these same drills on a daily basis until the player is able to perform them without any problems. Only then can the player return to practice without any restrictions.

Adapted with permission from UW Health, Madison, WI. Sports Link – Tim McGuine LAT. 2002 UW Hospitals and Clinics Authority.

Career Spotlight: Occupational Health Athletic Trainer

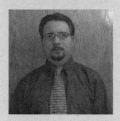

Daniel G. Trampf, LAT, CSCS

Industrial Rehabilitation Coordinator, Ripon Medical Center

Ripon, WI

My Position

I currently serve as the industrial rehabilitation coordinator at Ripon Medical Center. With this role, I coordinate and manage outreach occupational health/athletic training services to 4 major companies. Alliance Laundry Systems, Smuckers, Menasha Corporation, and Condon Companies are served on a either a daily or weekly basis with occupational health/athletic training services. Essentially, these companies total nearly 3000 employees and Condon Companies alone has 42 different conveniently located centers around Wisconsin.

The programming that I am involved with incorporates the idea of placing the "sports medicine model" into business and industry. The similar physical and psychosocial issues that face athletes also are present with the "industrial athlete." In addition, business and industry continues to struggle with musculoskeletal disorders (MSDs), and all the associated costs and employment issues that surround them. The Occupational Safety and Health Administration (OSHA) recommends proactive health care providers that are well-versed in the prevention, recognition, management, rehabilitation, and documentation of MSDs. The profession of athletic training fits well within this model and will significantly expand the role of the certified athletic trainer (ATC) in this setting. Currently, only a small percentage of ATCs are involved with the occupational/industrial setting; however, due to industry MSD concerns, OSHA mandates, and wellness initiatives, the opportunities will continue to expand for the ATC.

The industrial/occupational setting is unique in that the results of the proactive health care initiatives immediately show up on safety and health metrics. Decreased MSD injuries resulting in less restricted days at work, less days away from work, fewer costs to the comp and commercial carriers, increased productivity, and improved overall safety records are some of the immediate impacts of the ATC within business and industry.

Unique or Desired Qualifications

The special qualifications for this position require knowledge in industry environmental health and safety. I would also recommend a background in community health programs. Ergonomic degrees and certifications are preferred but not required. Biomechanics and/or kinesiology are required. A strong background in workers' compensation programs and law are required. Each state has different licensure requirements that may or may not allow the ATC to practice only certain aspects of athletic training in the occupational setting.

Favorite Aspect of My Job

The favorite aspect of this setting is the fact that I am able to learn and become a better ATC each day. I am exposed to a wide variety of health and safety situations, which require many skills of the ATC and some that I would strongly recommend. Leadership, excellent communication skills, problem solving ability, and "out of the box" thinking are some additional skills that make the ATC successful in this setting.

Advice

Continue to learn and challenge yourself to provide outstanding customer service, leadership, and communication. These are what will make you quickly successful in the occupational setting.

CHAPTER 7

COMMON INJURIES
TO THE UPPER EXTREMITY

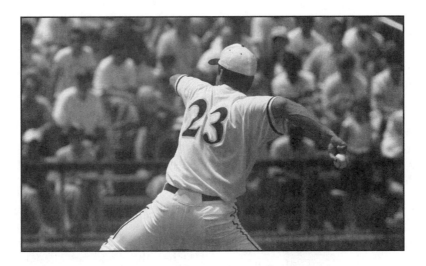

Good athletic trainers are bright and they know where to go when they don't know something. I think good athletic trainers have a great deal of common sense and you have to have that when you are thrown into situations when you have to make decisions very quickly and use good judgment. Good athletic trainers work hard while being efficient in that work. I think good athletic trainers are also very creative.

Paula Sammarone-Turocy, EdD, ATC
Department Chairperson and Associate Professor
Department of Athletic Training, Duquesne University

Somewhere along the evolutionary path, we moved upright. Humans, as upright walkers, have developed a nice, freely movable upper extremity. Unlike most 4-legged mammals, humans have the advantage of moveable upper extremities with a wide ROM, hands with opposable thumbs, highly advanced CNSs, and hand and eye relationships that allow us, not just to function, but also to use our limbs for recreation and competition. From pitching a baseball to grasping the tennis racquet, we owe a great deal to evolution for providing us with that mobile upper extremity. Humans can reach, grab, push, pull, throw, catch, swing, spike, dunk, and perform countless other motions; advanced evolution indeed. However, this upper extremity mobility can lead to problems.

If the lower extremity (namely the hip) requires great strength and stability so that we may stand upright, the upper extremity is just the opposite. We sacrifice some stability in the interest of mobility. This increased mobility allows us to perform many

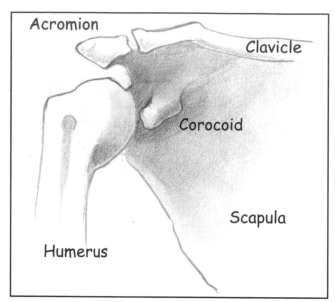

Figure 7-1. Bones of the shoulder girdle (sternum is not shown).

activities, but sometimes at the expense of stability. Injuries to the upper extremity are common and can account for approximately 20% of the injuries seen in the sports medicine environment.[1] That rate may be much higher for specific sports. The repetitive demands of overhead sports can create unique chronic injuries for the shoulder and elbow. In addition, the natural tendency to place our hand out to break our fall can create a number of injury scenarios for the upper extremity, particularly at the wrist and elbow.

This chapter discusses general anatomy of the upper extremity and presents some injuries commonly seen in physically active individuals. While some information is provided on immediate care, a discussion of treatment and rehabilitation of specific injuries is beyond the goal of this text.

Upon completion of this chapter, the student will be able to:

✓ Identify general musculoskeletal anatomy of the upper extremity, including specific articulations at the shoulder girdle, elbow, wrist, and hand

✓ Describe injuries and conditions common to the upper extremity

✓ Explain common mechanisms of upper extremity injury

✓ Discuss the athletic trainer's role in assessment and referral

ANATOMY

SHOULDER GIRDLE

The shoulder is a hypermobile joint that allows the upper extremity to assume a wide range of positions. However, the shoulder exchanges stability for mobility. The increased mobility often places the articulations and associated soft tissue structures at risk for injury. The motions of the shoulder include flexion, extension, abduction, adduction, circumduction, internal rotation and external rotation, and horizontal flexion and extension. Understanding the anatomical structures and their function will provide the athletic training student with a foundation to learn about common injuries and conditions of the shoulder girdle.

The shoulder girdle is composed of 4 bones: the sternum, clavicle, scapula, and humerus (Figure 7-1); this girdle attaches the upper extremity to the axial skeleton. Four articulations reside at the shoulder girdle: the sternoclavicular (SC) joint, the acromioclavicular (AC) joint, the glenohumeral (GH) joint, and the scapulothoracic articulation. The SC, AC, and GH joints are true bony articulations while the scapulothoracic articulation allows the scapula to glide on the rib cage. The scapula must be able to move and adjust its position to allow the humerus to be properly positioned for optimal function.

The SC joint is a stable joint with little mobility that attaches the proximal clavicle to the sternum. The clavicle is an S-shaped bone that articulates distally with the acromion at the AC joint and supports the shoulder joint by serving as an attachment for the scapula. A very superficial bone, the clavicle is easily palpated. The AC joint is supported by a group of ligaments that attach the clavicle to the scapula. The AC ligament and the conoid ligament offer support to the AC joint. This joint is the site of frequent sprain injuries (Figure 7-2). The coracoacromial ligament does not directly support the AC joint; however, its proximity to the tendons of the rotator cuff cause it to play a role in overuse injuries. The acromion is 1 of 2 unique-shaped projections (the other is the coracoid) that arise from the scapula. The AC joint can be found by following the clavicle distally until you reach the bumpy projection of the AC joint. This joint may be quite prominent in individuals who have a history of AC joint injury. The movement and orientation of the scapula are critical to proper function of the shoulder girdle. In addition to muscular control, this motion is

Articulations of the Upper Extremity

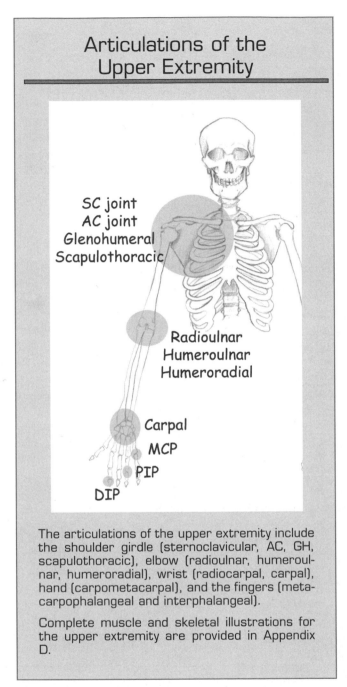

The articulations of the upper extremity include the shoulder girdle (sternoclavicular, AC, GH, scapulothoracic), elbow (radioulnar, humeroulnar, humeroradial), wrist (radiocarpal, carpal), hand (carpometacarpal), and the fingers (metacarpophalangeal and interphalangeal).

Complete muscle and skeletal illustrations for the upper extremity are provided in Appendix D.

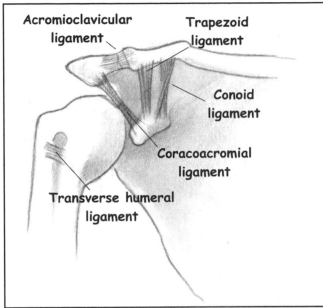

Figure 7-2. Ligaments of the AC joint.

that help the scapula maintain its proper position. Special consideration is given to the rotator cuff, a group of 4 muscles that arise from the scapula and insert on the humerus.

Dynamic Versus Static Stability

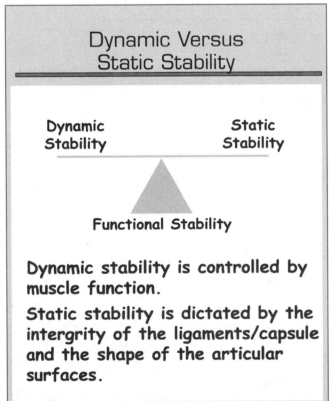

Dynamic stability is controlled by muscle function.

Static stability is dictated by the intergrity of the ligaments/capsule and the shape of the articular surfaces.

dependent upon movement from both the AC and SC joints.

The GH joint articulates with the scapula at a region called the glenoid. The glenoid is a slightly concave surface that articulates with the round head of the humerus. This flat surface gains some depth from the fibrous ring that surrounds the glenoid called the glenoid labrum. Students can think of the GH joint like a golf ball (the humerus) sitting on a golf tee (the glenoid). Since the bony and ligamentous structures provide little static stability, the shoulder girdle must rely on the dynamic stability of the muscles that support the shoulder (Table 7-1).[2] These muscles can be thought of as those that act on the humerus and those

Table 7-1

Major Muscles, Primary Actions, and Innervations of the Shoulder

Muscles That Act on the Humerus

Muscles	Action	Innervation
Deltoid	Abduction/flexion/extension	Axillary
Biceps brachii	Flexion	Musculocutaneous
Triceps brachii	Extension/horizontal adduction	Radial
Coracobrachialis	Flexion/horizontal adduction	Musculocutaneous

Rotator cuff
  Supraspinatus
  Infraspinatus
  Teres minor
  Subscapularis
	Collectively provide GH stability
	Abduction
	External rotation/horizontal abduction
	External rotation/horizontal abduction
	Internal rotation
		
		Suprascapular
		Suprascapular
		Axillary
		Subscapular

Pectoralis major Upper fibers Lower fibers	 Internal rotation/horizontal adduction/ flexion/abduction (above 90 degrees)/ abduction (below 90 degrees) Internal rotation/horizontal adduction/ extension/adduction of GH joint	 Lateral pectoral Medial pectoral
Latissimus dorsi	Adduction/extension/internal rotation/ depression of shoulder girdle/horizontal abduction	Thoracodorsal
Teres major	Extension/internal rotation/adduction	Subscapular

Muscles That Control the Scapula

Muscles	Action	Innervation
Rhomboids (major and minor)	Stabilization/elevation/retraction/down- ward rotation	Dorsal scapular
Levator scapulae	Elevation	Dorsal scapular

Muscles That Control the Scapula

Muscles	Action	Innervation
Serratus anterior	Upward rotation/protraction/depression	Long thoracic

Trapezius
  Upper fibers
  Middle fibers
  Lower fibers
	
	Elevation/extension of head and neck
	Elevation/upward rotation/retraction
	Depression/retraction/upward rotation
		Spinal accessory

ELBOW

Three bones make up the elbow: the distal humerus, proximal radius, and the proximal ulna (Figure 7-3). The movements that take place at the elbow are flexion and extension. Three distinct articulations make up the joint: the humeroulnar, humeroradial, and radioulnar (Figures 7-4 and 7-5). Pronation and supination are movements of the forearm that are facilitated by the radioulnar and humeroradial joints. The humeroradial joint allows for the radial head to spin when the forearm is pronated and supinated.

The rounded head of the radius is well suited for this purpose. The head of the radius is held in place by the annular ligament. Acting like a hinge, the humeroulnar joint allows for flexion and extension. The proximal ulna has a significant bony prominence called the olecranon process. The olecranon process is the pointy portion of the elbow and a common site for contusions and abrasions. The elbow is supported on each side by the medial and lateral collateral ligaments and its bony configuration. These elements combine to make the elbow quite stable.

Rotator Cuff

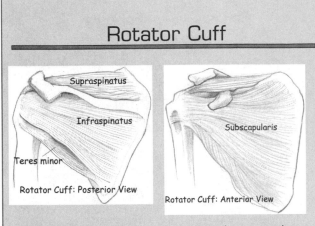

Supraspinatus

Infraspinatus

Teres minor

Rotator Cuff: Posterior View

Subscapularis

Rotator Cuff: Anterior View

The rotator cuff is a unique muscle group that collectively provides stability to the GH joint. The importance of these 4 small muscles cannot be overstated. The tendons of the rotator cuff pass beneath the subacromial arch and are a frequent site of inflammation. The muscles of the rotator cuff are often loaded in an eccentric fashion as the upper extremity participates in overhead activities, particularly during follow-through motions such as throwing a ball. The muscles of the rotator cuff can be easily remembered by the acronym SITS. The cuff SITS on the humerus. The muscles of the rotator cuff include the following:

Muscles	Primary Action
Supraspinatus	Abduction
Infraspinatus	External rotation/ horizontal abduction
Teres minor	External rotation/ horizontal abduction
Subscapularis	Internal rotation

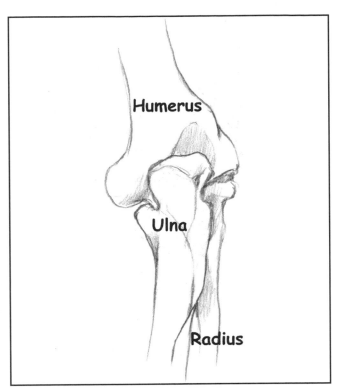

Figure 7-3. Bones of the elbow.

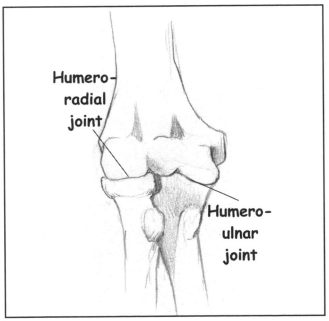

Figure 7-5. Distinct articulations of the humerus with radius and ulna.

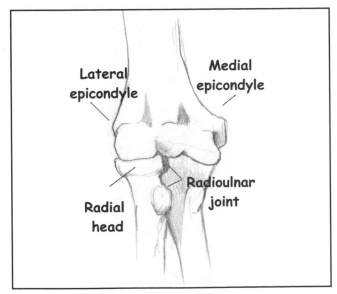

Figure 7-4. Landmarks of the elbow.

The distal humerus serves as the origin of 2 distinct muscle groups that cross the elbow joint and act on the wrist: the flexor and extensor groups. Chronic injury often associated with throwing sports can originate from these flexor and extensor muscle groups (Figures 7-6 and 7-7). The biceps brachii and triceps brachii muscles act as the primary flexors and

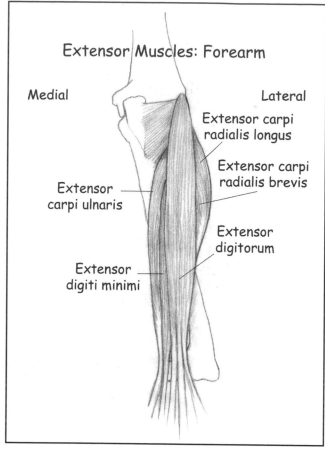

Figure 7-6. Extensor muscle group of the forearm.

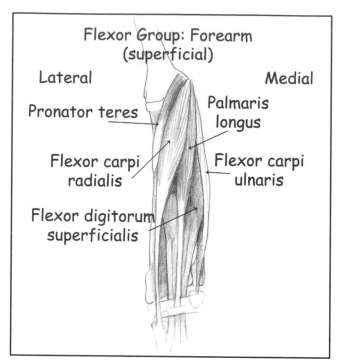

Figure 7-7. Flexor muscle group of the forearm.

extensors of the elbow, respectively. Table 7-2 lists the muscles that act on the elbow joint. Injuries to the elbow can sometimes be complicated by the superficial neurovascular structures that pass through it. Anyone who has hit their "funny bone" or ulnar nerve knows how superficial these structures can be. Another common neurovascular structure is the antecubital vein. The superficial nature of this vein makes it a frequent location for drawing blood. The athletic trainer must be knowledgeable of these neurovascular structures and recognize their potential injury and the secondary complications that can arise following a traumatic injury to the elbow.

WRIST AND HAND

Injuries of the wrist and hand run the spectrum of minor to potentially debilitating. I jokingly talked about the value of the opposable thumb earlier. In all seriousness, maintaining proper function of the hand and fingers is essential for daily function, therefore all injuries to the wrist and hand must be taken seriously. Two rows of carpal bones are present in the wrist. The proximal wrist bones articulate with the distal radius and ulna. The proximal row of bones (lateral to

medial from anatomical position) includes the scaphoid, lunate, triquetral, and pisiform. The distal row articulates with the metacarpal bones of the hand and includes the trapezium, trapezoid, capitate, and hamate. All total, there are 27 bones in the wrist and hand that include 8 carpal bones (wrist), 5 metacarpal bones (hand), and 14 phalanges (fingers). There are over 30 individual articulations in the wrist and hand (Figure 7-8).

An assortment of articulations allow for movement at the wrist and hand. The available ROM for the wrist includes flexion, extension, radial deviation, and ulnar deviation. Joints of the wrist and hand are named based on their location, shape, , and the bones with which they articulate. The carpal bones must articulate either with the radius and ulna, other carpal bones, or metacarpal bones of the hand. The joints of the wrist and hand include the following:

- ✓ Wrist (Carpals)
  - ○ Radiocarpal
  - ○ Midcarpal
  - ○ Carpometacarpal
  - ○ Intercarpal
  - ○ Radioulnar
  - ○ Carpometacarpal
- ✓ Phalanges (fingers)
  - ○ Metacarpophalangeal (MCP)
  - ○ Proximal interphalangeal (PIP)
  - ○ Distal interphalangeal (DIP)

Table 7-2

Major Muscles, Primary Actions, and Innervations of the Elbow and Wrist

Muscles That Control the Elbow and Forearm

Muscles	Action	Innervation
Biceps	Elbow flexion/forearm supination	Musculocutaneous
Triceps	Elbow extension	Radial
Brachialis	Elbow flexion/forearm supination	Musculocutaneous/radial
Anconeus	Elbow extension/stabilize ulna (with pronation and supination)	Radial
Brachioradialis	Elbow flexion/forearm pronation	Radial
Supinator	Forearm supination	Radial
Pronator teres	Forearm pronation, elbow flexion	Median
Pronator quadratus	Forearm pronation	Median
Flexor Group		
Flexor carpi radialis	Wrist flexion/forearm pronation/wrist deviation (radial)/elbow flexion	Median
Flexor carpi ulnaris	Wrist flexion/wrist deviation (ulnar)/elbow flexion	Ulnar
Flexor digitorum profundus	Assist wrist flexion	Median/ulnar
Flexor digitorum superficialis	Assist wrist flexion	Median
Palmaris longus	Wrist flexion	Median
Flexor pollicis longus	Assist wrist flexion	Median
Extensor Group		
Extensor digitorum communis	Assist wrist extension	Radial
Extensor carpi radialis brevis	Wrist extension/wrist deviation (radial)	Radial
Extensor carpi radialis longus	Wrist extension/wrist deviation (radial)	Radial
Extensor carpi ulnaris	Wrist extension/wrist deviation (ulnar)	Radial
Extensor pollicis brevis	Assist wrist extension	Radial

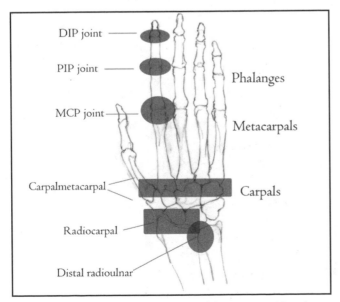

Figure 7-8. Bones and articulations of the wrist and hand.

Several muscles that act on the wrist originate at the elbow. Some of these muscles cross the wrist joint and act to flex and extend the phalanges. Table 7-3 lists the muscles and functions for the wrist and hand.

COMMON INJURIES TO THE SHOULDER

The shoulder girdle is a commonly injured region of the body. Falls and direct contact are common mechanisms for acute injury with overuse and sport-specific motions common contributors to chronic injury. A wrestler who is pounded into the mat on the point of the shoulder may very well injure the AC joint, while a baseball pitcher with poor mechanics or a weak rotator cuff is susceptible to tendonitis or impingement problems. The athletic trainer must

Table 7-3

Major Muscles, Primary Actions, and Innervations of the Hand and Fingers

Muscles	Action	Innervation
Abductor pollicis longus	Thumb abduction (CMC) assists radial deviation	Radial
Adductor pollicis	CMC adduction/thumb flexion (MCP)	Ulnar
Extensor pollicis brevis	Thumb extension (MCP, CMC)	Radial
Flexor pollicis longus	Thumb flexion (MCP, IP)	Median
Flexor digitorum profundus	Flexion of MCP, DIP, and PIP 2nd to 5th digits	Median/ulnar
Flexor digitorum superficialis	Flexion of the MCP and PIP	Median
Extensor digitorum communis	Extension MCP and PIP	Radial
Extensor digiti minimi	Extension of the 5th digit at MCP	Radial
Extensor indicis	Extension of the 2nd digit at MCP	Radial
Intrinsic Muscles of the Hand		
Abductor digiti minimi	MCP abduction 5th digit	Ulnar
Flexor digiti minimi	MCP flexion 5th digit	Ulnar
Opponens pollicis	CMC opposition—thumb	Median
Opponens digiti minimi	MCP opposition of 5th digit	Ulnar
Dorsal interossei	MCP flexion/abduction and PIP and DIP extension of 2nd to 4th digits	Ulnar, palmar branch
Palmar interossei	MCP adduction of the 2nd, 4th, and 5th digits	Ulnar
Lumbricales	Flexion of the 2nd to 5th MCP/extension of PIP and DIP	Median/ulnar

Key

CMC = carpometacarpal, MCP = metacarpophalangeal, PIP = proximal interphalangeal, DIP = distal interphalangeal.

 ## Remembering the Bones of the Wrist

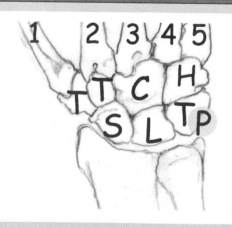

Remembering the bones of the wrist joint can be a challenge for the new athletic training student. Many a mnemonic has been developed to assist with memorization of anatomical structures. Some are these are "G" rated and others, well not so much. Some commonly used for the wrist include:

Sally Left The Party/To Take Cathy Home

or

Some Lovers Try Positions/That They Can't Handle

These will help you remember:

Scaphoid, Lunate, Triquetral, Pisiform/Trapezium, Trapezoid, Capitate, and Hamate.

Authors note: Positions of course refer to jobs (eg, employment).

be able to recognize the underlying mechanisms of injury, the relationship between injured tissue and dysfunction, and the demands placed on the patient by his or her specific activity. If the athletic trainer can understand these items, he or she will be well prepared to recognize, manage, and properly refer the injuries that he or she encounters.

FRACTURES AND INJURIES TO BONE

The clavicle is commonly fractured in active participants. The most common mechanisms of injury include direct blows, indirect forces from a fall on the point of the shoulder, or a fall on an outstretched hand (FOOSH). Easily palpated, the clavicle is quite superficial and commonly fractures in the middle third of the bone. This injury may present with an obvious deformity and pain for the patient. Not all fractures will have an obvious deformity, therefore if a patient has point tenderness over the bone, he or she should be referred for a radiograph. The clavicle fracture is treated with a sling or a figure-of-8 brace for a period of 4 to 8 weeks. The clavicle, in general, heals well; however, in cases where the fracture is on the most lateral aspect of the bone or the ends of the fracture site threaten to penetrate the skin, surgical fixation may be required.

The scapula and humerus are other possible locations for fracture in the shoulder region. Fractures of the humerus and scapula are less common than injuries to the clavicle. Direct blows and FOOSH are the most common mechanisms of injury. Fractures of the humerus occur most frequently through the surgical neck of the humerus (the area just below the humeral head) and the mid shaft. Avulsion fractures of the greater tubercle (insertion of supraspinatus) and lesser tubercle (insertion of the subscapularis) sometimes occur. When evaluating the humerus, the soft tissue covering these structures may make direct palpation of the bone difficult. Pain, deformity, and loss of function are common signs of a fracture. Fractures to the humerus have the potential to impact the long-term use of the GH joint. The athletic trainer must immobilize and transport this patient for immediate evaluation. Stress fractures, while uncommon, can occasionally occur in the humerus. Javelin throwers and other overhead-throwing athletes are most susceptible.

SOFT TISSUE INJURIES

Sprains, Subluxations, and Dislocations

Common sprains at the shoulder girdle include injuries to the SC, AC, and GH joints. A sprain to the SC joint results from an indirect force transmitted along the clavicle to the ligaments that support the articulation between the sternum and the proximal clavicle. A sprain to the SC joint is less common than those to the AC joint; however, they can occur in sports where forces are applied to the point of the shoulder. SC joint sprains are tender to palpation and may present with a deformity at the proximal clavicle. In uncommon situations, the proximal clavicle can become separated from the sternum. If the clavicle is displaced backwards (posteriorly), it can interfere with the subclavian artery and vein and create a life-threatening situation. These cases must receive a full evaluation. Most stable SC sprains heal well with a period of rest and immobilization. Unstable SC sprains may require surgical repair.

The AC joint sprain is often referred to by laypersons as a "separation" of the shoulder. The degree of injury and resulting deformity of the AC joint correlates with which ligaments have been injured and the amount of damage to each. Patients who have sustained an AC sprain will often have an observable deformity on the top of the shoulder due to swelling or the distal clavicle riding higher than normal. An AC joint sprain will be painful and the pain will increase with movement (particularly when the arm is moved across the body [ie, horizontal adduction]). Swelling at the joint and obvious deformity may accompany an AC sprain. The athletic trainer may be able to depress the distal clavicle and note the amount of movement. AC sprains are graded by degrees with a 1st-degree sprain being the least severe and a 3rd-degree sprain involving a complete disruption of the ligaments securing the acromion and distal clavicle the worst. Patients with an AC sprain should follow a program of PRICE with protection coming in the form of a sling. A physician should evaluate the injured AC joint to rule out a fracture and determine the severity of the injury. Most AC sprains will respond to a program of mobilization and symptomatic care.

The GH joint allows for a wide ROM at the shoulder. The shallow glenoid portion of the scapula provides great mobility at the expense of stability. The ligaments supporting the GH joint include the capsular (or GH ligament), coracohumeral, and inferior GH ligaments. These ligaments are consistent with the joint capsule, and the tension on each ligament changes depending upon the position of the arm. If excessive stress is placed on the GH joint, these ligaments can be sprained. The GH joint is most vulnerable when the arm is abducted and externally rotated. If the joint is forced beyond its limits in this direction, the capsular ligament can fail and the humerus will slide in an anterior and inferior direction and out of the "socket" of the glenoid, resulting in dislocation. The dislocation injury is relatively common in sports.

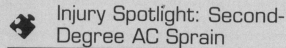

Injury Spotlight: Second-Degree AC Sprain

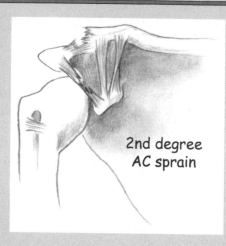

2nd degree
AC sprain

Mechanism of Injury

Direct blow to the point of the shoulder, contact with the ground or other object with point of the shoulder, or FOOSH.

Affected Structures

Rupture of the AC and coracoclavicular ligaments.

Signs and Symptoms

Pain, gross deformity from the upward displacement of the clavicle, pain with active movement (horizontal flexion [across the body]) in particular.

Initial Care

PRICE is the best course of action. Ice should be applied gently and held in place with an elastic bandage. The patient should be placed in a sling and referred to the physician for evaluation.

This injury is 3 times more common in men between the ages of 20 to 30 than in persons over 30; the male to female ratio for this injury is 9:1.[3] While anterior/inferior dislocations are the most common, posterior dislocations do occur.

GH dislocations can cause damage to the associated structures of the joint. The fibrous cartilage labrum that sits on the glenoid of the scapula can be avulsed from the glenoid rim and is called a Bankart lesion. A Bankart lesion is the most common cause of recurrent dislocation of the GH joint. The joint capsule can be stretched to varying degrees during a dislocation episode. Repeated injury can lead to excessive laxity of the capsule and therefore recurrent injury. Significant muscle lesions are not common following

a dislocation; however, a bony lesion can occur from the compression of the posterior humeral head against the anterior rim of the glenoid. This lesion is called a Hill-Sachs lesion (compression injury to the humeral head). This lesion can occur with a single dislocation or with recurrent dislocations. This bony lesion usually heals fine as long as the underlying instability of the shoulder is addressed. Patients with this dislocation will have significant pain while the joint is dislocated. The contour of the deltoid may look flat and the arm will hang near the side. The round humeral head may be palpable in the axilla (armpit). The patient should be immobilized and taken to a physician for reduction of the joint and a full evaluation, including associated radiographs.

If the GH joint only partially slides out of position, it is referred to as a subluxation. Sprains to the joint capsule and ligaments can result in increased laxity to the joint as a whole. As laxity increases, the demands placed on the supporting musculature (namely the rotator cuff) to provide dynamic support are increased. There is a direct relationship between laxity in the GH joint and overuse problems of the rotator cuff.[4]

Muscle-Tendon Injuries

Several muscles act on the upper extremity to allow for the wide ROM available at the shoulder girdle. During the course of these motions, any one of these muscle groups may be subject to a muscle strain injury. The nature of muscle strain injury is often sport specific. Muscle injuries are classified as 1st thru 3rd degree. These injuries often present with pain, stiffness in the muscle group, discomfort with activity, and weakness. Any discussion of the shoulder must give special consideration to the muscles commonly injured in overhand sport activities. Throwing a football, pitching a baseball, serving in tennis, swimming, and spiking the volleyball are common sport-specific activities that often involve strain and overuse problems with the rotator cuff muscle group.

The rotator cuff is responsible for providing dynamic stability to the GH joint. If the GH joint is unstable, the rotator cuff must work harder to hold the humerus in place. In this situation, the muscles of the rotator cuff are susceptible to overload and strain injuries (muscle-tendon strains and tendonitis). The nature of the throwing motion requires rapid acceleration and deceleration of the upper arm. It is in this deceleration phase that the rotator cuff must contract while being lengthened. Such a contraction is called an eccentric contraction. Eccentric contractions are commonly associated with muscle strain injury and tendonitis. When rotator cuff strains occur, the athletic trainer must look at the big picture of shoulder function. As noted above, there is a direct relationship

Injury Spotlight: Glenohumeral Dislocation

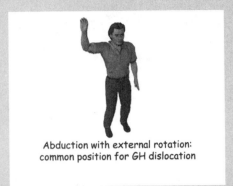

Abduction with external rotation: common position for GH dislocation

Mechanism of Injury

Forced abduction and external rotation of the humerus is the most common MOI leading to anterior/inferior dislocations.

Affected Structures

The round humeral head disarticulates from the shallow glenoid fossa of the scapula. In the process, the glenoid labrum and its bony attachment may be damaged (Bankart lesion) or the head of the humerus may sustain a compression fracture (Hill-Sachs lesion).

Signs and Symptoms

Pain, especially if a first-time dislocation. Subsequent dislocations will not be as painful. The shoulder will appear flat and not have the usual smooth contour over the deltoid. Patient will resist motion and will support the arm with the unaffected hand. The humeral head may be palpable in the axilla.

Initial Care

Do not try to reduce the GH joint. Place a bag of ice gently over the shoulder. Hold the ice in place with a compression wrap, place in a sling, and transport to a medical facility for reduction and evaluation. Monitor a distal pulse (radial) and check for numbness and tingling in the upper extremity.

Injury Spotlight: Impingement Syndrome

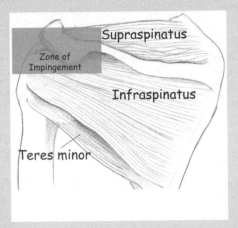

Mechanism of Injury

Chronic overuse injury that develops over time. Common to overhead sports such as swimming, baseball, softball, volleyball, and tennis.

Affected Structures

The area below the acromial arch. The tendons of the rotator cuff, subacromial bursa, biceps tendon, and coracoacromial ligament may all be involved.

Signs and Symptoms

Pain with raising the arm to shoulder level or above. Pain following activity, pain at night, and pain deep in the shoulder are all common signs of impingement syndrome.

Initial Care

Impingement syndrome is a chronic injury. Common treatment includes decreasing the inflammation that is present through ice and nonsteroidal anti-inflammatory medications. Treatment must include proper strengthening of the muscles of the rotator cuff and those that control the scapula. Some cases may require arthroscopic surgery to decompress the coracoacromial ligament and remove any spurs from the underside of the acromion. A section of the acromion may also be resected to create more space below the arch.

between laxity in the GH joint and overuse injuries of the rotator cuff.[4]

Another common injury that affects the shoulder is an impingement syndrome. A syndrome is a collection of symptoms. The anatomy of the shoulder requires that the tendons of the rotator cuff slide beneath the acromial arch. Space beneath the acromion must be sufficient to allow for movement of the tendons of the rotator cuff, as well as the subacromial bursae and the ligaments that support the AC joint. Impingement syndrome occurs if any of these structures are inflamed. The space may be compromised and cause pain for the patient with movements (eg, rotator cuff tendonitis, subacromial bursitis). While most impingement problems are chronic, an acute impingement injury can occur when the head of the humerus is jammed up against the acromial arch. This can occur with a FOOSH mechanism. Anatomical variations in the shape of the acromion can also contribute to impingement problems.[4] The space is further compromised when the humerus is internally rotated and flexed. Athletes with an impingement syndrome will present with pain felt deep in the shoulder joint and describe an increase in pain with abduction and internal rotation of the humerus. Treatment of impingement syndrome includes decreasing the inflammation and pain while addressing underlying factors that promote inflammation to the structures. This most often includes biomechanical corrections in technique, improving strength, and maintaining flexibility.[5] Arthroscopic surgery is recommended in some cases to release the coracoacromial ligament and smooth the underside of the acromion.

The rotator cuff is not the only common location for tendonitis at the shoulder. The biceps tendon is also a frequent source of inflammation. The tendon of the long head of the biceps brachii helps depress and stabilize the head of the humerus during abduction. It originates from the area above the glenoid. While it is distinct from the actual GH joint, it does pass below the subacromial arch and can play a role in impingement. The signs and symptoms of biceps tendonitis are similar to those associated with impingement of other subacromial structures. This chronic injury has a gradual onset and is frequently found in overhead sport athletes. This tendon is held in place by the transverse humeral ligament. This ligament can become injured acutely and cause the tendon to sublux out of the bicipital groove.

Other Soft Tissue Injuries

Contusions are common soft tissue injuries that can occur to many areas of the body during physical activity. The shoulder frequently receives blows in many contact activities. The large deltoid muscle provides a great deal of protection for the GH joint. Other joints of the shoulder girdle are exposed and can be susceptible to contusion-type injuries. Direct blows from other players or objects (balls, etc) are the MOI for the contusion. Ecchymosis and edema are common findings, and the athletic trainer must take special care to insure that a fracture or serious injury (sprain) has not occurred to the underlying tissue. Contusions can be severe and may require support (sling) to allow for adequate rest and healing. A fall on the point of the shoulder that contuses the AC joint is referred to as a shoulder pointer. This injury should receive ice and compression to decrease the inflammation. Significant contusions can cause bleeding and pooling of blood in the muscle tissue. If left untreated, a secondary formation of calcium can take place. This is known as myositis ossificans. While more common

in the thigh, this injury can occur in the deltoid region along the humerus as well. If the athletic trainer is unsure as to the severity of a contusion, referral to a physician is warranted.

COMMON INJURIES TO THE ELBOW

FRACTURES AND INJURIES TO BONE

Several of the bones that make up the elbow joint are subject to fracture. While fractures of the elbow and upper arm do occur in sports, they are more often seen in the pediatric patient when compared to adults.[6] Common fracture locations at the elbow include the proximal ulna, radial head, medial epicondyle, and supracondylar fractures of the humerus. Common injury mechanisms include direct blows, FOOSH, and fractures secondary to dislocation. In young athletes, there is a common triad of fractures that can occur with a fall in full extension combined with a valgus force. This triad includes the fracture of the olecranon process, compression of the radial neck, and avulsion of the medial epicondyle.[6]

In addition to fractures, overuse injuries secondary to throwing can occur to the boney structures of the elbow. While skeletally immature athletes are susceptible to specific bone injuries related to throwing (see below), mature athletes are not immune from chronic bone injury at the elbow. Posterior elbow impingement is a condition involving the repeated contact between the medial olecranon process and the olecranon fossa. This injury is common among overhead throwers. Overhead motions place the elbow under stress through a valgus extension overload (ie, rapidly moving from a valgus position to an extended position). The condition is also seen in football linemen who frequently force the elbow into extension during pass protection. Posterior impingement patients will often show decreases in throwing performance and have posteromedial elbow pain. On exam, they may have a loss of extension and have pain with valgus stress. Crepitus may be present and, in severe cases, locking (an inability to move the joint) can occur. X-rays are needed to determine the health of the joint surfaces and to look for osteophytes and loose bodies in the joint. The ulnar collateral ligament has a resulting instability because of the repetitive valgus stress. In addition, a stress fracture to the tip of the olecranon can occur with this same MOI.

Treatment of elbow impingement involves rest and a gradual return to throwing with an emphasis on proper mechanics. A period of rehabilitation that includes ROM and strength exercises is essential. Repairing the ulnar collateral ligament to gain added elbow stability is a common surgical intervention to assist baseball players with this problem.

SOFT TISSUE INJURIES

Sprains, Subluxations, and Dislocations

Collateral ligaments support the elbow and protect the elbow from excessive varus and valgus stress. Like all ligaments, they are subject to sprain injury and are graded as 1st thru 3rd degree. Common injury mechanisms for sprains of the elbow ligaments include a FOOSH combined with a varus or valgus force, hyperextension, or repetitive overload on the medial aspect of the elbow. Sprain injuries commonly produce pain, joint laxity with activity or on examination, and in severe cases loss of function. Rest and rehabilitation are the primary courses of treatment for sprains at the elbow. Third-degree cases may require surgical intervention depending on the desired outcome. Immediate care involves PRICE with protection in the form of a sling.

Dislocations of the elbow can occur when the humeroulnar joint is separated. The common mechanism is again the FOOSH with the elbow extended. The elbow will dislocate posteriorly, causing the olecranon process to sit well behind the distal humerus. The resulting deformity is significant. An athlete who has dislocated the elbow may have complications to neurovascular structures. He or she should have immediate application of a splint with ice and gentle compression. This patient should be transported for medical attention immediately, keeping in mind that he or she may need to be treated for shock.

Muscle-Tendon Injuries

Two common musculotendinous injuries that happen at the elbow are medial and lateral epicondylitis. On the medial aspect of the elbow, the prominent medial epicondyle serves as the origin for the muscles that flex the wrist. On the lateral side of the elbow, the lateral epicondyle serves as the origin for the muscles that extend the wrist. Medial epicondylitis is commonly known as golfer's elbow and is less common than lateral epicondylitis also known as tennis elbow. Tennis elbow is caused by strong forceful eccentric contractions of the extensor muscle group. Sports that use racquets are the most common activities that promote lateral epicondylitis, thus the tennis elbow moniker; however, any repetitive activity that involves wrist extension can induce "tennis" elbow. Patients

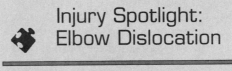

Injury Spotlight: Elbow Dislocation

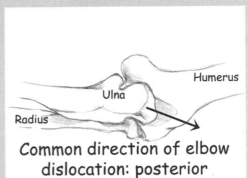

Common direction of elbow dislocation: posterior

Mechanism of Injury
FOOSH with hyperextension of elbow.

Affected Structures
A dislocation occurs when the olecranon is forced posteriorly away from its articulation with the humerus.

Signs and Symptoms
Severe pain, gross deformity with radius and ulna forced posterior behind humerus with complete loss of function at the joint.

Initial Care
The elbow dislocation may compromise both vascular and nerve structures. The patient should be splinted with application of ice and compression. The patient must be transported to a medical facility for reduction and evaluation.

with lateral epicondylitis will have pain, may have swelling over the epicondyle, and active extension of the wrist or reproduction of an eccentric contraction will be painful. This condition is more common in novice tennis players and there is a 30% to 50% lifetime prevalence in recreational players with the peak incidence occurring to players between 35 to 55 years of age.[7]

Medial epicondylitis is common to activities that require pronation of the forearm and strong flexion of the wrist. Throwing activities and the follow-through motion in golf can lead to medial epicondylitis. While the name implies that these injuries are a straight forward inflammation (-itis) of muscle groups that originate at the epicondyles, literature suggests that golfer's elbow and tennis elbow are better described as a tendinosis or epicondylosis that represents a condition of the tendon rather than a description of inflammation.[7] Irritations to the medical epicondyle must be treated with care due to the anatomical proximity of the ulnar nerve. Any patient with medial elbow pain should be examined for neurovascular involvement.

Treatment of injuries to the epicondyle must decrease aggravating activities, use ice and anti-inflammatory medications for local symptoms, and promote flexibility and strength to tolerate the loads placed on the muscles. Use of a counter force brace may be helpful to decrease the loads on the extensor muscles. Return to activity for epicondylitis should follow a slow progressive treatment plan. Analysis of sport mechanics can be helpful to avoid recurrence of symptoms.

Other Soft Tissue Injuries

Contusions can occur at the elbow due to the prominence of the olecranon on the proximal ulna. A common acute injury associated with a contusion of the olecranon is the development of olecranon bursitis. This acute injury can cause the bursa to swell and create a significant deformity to the elbow. Swelling can impair ROM and the size of the olecranon bursa may interfere with clothing or protective equipment. The athletic trainer must be aware that the olecranon bursa is susceptible to infection. Any athlete who sustains an injury to this region should be followed closely. A contusion to the medial or posterior aspect of the elbow can also irritate the ulnar nerve. This is the common experience of "hitting your funny bone."

NEUROVASCULAR INJURIES

The majority of nerve injuries seen in active populations can be described as a neuropraxia, which is the mildest form of nerve injury. These include injuries that do not disrupt the integrity of the nerve tissue. Friction, compression, contusion, and tension (or combinations thereof) are the most common mechanisms. Nerve tissue can also be damaged by stretch mechanisms secondary to trauma like fracture or dislocation. In the event of such trauma, the athletic trainer must assess the function of the associated nerves. The athletic trainer assesses neurovascular function by testing the athlete's muscle strength, sensation, and reflexes.

Three of the main peripheral nerves of the upper extremity cross the elbow joint. These are the ulnar, median, and radial nerve. The ulnar nerve is commonly irritated in conjunction with injuries that involve the medial aspect of the elbow (ie, sprains, medial epicondylitis, fractures). Entrapment of the ulnar nerve (ulnar neuritis) can be found distal to the medial epicondyle where the nerve enters the forearm. Entrapments can sometimes be found secondary to

elbow instability, bone spurs, and thickening of the synovium.[3] In addition, the ulnar nerve is vulnerable to stress during the valgus overload of the elbow common with overhand activities. The median nerve is located more toward the middle of the forearm and can sometimes become compressed under the pronator teres muscle. This injury is called pronator teres syndrome and could cause numbness, pain, and discomfort for the patient. The radial nerve can be entrapped and sometimes injured if it becomes compressed by the supinator musculature in the forearm. The pain is similar to the tennis elbow injury; however, the tenderness is more distal below the epicondyle over the area of the nerve entrapment. If rest, activity modification, and symptomatic care do not alleviate symptoms, surgical release of the entrapped nerve is sometimes indicated.

CONSIDERATIONS FOR THE SKELETALLY IMMATURE PATIENT

Special consideration must be given to the skeletally immature athlete when discussing injuries and conditions of the elbow. There are 6 ossification centers (apophyses) around the elbow. These growth areas usually fuse, or "close," in adolescents anywhere between 14 and 16 years of age. However, there is some variation timing of appearance of closure of these apophyses between males and females. In growing athletes, these unfused or "open" areas are common sites of injury, particularly in athletes who take part in repetitive overhand throwing activities. High repetitions of multidirectional mechanical forces at the elbow can result in bony and/or soft tissue overload and injury.[8] When these occur in a young thrower, the result can be specific injuries that are not seen in the skeletally mature patient.

Little Leaguer's elbow is a term that was coined in the 1960s to describe the spectrum of bony changes at the elbow that are caused by medial stress and lateral compression to the elbow. The consistent variables to this condition include throwing, elbow pain, and skeletal immaturity. It may be unfair to Little League Inc to use their name to discuss such conditions in vague terms. Recognizing the specific conditions that fall under this umbrella term is more appropriate for health care professionals like athletic trainers. In fact, Little League Inc has played an active role in studying these injuries as well as establishing guidelines for safe participation in throwing sports by young athletes.[8] The 3 injuries identified below are examples of such age-dependent conditions in the elbow.

Medial Epicondylar Apophysitis

Medial epicondylar apophysitis can develop due to repetitive stress to the medial epicondyle of the humerus at the origin of the flexor and pronator muscles. This is an example of a traction apophysitis. Repetitive microtrauma to this region may ultimately lead to a stress fracture failure of the tissue. It is also possible for an avulsion injury to develop. The medial epicondylar apophysitis (see injury spotlight) is the classic injury most often called "Little Leaguer's elbow." Patients with this condition will present with progressively worsening medial elbow pain brought on by throwing and/or pitching. This pain tends to occur during the late cocking and early acceleration phases of pitching when maximum valgus stress (also called valgus stress overload) occurs at the elbow.

Olecranon Apophysitis

Olecranon apophysitis occurs at the insertion of the triceps tendon at the olecranon apophysis. Pain at this posterior region of the elbow is caused by rapid and repetitive acceleration and deceleration during throwing and/or pitching. These young patients will present with posterior elbow pain and decreased ROM, and they may or may not have swelling. The posterior elbow will be tender to palpation, and activating the triceps against resistance (resisted extension) will be painful. Radiographs may show widening or changes at the apophysis. Cases that do not respond to conservative therapy (activity modification, ROM, strength, proper mechanics, etc) may require surgical repair.

Osteochondritis Dissecans

OCD is not a true inflammatory process despite the *itis* suffix. OCD is a focal injury to subchondral bone and can result in degeneration of the overlying articular cartilage. In the skeletally immature thrower or pitcher, this injury is often the cause of lateral elbow pain. OCD in the elbow is caused by repetitive stress and lateral compression to the humeroradial (radiocapitellar) joint. Compression on the lateral side of the elbow occurs opposite the traction seen on the medial aspect of the elbow with a repetitive valgus stress overload. It can be thought of as repeatedly banging together the joint surfaces of the radial head and the distal humerus. The injury presents with gradual onset lateral elbow pain that is worse with activity and better with rest. Patients will be tender to touch over the anterior and lateral aspect of the elbow. They may have varying degrees of crepitus or swelling. In advanced cases, patients will have loss of ROM in extension of the elbow or rotation of the forearm. Radiographs may not show any early changes of OCD. More advanced cases may show irregularities of the articular surface, loose bodies, subchondral cysts, radial head enlargement, or osteophytes. MRI may be required to fully evaluate the status of the injury.

 ### Injury Spotlight: Medial Epicondylar Apophysitis

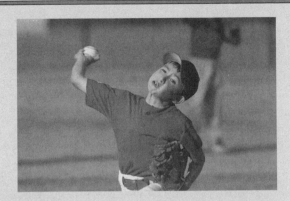

Mechanism of Injury

This injury is caused by repetitive microtrauma to the medial epicondylar apophysis of the elbow due to throwing and/or pitching in skeletally immature athletes (valgus extension overload).

Affected Structures

Medial epicondyle of the humerus at the origin of the flexor and pronator muscle groups. Valgus stress overload can lead to a stress reaction, widening of the apophysis, and a possible bony avulsion

Signs and Symptoms

Patients with this condition will have medial elbow pain, loss of throwing velocity or distance, diminished throwing effectiveness, and pain during the cocking and/or acceleration phases of pitching. Physical exam will reveal point tenderness at the medical epicondyle, a possible flexion contracture (inability to straighten the elbow), and pain with valgus stress and wrist flexion.

Initial Care

Treatment of medial epicondylar apophysitis includes elimination of the valgus stress overload, cessation of all throwing activities for 4 to 6 weeks (or just eliminate pitching), brief immobilization followed by rehabilitation that focuses on improved ROM and core strength exercises. Symptomatic care using ice may alleviate discomfort. Any return to throwing must by guided by pain. Returns to competitive pitching may take 12 weeks. During this recovery period, proper throwing and pitching mechanics must be addressed with any deficiencies corrected.

Treatment of OCD lesions in the elbow is dictated by the stability of the OCD lesion. Stabile lesions can be treated conservatively with activity modification and careful monitoring of healing. Return to activity must be carefully advanced following full resolution of all symptoms. More advanced unstable OCD lesions may require surgery to remove loose bodies, repair fragments, and address joint surface repairs if possible. The natural history of these injuries is difficult to predict.[9] Physicians may not be able to predict which will heal and which will develop joint incongruities. Those whose OCD lesions do not heal properly can suffer lifelong changes that result in pain and loss of motion.

 Progression of Osteochondritis Dissecans

OCD involves the combination of repetitive microtrauma combined with poor blood supply and can lead to subchondral osteonecrosis (bone death below the cartilage) in the joint. In the upper extremity, this condition is often seen as part of the spectrum of elbow pain found in skeletally immature patients.

The natural progression of the injury is as follows:

Microtrauma

Subchondral bone is weakened

Fatigue fracture

Osseous repair fails

Bone resorption

Altered subchondral architecture cannot support overlying articular cartilage

Articular cartilage is vulnerable to shear stress and further degeneration

---

COMMON INJURIES TO THE WRIST AND HAND

The wrist and the hand make up one of the most important regions in our body. The ability to reach, grasp, and use our opposable thumb is a human trait that has allowed for great advancement. Try to go a day without using your thumb or bending your wrist. With this in mind, the athletic trainer must take great care in properly identifying, treating, and referring injuries to this region. The incidence of hand and wrist injuries makes up between 3% and 9% of all injuries reported in sport.[10] Specific activities are often associated with very specific injuries to the wrist

and hand. In fact, physicians are encouraged to have an increased suspicion of bone injury simply at the mention of sport as a possible mechanism.[10]

FRACTURES AND INJURIES TO BONE

When bone injuries occur in the upper extremity, the most common mechanisms of injury involve direct blows, compression injuries (striking and punching), and falling with the wrist outstretched. In fact, if you review this chapter, you will find that the FOOSH injury mechanism is widely responsible for several injuries. Falling and trying to break the fall by putting our hand out is the culprit in many fractures to the wrist and forearm. Common bony injuries include fractures to the distal radius and ulna, carpal bones, and metacarpals. A fracture to the upper extremity that pushes the wrist back over the fracture and creates a silver fork deformity is called a Colles' fracture. This fracture is common for any active individual who falls on the outstretched hand. This fracture may involve just the radius or the ulna as well. The deformity is significant and the patient with a Colles' fracture will experience severe pain. The reverse Colles' or Smith's fracture involves falling on an outstretched hand with the wrist flexed. The resulting deformity is the opposite of the silver fork deformity. The immediate care is the same for both injuries. Splinting, compression, and elevation followed by immediate referral are the appropriate actions for this injury. Care should be taken to monitor blood supply and nerve function. Ice can be used for pain but should be avoided if there is a concern about the blood supply or nerve function. The patient should also be monitored for shock.

The scaphoid (navicular) is a bone in the first row of the carpal bones that articulates with the distal radius. The scaphoid is frequently injured in FOOSH mechanisms and activities that require forceful wrist extension and impact (ie, pass blocking for the football lineman). The scaphoid can be gently palpated by pressing into the anatomical snuffbox. Extensor tendons that control the thumb make up the borders of this anatomical landmark (Figure 7-9). Pain with palpation in the anatomical snuffbox warrants a referral to the physician. The scaphoid fracture represents 60% to 70% of all bone injuries to the carpals.[10] The hook of the hamate bone is another common site of fractures in the wrist. The hamate bone sits in the distal row of the carpal bones and its unique shape makes it a common fracture location. The hamate is involved in 2% to 4% of all carpal bone fractures. The hamate is susceptible in sports that involve racquets, sticks (eg, lacrosse, field hockey), and clubs (golf). The common MOI involves the handle of the implement placing direct compression against the hook of the

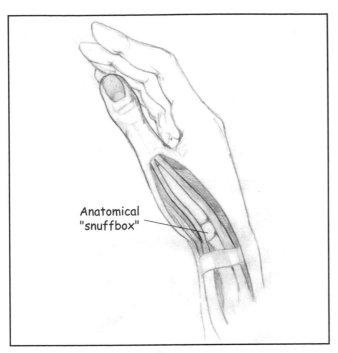

Figure 7-9. Anatomical "snuffbox."

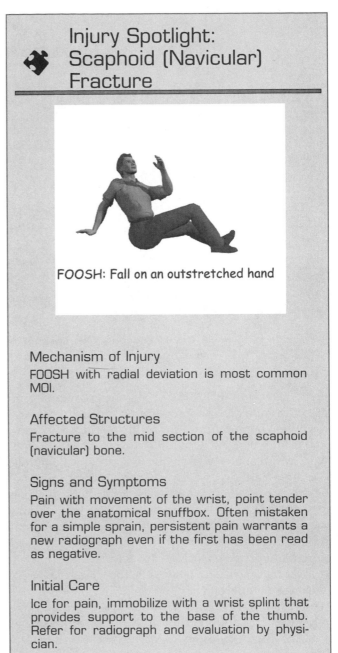

FOOSH: Fall on an outstretched hand

Mechanism of Injury
FOOSH with radial deviation is most common MOI.

Affected Structures
Fracture to the mid section of the scaphoid (navicular) bone.

Signs and Symptoms
Pain with movement of the wrist, point tender over the anatomical snuffbox. Often mistaken for a simple sprain, persistent pain warrants a new radiograph even if the first has been read as negative.

Initial Care
Ice for pain, immobilize with a wrist splint that provides support to the base of the thumb. Refer for radiograph and evaluation by physician.

hamate. In addition, contraction of the hypothenar musculature (the fleshy part at the base of the hand) and flexion of the wrist can also contribute to this fracture.[10] In implement sports (eg, racquets, hockey sticks, lacrosse sticks), the wrist nearest the handle is most susceptible for this injury. Other carpal bones are also susceptible to injury. See Table 7-4 for an overview of their frequency.

Fractures can also occur in the bones of the hand. The most common are those associated with direct blows, secondary to dislocation of the fingers, or associated with avulsions of tendons or ligaments. A boxer's fracture occurs from a blow with a closed fist. This fracture is common to the 4th and 5th metacarpal. A Bennett's fracture is a fracture at the base of the first metacarpal near the articulation of the carpometacarpal articulation.[6] This fracture may cause the thumb to appear shorter when compared to the opposite side. An athlete with this fracture will have pain and swelling at the base of the thumb and a loss of function. This fracture will often require surgical repair to insure adequate function of the thumb.

Other fractures to the phalanges (fingers) can occur when the joint is dislocated. The force associated with a dislocation (usually of the PIP joint) may cause a fracture to the articular region of the phalanx. This is a serious injury. Any fracture that extends into the articular surface is called an osteochondral fracture. These injuries can compromise the long-term health of the joint. All dislocations should be evaluated and a radiograph taken to examine the integrity of the joint surfaces. Avulsion fractures in the fingers can also occur if small pieces of bone are avulsed in conjunction with a ligamentous (sprain) injury or tendon avulsion.

SOFT TISSUE INJURIES

Sprains, Subluxations, and Dislocations

An extensive system of ligaments supports the carpal bones that comprise the wrist joint. The palmar radiocarpal ligament and the dorsal radiocarpal ligament support the radiocarpal (wrist) joint at the distal radius. This complex of ligaments is subject to sprain injuries most often associated with falls.

Table 7-4

Carpal Fractures in Athletes

Type of Carpal Fracture	Percentage of All Bone Injuries to Carpals
Scaphoid	60% to 70%
Triquetral	3% to 4%
Hook of the hamate	2% to 4%
Trapezium	1% to 5%
Pisiform	1% to 3%
Capitate	1% to 2%
Trapezoid	<1%
Lunate	Isolated fractures are rare

Wrist injuries make up between 3% to 9% of all injuries in sport. The above table outlines specific carpal fractures and what percentage of total carpal fractures they represent.

Adapted from Geissler WB. Carpal fractures in athletes. *Clin Sports Med.* 2001;20(1):167-188.

Hyperextension (FOOSH) is the more common forced direction in a wrist sprain. Sprains to the wrist produce general soreness, pain with motion, and some loss of function. As noted in our discussion of scaphoid fractures, any wrist pain that does not improve warrants a radiograph. The scaphoid fracture may not be present on the first x-ray. The MOI that can generate a sprain can also cause a dislocation to one or more carpal bones. Suspected dislocations of a carpal bone should be referred for further evaluation.

An important structure for consideration when evaluating injuries to the wrist is the triangular fibrocartilage complex (TFCC). The TFCC is a disc-like structure that sits at the distal end of the ulna in the wrist joint. It supports the carpal bones on the ulnar side and also helps provide stability to the distal radioulnar joint. Trauma, overuse, and degeneration of the TFCC can cause tears to the TFCC.[3] While symptoms can vary and be vague with degenerative cases, injuries to the TFCC often involve clicking and ulnar side pain. Some cases will require surgical repair. Patients with suspected TFCC injury should be referred for orthopedic assessment.

The PIP and DIP joints are commonly sprained and dislocated in physical activity (Figure 7-10). Too often, the routine nature of the injury causes participants to minimize the seriousness. Athletes themselves will often instinctively apply traction and place the joint back into position.[11] Dislocations can result in underlying fractures and may compromise the health and function of the joint. Pieces of bone or ligament can also become lodged in the joint space following a dislocation. Untrained personnel should not attempt to relocate a dislocation to the interphalangeal (IP). The joint should be splinted on the palmar side of the injury with ice applied to the dorsal side of the injured joint and the athlete referred to a physician.[7]

Sprains to the collateral ligament of the IP joints are common. These joints are small and do not tolerate swelling very well. Individuals who have sprained these joints will often have difficulty with ROM. Regaining full active ROM is essential for proper hand function.

Muscle-Tendon Injuries

Specific injuries to tendons in the hand can lead to a group of finger pathologies that are identified by the resulting deformities they create. A jersey finger is an injury that involves the rupture or avulsion of the flexor digitorum profundus tendon away from the distal phalanx. It is named because of its common mechanism that involves grasping of a jersey and having the flexor tendon pulled away from the distal phalanx. An athlete with a jersey finger will be unable to flex the distal portion of the finger (Figure 7-11). An observable or palpable deformity of the avulsed tendon may be present.

A mallet finger can be thought of as the opposite of a jersey finger. A mallet finger occurs when the tendon of the extensor digitorum is avulsed from the insertion at the distal phalanx. The resultant deformity will cause the distal phalanx to fall into flexion and take on the appearance of a mallet. The athlete will be unable to extend the distal phalanx. Mallet

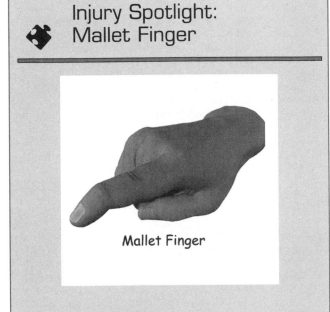

Mallet Finger

Mechanism of Injury

Hit on the end of the finger with a ball, often a baseball. That is why this injury is also called baseball finger.

Affected Structures

A mallet finger occurs when the extensor profundus tendon ruptures or is avulsed from the distal phalanx.

Signs and Symptoms

Pain, associated MOI, inability of patient to extend the distal phalanx when it is isolated.

Initial Care

Since this injury may be associated with an avulsion fracture at the same location, a radiograph is essential. Ice the finger, splint into an extended position, and refer for further evaluation.

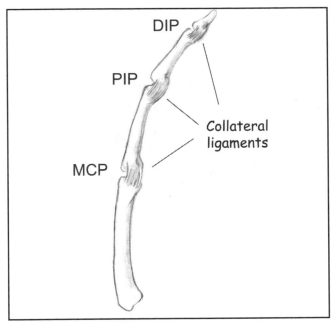

Figure 7-10. Collateral ligaments of the MCP, PIP, and DIP joints.

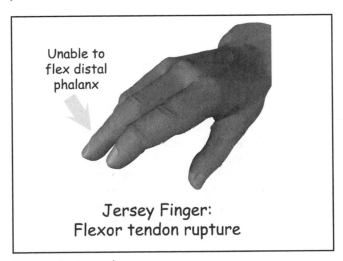

Jersey Finger:
Flexor tendon rupture

Figure 7-11. Jersey finger.

finger is sometimes called baseball finger because the mechanism involves trauma to the end of the finger (common when a ball is misplayed and hits the end of the finger).

A boutonniere deformity is an injury to the PIP joint (Figure 7-12). It occurs when there has been damage to a portion of the extensor digitorum tendon over the top of the PIP joint. The extensor tendon is made up of 2 lateral bands and a dorsal central slip band. A boutonniere injury occurs when hyperflexion of the PIP caused the central slip to rupture. If unattended, the lateral bands will fall to the side and will bowstring, causing the joint to be pulled into a flexion deformity. The boutonniere deformity is characterized by hyperextension at the MCP and DIP joints with flexion of the PIP. Boutonniere deformities must be splinted in

extension for long periods of time to allow for proper healing of the central slip.

NEUROVASCULAR INJURIES

The most common neurovascular injury to the wrist and hand is called carpal tunnel syndrome. Carpal tunnel syndrome is a chronic injury that involves an irritation to the median nerve as it travels through the carpal tunnel. The median nerve crosses the wrist and sits adjacent to the deep and superficial flexor tendons that assist with movement of the wrist and fingers. If you view the hand from the palm side, you can think of the floor of the carpal tunnel being formed by the carpal bones and the roof being formed by the transverse carpal ligament. Repetitive

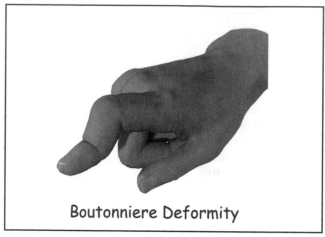

Boutonniere Deformity

Figure 7-12. Boutonniere deformity due to rupture of the central slip.

motion and holding the wrist in flexion for prolonged periods (ie, while sleeping) are common causes of this condition. Treatment involves improving flexibility, decreasing inflammation, and adjusting activities. Surgery is required in some cases to decrease the pressure placed on the median nerve by releasing the transverse carpal ligament.

SUMMARY

Injuries to the upper extremity may only make up approximately 20% of the total injuries in the sports medicine setting, but when you consider only throwing and overhead sports that number rises dramatically. This chapter provides an overview of many common athletic injuries to the upper extremity. As with the lower extremity, the athletic trainer must be able to evaluate; provide initial care; and properly refer, treat, and rehabilitate a wide variety of injuries and conditions for the upper extremity. The ability to understand the relationship between the anatomy, underlying dysfunction, and sport demands is what helps set the athletic trainer apart from other allied health professionals. Students in an athletic training education program must work diligently to understand these relationships. Those who do will be well prepared to care for the wide range of injuries they encounter.

REFERENCES

1. Powell JW, Barber-Foss, KD. Injury patterns in selected high school sports: a review of the 1995-1997 seasons. *Journal of Athletic Training.* 1999;34:277-284.
2. Glenn T, Chopp TM. Functional anatomy of the shoulder. *Journal of Athletic Training.* 2000;35:248-255.
3. Peterson L, Renstrom P. *Sports Injuries: Their Prevention and Treatment.* 3rd ed. Champaign, IL: Human Kinetics; 2001.
4. Warner JP, Boardman ND. Anatomy, biomechanics and pathophysiology of glenohumeral instability. In: Warren RF, Craig E, Altchek DW, eds. *The Unstable Shoulder.* Philadelphia, PA: Lippincott, Williams & Wilkins; 1998:52-55.
5. Williams GR, Kelley M. Management of rotator cuff and impingement injuries in the athlete. *Journal of Athletic Training.* 2000;35:300-315.
6. Sullivan AJ, Anderson SJ. *Care of the Young Athlete.* Oklahoma City, OK: American Academy of Orthopaedic Surgeons & American Academy of Pediatrics; 2000.
7. Hume PA, Reid D, Edwards T. Epicondylar injury in sport. *Sport Med.* 2006;36(2):151-170.
8. Benjamin HJ, Briner WW. Little League elbow. *Clin J Sports Med.* 2005;15(1):37-40.
9. Bauer M, Jonsson , Josefsson PO, Linden B. Osteochondritis dissecans of the elbow: a long-term follow-up study. *Clin Orthop Relat Res.* 1992;284:156-160.
10. Geissler WB. Carpal fractures in athletes. *Clin Sports Med.* 2001;20(1):167-188.
11. Starkey C, Ryan J. *Evaluation of Orthopedic and Athletic Injuries.* 2nd ed. Philadelphia, PA: FA Davis; 2002.

WEB RESOURCES

American Academy of Orthopaedic Surgeons
http://orthoinfo.aaos.org
The AAOS supports this site, which includes general injury information by body part, patient education materials, and information about locating an orthopaedic surgeon. The site also maintains links to sports medicine-related topics.

American Orthopedic Society for Sports Medicine
www.aossm.org
The AOSSM is a national organization of orthopaedic surgeons specializing in sports medicine, including national and international sports medicine leaders.

American Academy of Pediatrics
www.aap.org
The Web site for the AAP provides information regarding many aspects of providing care for children and adolescents. The professional publications sections allow for searches of current position statements and reports.

National Institutes of Health–Medline Plus
www.nlm.nih.gov/medlineplus
A Web site sponsored by the National Institute of Health that provides information on a range of health topics, including injuries, drug and pharmacology information, medical dictionaries, and access to search the Medline database.

Career Spotlight: Athletic Training Professor

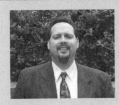

Jay Hertel, PhD, ATC

Associate Professor of Kinesiology

University of Virginia

My Position

As a tenure-track faculty member at a major research university, my job responsibilities fall into 3 primary categories: research, teaching, and service. Research tasks comprise about 50% of my job effort, while undergraduate and graduate teaching comprise about 40%, and institutional and professional service comprise about 10% of my effort. The research process includes development of sound research questions, designing and executing experiments to answer those questions, interpreting the results of the experiments, and disseminating the research results in both oral (conference presentations) and written (journal articles) formats. Another important component of the research process is pursuing grant funding from government, nonprofit, and industry sources to provide financial support for research endeavors.

My primary area of research deals with ankle sprains and instability, which I study from a broad perspective using diverse research methods ranging from laboratory-based assessments of biomechanics and motor control to evidence-based practice principles inherent to clinical epidemiology. While not every study I do has direct clinical application, my goal is to solve problems that impact the clinical practice of athletic trainers and the ability of athletes to participate safely in sports and exercise.

Unique or Desired Qualifications

To become an independent researcher in the university setting, a PhD degree is required. PhD programs typically take at least 4 years to complete beyond the master's degree and the relationship between the student and the advisor is critical as individual mentorship is the cornerstone of PhD-level education. When selecting a PhD program, potential applicants should find an advisor who is an expert in the area in which they want to do research. For example, the PhD students that I mentor are all interested in doing sports medicine-related lower extremity research.

Favorite Aspect of My Job

The favorite part of my job is solving complex clinical problems. Seeing a study through from the inception of the research question to the design of the experiment to the interpretation of the results is an incredibly rewarding process. Additionally, each study that is completed opens up new research questions that can be answered in future work.

Advice

Never be afraid to question assumptions. The only way that clinical practice advances are made is through someone asking the questions that most people do not want to ask.

CHAPTER 8

COMMON INJURIES TO THE HEAD, FACE, AND SPINE

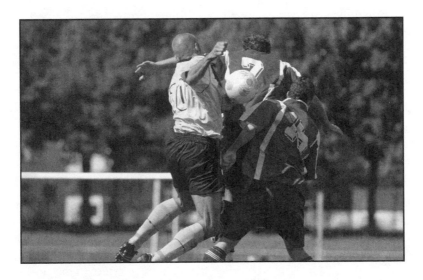

I was fortunate many years ago to have something published in an edition of Cramer's First Aider. *It was called "C" your way to success. To be successful in athletic training, one must rely on: conscientiousness—about responsibilities, competency—be skilled at your craft, and courtesy—treat everybody well. Now I would add another "C", continuing education. I think that is very important for long-term success.*

Thomas E. Abdenour, MA, ATC, CSCS
Athletic Trainer
National Basketball Association–Golden State Warriors

Our skull and spine house the CNS. That is a large responsibility; the center of all movement, thought, balance, emotion, and vital function sloshing around in fluid protected by your skull and a couple dozen or so vertebrae. It is quite an amazing system given the stress and strain we place upon it. The athletic trainer must be aware of the types of injuries that can happen to the head and spine. At times, these injuries may be routine and, at worst, catastrophic. The human skull weighs around 2.2 lbs and despite its thickness (no pun intended), injuries to the brain are commonplace, and they can be deadly if not properly detected. Epidemiology research suggests that over

300,000 sports-related concussions occur annually in the United States.[1] Recent studies suggest that players with a history of previous concussions are more likely to have future concussive injuries than those with no history and that previous concussion may be associated with slower recovery of neurological function.[2] The potential for lifelong disability or even death should give us great pause as care providers when dealing with brain injury—both mild and traumatic.

The spine is equally subject to both mild and catastrophic injury. In Chapter 6, emphasis was placed on the fact that humans walk upright, which contributes to some of our lower extremity problems. However, all adaptations to bipedal motion are not perfect. Our spine evolved from distant ancestors who did not walk upright. In fact, humans are the only species that made this a habitual posture. For our evolutionary ancestors, the spine was like a suspension bridge that supported the body's organs and it was well suited for the role. As we have evolved, the human spine has been transformed into a weight-bearing column that has required us to develop different curvatures and put it under stress. Our evolutionary history has not been kind to the back. Our upright posture has doomed us to the likelihood of back injuries and pain.[3] It is estimated that 60% to 80% of all individuals will experience back pain at some point in their lives.[4] Athletic trainers will see a variety of athletic injuries that involve the spine. While most are not serious, the potential for catastrophic injury serves as a reminder to evaluate and treat with great care.

This chapter also explores other injuries to the face and head that are frequently encountered in active settings. Sticking with our theme, these facial injuries run from the routine laceration to life-altering eye injuries. Again, athletic trainers must be keenly aware of the potential seriousness of these injuries and be prepared to evaluate and refer as needed.

Upon completion of this chapter, the student will be able to:
- ✓ Identify the basic anatomical structures of the skull and spine
- ✓ Describe signs and symptoms of a cerebral concussion
- ✓ List common signs and symptoms of mild and traumatic brain injury
- ✓ Explain the components of a head injury referral checklist
- ✓ Discuss the importance of home care and follow-up in treating head injuries
- ✓ Identify common injuries to the face and head
- ✓ List specific factors that predispose individuals to back pain
- ✓ Explain the signs and symptoms of common spine injuries
- ✓ Discuss the potential for catastrophic injury when dealing with the head and spine

ANATOMY

FACE AND SKULL

Twenty-two individual bones make up the skull (Figure 8-1). There are 8 cranial bones and 14 facial bones. The bones of the skull are fused together in a

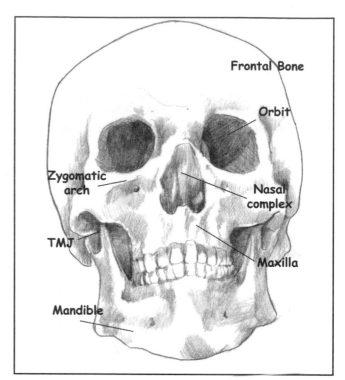

Figure 8-1. Anterior view, skull.

collection of immovable joints. These joints are called sutures. The jawbone or mandible is the only movable bone in the skull. The mandible is attached to the skull at the temporomandibular joint (TMJ). The skull is covered with layers of tissue that make up the scalp. The cranium refers to the portion of the skull that protects the brain. As we discuss injuries to the head, we will discuss the cranium and face separately.

The brain and the spinal cord make up the CNS. The cerebrum, cerebellum, and brainstem (pons and medulla oblongata) make up the main sections of the brain. Our brain controls mental function, complex movements, memory, emotion, balance, sleep, and countless vital functions. Table 8-1 outlines the various functions of different regions of the brain. Twelve pairs of cranial nerves are attached to the base of the brain and leave the CNS to control various functions. Smiling, frowning, hearing, vision, eye movement, taste, smell, and several other functions are directly controlled by the cranial nerves. The CNS has a very good blood supply.

Layers of membrane surround and protect our brain and spinal cord. These membranes are known as meninges. These include the dura mater, arachnoid, and pia mater. The space between the dura mater and the skull is called the epidural space. Any injury below the dura mater is considered sub dural or below the dura. Cerebrospinal fluid (CSF) is contained in the space below the arachnoid layer. CSF protects the brain and spinal cord. The brain is suspended in this

Table 8-1

Main Regions of the Brain

Region	Function
Cerebrum (Hemispheres)	Four lobes: frontal, temporal, parietal, and occipital
	The cerebrum coordinates voluntary movements, interprets sensory information, controls higher-level brain function (intelligence, reason, emotion, etc)
Cerebellum	Second largest area of the brain connected to the brainstem
	Essential to balance, equilibrium, and voluntary muscle movements
Brainstem	Sits deep in the brain and leads to the spinal cord. Controls breathing, heart rate, swallowing, reflexes to seeing and hearing, sweating, blood pressure, digestion, temperature, alertness, and sleep
	The pons is part of the brainstem that contains the origin of the 5th through 8th cranial nerves
	The medulla oblongata is part of the brainstem that contains the origins of the 9th through 12th cranial nerves

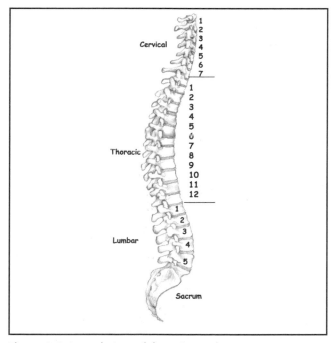

Figure 8-2. Lateral view of the spine.

fluid, which serves to protect the brain as the head moves or comes into contact with an object. Steady delivery of oxygen is required for optimal function of the CNS and the CNS has an extensive blood supply. Disruptions in this blood flow or change in oxygen level can cause irreparable damage after just a few minutes time.

Spine

The spine is divided into 4 regions: cervical, thoracic, lumbar, and sacral (Figure 8-2). There are 7 cer-

vical vertebrae. The cervical spine provides support for the skull and allows for rotation of the neck. The first 2 vertebrae are unique. While the skull articulates with C-1 also known as the atlas, C-2 is known as the axis. They combine to form the atlantoaxial joint. As you travel from the skull to the base of the spine, the vertebrae get progressively larger. This is due to the spines evolution as a weight-bearing column. Paired spinal nerves depart the spinal cord at the level between each vertebra. These nerves transmit sensory impulses from the periphery and carry motor impulses to the periphery. The upper cervical spinal nerves (1st through 3rd) are responsible for providing sensations to the head and face. The nerves from the mid and lower cervical spine combine to form the brachial plexus, a collection of nerves that innervate the arms. The cervical spine allows for the movements of flexion, extension, rotation, and lateral flexion.

Twelve vertebrae make up the thoracic spine. The thoracic spine sits below the cervical region and allows for the articulation with the 12 pairs of ribs. The ribs articulate with either the sternum or costal cartilage. Collectively, the thoracic vertebrae, ribs, and sternum make up the rib cage (thoracic cage). The movement of the thoracic spine is limited. Most of the available rotation of the spine takes place at the thoracic level. Most movement of the rib cage allows for inspiration and expiration.

The lumbar spine consists of 5 vertebrae that sit below the thoracic vertebrae. The lumbar vertebrae are the largest of the vertebrae. The movements of the lumbar spine include flexion, extension, and lateral flexion.

Sitting between each of the vertebrae are intervertebral disks that act as shock absorbers. They have often been compared to jelly donuts due to their viscous center and tough fibrous outer material. The inner region of the disc is known as the nucleus pulposus and the outer edge is known as the annulus fibrosus. Each intervertebral disk has very high water content. As we age, the disks will lose some of this water content and become more susceptible to injury. If the outer ring of the disk deteriorates, the nucleus will protrude outward and put pressure on the adjacent spinal nerves. Pressure on the disks increases with flexion. If there is deterioration in tissue, this will cause pain.

The vertebrae (cervical, thoracic, and lumbar) are stabilized by ligaments that travel the length of the spinal column: the anterior and posterior longitudinal ligament. This ligament helps provide stability during flexion and extension movements. The vertebrae have articulations above and below called facet joints. The facets, like all joints, have articular surfaces and are subject to irritations and sprain-type injuries. The facet surfaces at the cervical spine are in a more transverse plane and become more upright as you travel toward the lumbar vertebrae.

The sacrum is a group of 5 fused vertebrae. The sacrum articulates with the ilium of the pelvis to form the SI joints. Strong ligaments that bind the sacrum to the pelvis hold the SI joints. The SI joint is a common site of lumbar/pelvic pain. The SI joint binds our axial and lower appendicular skeletons together. A small pointed bone that hangs off the end of the sacrum is called the coccyx (sometimes referred to as the tailbone).

Several muscle groups act on the various regions of the spine. Groups of muscles sit on each side of the spinal column and are referred to as the paraspinal muscle groups. They include the erector spinae group, which helps support the spinal column and contributes to extension movements of the spine. The spinal column is also stabilized and supported by the muscles of the trunk, abdomen, and hip/trunk flexors. These muscles collectively help stabilize vertebrae during a variety of movements. Table 8-2 presents some of the major muscles of the trunk and their respective function.

INJURIES TO THE HEAD AND SPINE

CONCUSSIONS—MILD TRAUMATIC BRAIN INJURY

The Consumer Product Safety Commission maintains the National Electronic Injury Surveillance System, which estimated that over 54,000 teenagers were treated for concussions in 2007 with over half of those being related to recreation and sport.[5] This injury database is maintained by a representative sample of clinics, hospitals, and emergency facilities nationwide. When you consider that head injury, specifically mild traumatic head injury, is likely to be underreported[6] the potential scope of the problem is even larger.

The most common sports injury involving the brain is the concussion. The terms *concussion* and *mild traumatic brain injury* (MTBI) are sometimes used synonymously. While the medical community has not completely agreed on a consistent way to define concussions or to classify their severity, the definition of concussion has evolved in recent years. The most widely used definition to date is provided by the Congress of Neurologic Surgeons. In 1966, it stated that[7]:

> *...a concussion is a collection of signs and symptoms (clinical syndrome) characterized by an immediate and transient impairment of neural functions, such as alteration of consciousness, disturbance of vision and equilibrium due to brainstem involvement.*

Currently, there is agreement that the 1966 definition failed to address key factors. While there may not be complete agreement on the definition or nature of concussions, there is consensus on several features of concussion that incorporate clinical, pathologic, and biomechanical injury constructs associated with head injury.[8] A concussion may:

✓ Be caused by a direct blow to the head or elsewhere on the body from an "impulsive" force transmission to the head.

✓ Cause an immediate and short-lived impairment of neurologic function.

✓ Cause neuropathologic changes; however, the acute clinical symptoms largely reflect a functional disturbance rather than a structural injury.

Table 8-2

Major Muscles, Primary Actions, and Innervations of the Trunk and Spine

Deep Muscles of the Trunk and Spine

Muscles	Action	Innervation
Splenius Muscles		

Splenius capitus
Splenius cervicis
	Bilateral contraction:
	    Extension of the head and neck
	Unilateral contraction:
	    Rotation and lateral flexion
		Dorsal rami of the lower and middle cervical spinal nerves

Erector Spinae Muscles The actions are the same for all of the erector spinae muscles		

Iliocostalis lumborum
Iliocostalis thoracis
Iliocostalis cervicis
Longissimus thoracis
Longissimus cervicis
Longissimus capitis
Spinalis thoracis
Spinalis cervicis
Spinalis capitis
	Bilateral contraction:
	    Extension of the vertebral column
	    Maintenance of correct posture
	    Stabilization of the vertebral column during
	        flexion, act in contrast to the abdominal
	        muscles and to gravity
	Unilateral contraction:
	    Rotation and lateral flexion (same side)
		Dorsal rami of the spinal nerves

Transversospinal Muscles		
Semispinalis thoracis Semispinalis cervicis Semispinalis capitis	Bilateral extension of the vertebral column (primarily head and neck) Eccentric control of lateral flexion to opposite side Maintain head posture	Dorsal rami of the spinal nerves
Multifidus	Bilateral extension of the vertebral column Eccentric control of lateral flexion to opposite side Unilateral rotation of vertebral bodies (column)	Dorsal rami of the spinal nerves
Long and short rotators	Bilateral extension and rotation to opposite side	Dorsal rami of the spinal nerves
Segmental Muscles		
Interspinales Intertransversi	Extension of the vertebrae segments Lateral flexion of the transverse process immediately above Stability via eccentric contraction	Ventral and dorsal rami of the spinal nerves

✓ Cause a gradient of clinical syndromes that may or may not involve loss of consciousness (LOC). Resolution of the clinical and cognitive symptoms typically follows a sequential course.

✓ Often be associated with normal tests on conventional neuroimaging studies.[9]

The following signs and symptoms are associated with MTBI[10]:

✓ Headache

✓ Ringing in the ears

✓ Nausea

✓ Emotional changes (irritability)

✓ Confusion or disorientation

✓ LOC

✓ Dizziness

✓ Amnesia

   o Retrograde—forgetting items before the injury

   o Anterograde—forgetting items after the injury

✓ Difficulty with concentration

✓ Motor imbalances

✓ Blurred vision

✓ LOC is not required to sustain a concussion.

Signs and symptoms can differ greatly from one individual to the next. It is essential that the athletic trainer be proficient at evaluating possible concussions for the purpose of appropriate referral.

No athlete with signs and symptoms of a head injury should be permitted to return to play.

The majority of grading systems classify the severity of MTBI based on LOC, presence of amnesia, or other symptoms.[11] Determining the severity and grading of concussions is a point of disagreement among medical professionals and researchers. The most common approaches have focused on LOC, post-traumatic amnesia, and postconcussion signs and symptoms. Reliance on LOC as a grade of severity has not been shown to be predictive of recovery from brain injury.[11] An approach has been presented to this grading-scale dilemma and that is not to use a grading scale at all. Care providers should focus attention on the athlete's recovery via symptoms, neuropsychological tests, and postural stability tests. This removed the attention from trying to fit the patient's symptoms into a grading system and put the focus on whether the athlete is symptomatic or symptom free. Once symptom free, a progressive return to activity can be monitored. This multitiered approach was summarized and supported by consensus at the 2001 Vienna Conference on Concussion in Sport.[8,9]

Once the athlete is evaluated by a physician, the athletic trainer and physician can work together in developing logical criteria for return to competition. The athletic trainer can be a vital resource since he or she likely has more consistent interaction with the athlete than the physician. The athletic trainer knows the athlete's behavior on a daily basis and can be a good judge of how the postconcussive patient is responding. Decisions on return to play and release from care fall to the physician, but the best care requires a team approach.

Issues surrounding the classification, management, and return to play following MTBI are receiving significant attention from sports medicine researchers.[2,8,10,12,13] The use of objective measures rather than subjective observations is improving our understanding of how to recognize signs and symptoms of concussion to facilitate referral and assure safe return to play.[12] The Standardized Assessment of Concussions (SAC) test was developed to evaluate orientation, immediate memory, concentration, delayed recall, and symptoms with light exertion in a simple format that can be used in a sideline situation.[13] The advantage of such a test is the ability to take preseason measures thus creating a baseline for comparison. While research continues, early indications are that such tests can be useful in a variety of athletic training situations.

Neuropsychological testing can be used to establish baseline evaluation of specific cognitive domains that often are disrupted with a MTBI. The use of these tests to evaluate the cognitive effects and recovery of concussion has been shown to be a valuable tool. The nature of the tests and the 20- to 30-minute administration time do not make them a sideline assessment tool but rather a baseline measure to which progress can be compared. Properly trained individuals must administer and interpret these tests. Computerized neuropsychological tests are gaining popularity due to their ease of application. However, further research is needed in this area to address a variety of issues (eg, test reliability, validity, sensitivity, interpretation, practice effects).[8]

TRAUMATIC BRAIN INJURIES

The brain is suspended in the skull in CSF and can be injured either by a direct blow from a moving object to the skull (a coup injury) or the skull moving and hitting a stationary object (a contrecoup injury) as happens when someone falls to the ground (Figures 8-3 and 8-4). A coup mechanism usually results in an injury at the site of the contact, while a contrecoup injury can occur on the opposite side of the brain from the movement and contact. A shaking of the brain, direct blow, or indirect contact can cause a concussion. The concussion may be a bruising or contusion to the brain or it may include actual intracranial bleeding.

While most concussions are mild, a variety of serious traumatic brain injuries (TBI) can be seen. TBI can be classified into 2 types: focal and diffuse. Focal lesions include subdural hematomas, epidural hematomas, cerebral contusions, and intracranial hemorrhages and hematomas.[8]

These focal injuries can cause bleeding and swelling in the brain that is problematic due to the fact that the brain is encased within the skull. There is little room for edema to dissipate. An epidural hematoma can form if arteries in the membranes near the dura matter are torn due to the MOI or force of contact. An athlete with an epidural hematoma may briefly appear normal and then collapse. Epidural hematomas form rapidly secondary to arterial bleeding. This patient requires immediate referral to a trauma center. If untreated, an epidural hematoma can cause permanent damage to the brain or death. A subdural hematoma can occur acutely or may develop slowly following a concussive event. Subdural hematomas are most often associated with venous bleeding or edema that forms more slowly, thus causing a slower development of symptoms.

Proper Helmet Fitting

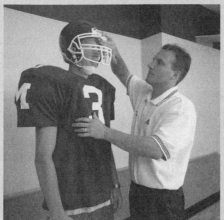

The ability to properly fit a football helmet is an essential skill for the certified athletic trainer. The proper fit of the helmet is essential for maximum player protection. Studies have shown that multiple errors in helmet fitting occur at the secondary school level when players and coaches fit their own helmet.[1,2] While a full discussion of protective equipment is beyond the scope of this text, knowing the appropriate steps to fit a helmet is a perfect first step for the athletic training student.

Helmet Fitting Steps

- A circumference measurement of the head with the tape 1 inch above the eyebrow will help determine the general size needed. Since sizes vary among manufacturers, this should only be used as a starting point for the steps below.
- Manufacturers recommend a shorter hair style during the season when using the helmet. Changes in hair length may require a new fitting.
- Follow the 7 criteria below:
  - 1-inch spacing above the eyebrows—downward pressure should be felt on the crown of the head and not the brow
  - 2-inch clearance from the nose to the face mask
  - Chinstrap centered and taught (all 4 points buckled)
  - Jaw pads snug to the face
  - Ear holes aligned with the ears
  - Adequate coverage over the base of the skull
  - Minimal movement of the shell with anterior, posterior, or lateral pressure
- Helmets should be inspected at regular intervals
- Only helmets that meet the National Operating Committee on Standards for Athletic Equipment (NOCSAE) standard for safety should be used. Each helmet should contain the NOCSAE stamp or sticker.

References

1. McGuine T, Nass S. Football helmet fitting errors in Wisconsin High School Players: safety in American football, ASTM STP 1305. In: Hoerner EF, ed. *American Society for Testing and Materials*. West Conshohocken, PA: Author; 1996;83-88.
2. Hong E, Covassin T. Relationship between football helmet fitting techniques and concussions in high school football athletes: paper presented at the American College of Sports Medicine. *Am J Sports Med.* 2006;38(5):S437.

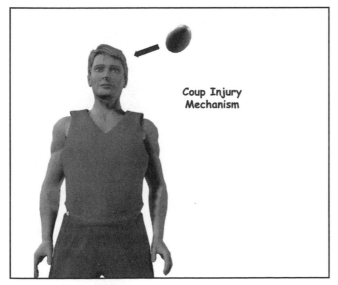

Figure 8-3. Coup MOI.

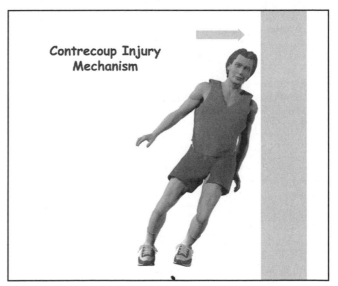

Figure 8-4. Contrecoup MOI.

Patients with focal injuries as described previously will show signs of increasing intracranial pressure associated with a clinical deterioration with worsening symptoms, which include the following[8]:
- ✓ LOC
- ✓ Cranial nerve deficits
- ✓ Mental status disorientation
- ✓ Worsening symptoms
  - o Persistent or increasing headache
  - o Headache with concentrated thought
  - o Nausea and vomiting
  - o Confusion or disorientation
  - o Changes in pupil size (unequal)
  - o Motor impairments
  - o Slowing of the pulse

Increasing intracranial pressure that is undetected can be fatal because the pressure pushes downward on the brainstem and vital functions can be compromised. Patients who have sustained concussions are often hospitalized for observation of intracranial pressure. Short of hospitalization, it is good practice to provide home instruction to parents, spouses, and roommates regarding these signs and symptoms. There is no such thing as a "minor concussion." Follow-up care is essential for a successful outcome following a head injury.

 Proper Terminology

Any fan who has ever watched a football game on television has heard the lingo after a hard hit, "Boy, did he get his bell rung." or "He will be ok. He just got dinged." We might sit up and take better notice if they appropriately reported that the player sustained a brain injury. The use of these terms should be discouraged. An athlete in a confused state after a hard blow has sustained a concussion, resulting in symptoms. Even if these symptoms are brief, they need to be assessed and re-evaluated frequently. The full signs of a concussion may not present right away (minutes or hours later). We cannot be dismissive of injuries to the brain. Allied health professions (and those in training) should use the proper vocabulary. Let us discard the "ding."

No athlete should be allowed to return to play unless the signs and symptoms of a concussion have completely cleared. If the athlete returns too soon, he or she risks a second impact syndrome. Second impact syndrome occurs due to rapid swelling and herniation of the brain after a second head injury that takes place before a previous head injury has resolved.[14] The previous head injury need not be serious. Second impact syndrome can occur following a minor head injury. These injuries have a rapid onset and the athlete's condition will deteriorate quickly. The mortality rate for second impact syndrome is high. Immediate activation of an emergency plan and immediate transport to a trauma center are essential.

CONCUSSION ASSESSMENT

The outline below provides considerations for evaluating a patient with a concussion. The following must be taken into account:
- ✓ Primary survey to determine proper airway and circulation
- ✓ Establish level of consciousness
- ✓ Obtain a history regarding:
  - o LOC
  - o Orientation to surroundings
  - o Amnesia
- ✓ Presence of postconcussion symptoms[6]:
  - o Headache
  - o Nausea
  - o Vomiting
  - o Dizziness
  - o Balance
  - o Sensitivity to noise
  - o Ringing in the ears
  - o Blurred vision
  - o Sensitivity to light
  - o Concentration
  - o Memory
  - o Drowsiness
  - o Fatigue
  - o Emotional state (sadness/depression)
  - o Irritability
  - o Neck pain
- ✓ Cranial nerve assessment (Table 8-3)
- ✓ Vital signs
  - o Pulse
  - o Respiration
  - o Blood pressure
- ✓ Objective measures of balance
- ✓ Standardized assessment

Information gathered from the evaluation is too often subjective and difficult to follow. Any effort to standardize evaluative findings, use objective measures of balance, or a standardized assessment test

Table 8-3
Cranial Nerves

Nerve (Number/Name)	Primary Function to Evaluate
I Olfactory	Smell
II Optic	Vision
III Oculomotor	Eye movement / pupil size
IV Trochlear	Eye movement
V Trigeminal	Facial sensations, jaw movements
VI Abducens	Movement of eye muscles (lateral)
VII Facial	Facial movements
VIII Vestibulocochlear	Hearing and equilibrium
IX Glossopharyngeal	Taste, throat movement
X Valgus	Swallowing, taste
XI Accessory	Movement of neck and shoulders
XII Hypoglossal	Movement of the tongue, swallowing

will be of value to the athletic trainer and physician. Clinicians must take steps to eliminate subjective components as much as possible.

Evaluating a patient for a concussion will follow a thorough evaluation that includes a history, observation (including pupil responses), palpation, and functional testing. Functional testing includes simple tests for memory, concentration, coordination, and cranial nerve assessment. The NATA Position Statement on Management of Sport Related Concussion[8] recommends using a graded symptom checklist (GSC) for keeping track of concussion symptoms in a serial fashion (Figure 8-5) from initial injury and at various time intervals.

Given the potential of serious injury, athletic trainers should have a low tolerance for referral for assessment by a physician for any head injury. It is standard practice to provide proper instructions for home care after a concussion has been properly evaluated. Despite this widespread practice, there is little scientific evidence on the support of these instructions.[8] Instructions should be provided to a responsible adult who will have direct contact with the patient during the 24 hours postinjury. The form provides a list of signs and symptoms to watch for and provides recommendations for follow-up care. Figures 8-6 and 8-7 provide examples of referral sheets and home care instructions.

RETURN TO PLAY FOLLOWING MILD TRAUMATIC BRAIN INJURY

Determining when to return a participant to full physical activity following a concussion is a challenging decision for the sports medicine physician. It has been reported that 30% of all high school and collegiate football players sustaining a concussion return the same day, with the remaining 70% averaging 4 days prior to returning to participation.[10] Many return-to-play guidelines call for the patient to be symptom free for 7 days prior to returning from a grade 1 or grade 2 concussion. Guskiewicz et al[2] suggest that the 7-day wait may minimize the risk of recurrent injury. The nature of repeat injury is a concern for care providers. It is suggested that same-season repeat injuries typically take place within a short window of time, 7 to 10 days after the first concussion.[2] This supports the idea that the brain may be more vulnerable for injury during that period.

After an athlete is symptom free, a step-wise progression of activity should be used to determine his or her ability to return to participation. All signs and symptoms must be evaluated using a GSC (see Figure 8-5) or similar tool. Follow-up assessments should be done at rest and after exertional activities such as biking, jogging, sit-ups, and push-ups.[8]

Graded Symptom Checklist (GSC)

Symptom	Time of Injury	2 to 3 Hours Postinjury	24 Hours Postinjury	48 Hours Postinjury	72 Hours Postinjury
Blurred vision					
Dizziness					
Drowsiness					
Excess sleep					
Easily distracted					
Fatigue					
Feel "in a fog"					
Feel "slowed down"					
Headache					
Inappropriate emotions					
Irritability					
Loss of consciousness					
Loss of orientation					
Memory problems					
Nausea					
Nervousness					
Personality change					
Poor balance/coordination					
Poor concentration					
Ringing in ears					
Sadness					
Seeing stars					
Sensitivity to light					
Sensitivity to noise					
Sleep disturbance					
Vacant stare/glassy eyed					
Vomiting					

Note: The GSC should be used not only for the initial evaluation but for each subsequent follow-up assessment until all signs and symptoms have cleared at rest and during physical exertion. In lieu of simply checking each symptom present, the ATC can ask the athlete to grade or score the severity of the symptom on a scale of 0 to 6, where 0 = not present, 1 = mild, 3 = moderate, and 6 = most severe.

Figure 8-5. Graded symptom checklist (GSC). (Reprinted with permission from Guskiewicz KM, Bruce SL, Cantu RC, et al. National Athletic Trainers' Association position statement: management of sport-related concussion. *Journal of Athletic Training.* 2004;39(3):280-297.)

Day-of-Injury Referral

Refer if any of the following are present:
- Loss of consciousness on the field
- Amnesia lasting longer than 15 min
- Deterioration of neurologic function*
- Decreasing level of consciousness*
- Decrease or irregularity in respirations*
- Decrease or irregularity in pulse*
- Increase in blood pressure
- Unequal, dilated, or unreactive pupils*
- Cranial nerve deficits
- Any signs or symptoms of associated injuries, spine or skull fracture, or bleeding*
- Mental status changes: lethargy, difficulty maintaining arousal, confusion, or agitation*
- Seizure activity*
- Vomiting
- Motor deficits subsequent to initial on-field assessment
- Sensory deficits subsequent to initial on-field assessment
- Balance deficits subsequent to initial on-field assessment
- Cranial nerve deficits subsequent to initial on-field assessment
- Postconcussion symptoms that worsen
- Additional postconcussion symptoms as compared with those on the field
- Athlete is still symptomatic at the end of the game (especially at high school level)

*Requires that the athlete be transported immediately to the nearest emergency department.

Delayed Referral (After the Day of Injury)

- Any of the findings in the day-of-injury referral category
- Postconcussion symptoms worsen or do not improve over time
- Increase in the number of postconcussion symptoms reported
- Postconcussion symptoms begin to interfere with the athlete's daily activities (i.e., sleep disturbances or cognitive difficulties)

Figure 8-6. Physician referral checklist. (Reprinted with permission from Guskiewicz KM, Bruce SL, Cantu RC, et al. National Athletic Trainers' association position statement: management of sport-related concussion. *Journal of Athletic Training.* 2004;39(3):280-297.)

Neuropsychological baselines and postural stability measures are recommended for comparing with postinjury measures. If an athlete can tolerate exertional activities without recurrent symptoms, then he or she resumes limited practice provided there is no risk of recurrent head injury. Athletes should not return to full contact participation until they are symptom free and fully tolerate limited practice activities. Neuropsychological and postural assessments should be repeated if available to determine if all scores have returned to baseline. It is strongly recommended that if an athlete has a recurrent injury,

especially a same-season injury, that the athlete be withheld from competition for an extended period of time (~7 days) after symptoms have resolved.[8]

A copy of the recommendations from the NATA Position Statement: Management of Sport Related Concussion appears at the end of this chapter.

POSTCONCUSSIVE SYNDROME

A postconcussive syndrome is a condition that occurs when signs and symptoms of concussion are persistent beyond the expected length of time. Postconcussive syndromes may be seen following

---

Concussion Home Instructions

I believe that _____ sustained a concussion on _____. To make sure he/she recovers, please follow the following important recommendations:

- Please remind _____ to report to the athletic training room tomorrow at _____ for a follow-up evaluation.

- Please review the items outlined on the enclosed Physician Referral Checklist. If any of these problems develop prior to his/her visit, please call _____ at _____ or contact the local emergency medical system or your family physician. Otherwise, you can follow the instructions outlined below.

It is OK to:	There is NO need to:	Do NOT:
• Use acetaminophen (Tylenol) for headaches	• Check eyes with flashlight	• Drink alcohol
• Use ice pack on head and neck as needed for comfort	• Wake up every hour	• Eat spicy foods
• Eat a light diet	• Test reflexes	
• Return to school	• Stay in bed	
• Go to sleep		
• Rest (no strenuous activity)		

Specific recommendations:

Recommendations provided to: _____

Recommendations provided by:_____ Date: _____ Time: _____

Please feel free to contact me if you have any questions. I can be reached at: _____

Signature: _____ Date: _____

Figure 8-7. Concussion: home care instruction form. (Reprinted with permission from Guskiewicz KM, Bruce SL, Cantu RC, et al. National Athletic Trainers' association position statement: management of sport-related concussion. *Journal of Athletic Training.* 2004;39(3):280-297.)

mild or severe head injuries. The signs and symptoms may include persistent headache, memory loss, fatigue, emotional instability, depression, increasing symptoms with activity, and persistent motor imbalances.[11] Postconcussive syndromes may last for months and may never fully resolve in severe injuries. Proper referral and follow-up care from a neurosurgeon are appropriate and testing administered and interpreted by a neuropsychologist may be recommended to monitor the progress of the postconcussive patient.

SKULL FRACTURES

Skull fractures may occur from a direct blow or blunt trauma from a bat, ball, racquet, or some other implement. Falls from a height (pole vault, equestrian sports, etc) provide a logical mechanism for a skull fracture. Patients who have sustained this injury will have pain, nausea, headache, and possibly a palpable

deformity. There may be bleeding from the nose (epistaxis), leakage of CSF from the ears (otorrhea) or nose (rhinorrhea), and the presence of a battle sign (discoloration behind the ear). Any patient with a suspected skull fracture must be transported for immediate evaluation.

FACIAL INJURIES

Several injuries can occur to the face. They range from the simple lacerations and hematomas to complex fractures. When dealing with injuries to the face, the athletic trainer must be acutely aware that injuries that can cause damage to the various tissues of the face may very well cause damage to the brain. Any athlete with a facial injury must be evaluated for the presence of brain trauma. The athletic trainer must remember to not be mislead by the obvious. If your

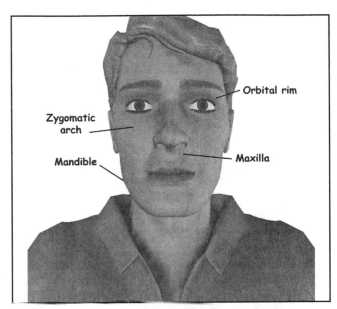

Figure 8-8. Common locations of facial injury.

player was hit hard enough for a nosebleed, hematoma, or laceration, he or she may well have been hit hard enough to injure the brain. Do not let the bleeding or obvious contusion detract from checking what lies beneath, the possible mild brain trauma.

FRACTURES

Three common bone injuries to the face include the orbital or blow out fracture, fractures to the zygomatic arch (cheek bone), and fractures to the mandible (jaw) (Figure 8-8). The most common mechanisms for each of these injuries is a punch or elbow to the face, hit by a ball or other spherical object, or blunt trauma. An orbital fracture occurs when the bones that support the eye are fractured due to one of the previously discussed mechanisms. The floor of the orbit can "blow out" and cause muscles that control eye movements to become entrapped at the fracture site.[15] Signs and symptoms of a blow out fracture include pain, swelling, double vision (diplopia), limits in eye motion, and sinking of the eye in the damaged socket. The athlete may feel some numbness on the check region due to compromise of the sensory nerve. Proper care includes an immediate referral for radiographs and a thorough medical evaluation.

Fractures to the zygomatic arch occur as a result of a direct blow. Getting hit by an errant elbow on a basketball rebound is a typical MOI. Swelling, deformity, and a defect with palpation are common with a fracture to this area. Associated nosebleeds, double vision, and numbness in the cheek may occur. Initial treatment should include the application of ice, and referral to a physician is the immediate course of action. Some fractures of this nature require surgical

repair and may require special protective equipment to avoid contact with the healing or repaired bone.

The fracture to the mandible is the most common facial fracture.[15] The mechanism is once again a direct blow. The jaw is susceptible to direct injury and has very little soft tissue protection. An athlete with a fracture to the mandible will have pain when biting down, misalignment of the teeth, point tenderness, and a possible deformity. The individual with a suspected fracture to the mandible must be referred for radiographs. The jaw may require fixation (usually wired shut once positioned) for a period of 6 to 8 weeks.[15] These athletes may be prone to weight loss due to an extended liquid diet. The consequences of such weight loss must be taken into consideration depending on the athlete's desired sport or activity.

SOFT TISSUE INJURIES

Several soft tissue injuries can occur to the face, most caused by direct blows or being hit by an object. Two types of hematomas are identified based on their location: the orbital hematoma and the auricular hematoma. An orbital hematoma is a "black eye" characterized by swelling near and around the orbital rim. Orbital hematomas are usually the result of a direct contact injury or often caused by a ball or object. The athletic trainer must take care to insure that there is not an underlying fracture and that the eye's vision has not been compromised. Initial care involves ice and proper referral. The auricular hematoma is an injury to the outer ear that can cause swelling and permanent damage to the appearance of the ear. An auricular hematoma that does not resolve properly can lead to cauliflower ear so named because of its bumpy, misshapen appearance. The cauliflower ear is common among wrestlers, rugby athletes, and boxers. Protective headgear can help prevent this injury. The cauliflower ear (Figure 8-9) was identified centuries ago. Statues of ancient Greek wrestlers depict them with cauliflower ears. The best course of treatment is to avoid the condition, therefore athletes must wear protective headgear. Should an athlete sustain an auricular hematoma, ice and compression are the immediate courses of action. If the swelling does not dissipate, the athlete should be referred to a physician to drain the fluid from the ear. This referral should be the same day if possible. The longer the time period between injury and aspiration, the greater the possibility of scarring, which can cause the cauliflower appearance. Constant pressure must be maintained on the ear after it has been aspirated.

Lacerations to the face and skull are common in athletic settings. Again, direct blows are the most common MOI. A laceration is characterized by jagged edges thus requiring careful closure to insure less of a

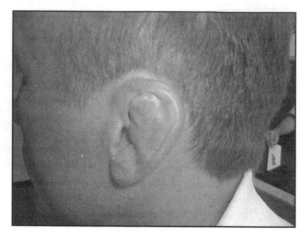

Figure 8-9. Cauliflower ear.

scar. The orbital rim and eyebrow region are common locations for lacerations. Even a small facial laceration may bleed profusely. The athletic trainer must use universal precautions, stop the bleeding, and refer the patient for sutures. Often a small facial laceration can be cared for without sutures; however, people can be quite sensitive about facial scars and their resulting appearance. Referral to the physician and closing the wound in such a way that will limit the scar are the preferred treatment options.

Nosebleeds can occur in several sport and recreation activities. A nosebleed occurs when one or more blood vessels in the nose have ruptured. Another term for a nosebleed is epistaxis. Care of the bleeding nose involves the following:

- ✓ Exercise universal precautions
- ✓ Sit the athlete upright
- ✓ Pinch the nostrils for 10 minutes with the head in an upright position
- ✓ A nose plug or cotton dressing may be used for about 1 hour
- ✓ Care should be taken to insure the plug is not too small and can easily be removed
- ✓ Tilting of the head back is contraindicated
- ✓ Persistent bleeding is cause for referral to the physician

If palpation produces pain or crepitus (a crunchy sensation with palpation) or a deformity is present, a nasal fracture or deviated septum should be suspected. Reduction of the deviation should not be done acutely as this may increase the amount of bleeding and soft tissue damage.[11] These patients should be referred for evaluation. Initial care requires the athletic trainer to control bleeding and apply ice to reduce pain. As previously mentioned, it is important to consider the possibility of an underlying brain injury when dealing with an obvious facial injury. Do not be mislead by the obvious.

The TMJ is prone to both acute and chronic injury. The TMJ connects the mandible to the skull and allows the jaw to move up and down. The TMJ may be the source of chronic pain due to changes at the joint surfaces or inflammation of the joint capsule. This chronic condition is referred to as TMJ syndrome. The TMJ joint may also dislocate with a forceful blow to an open jaw. This injury will produce significant pain, deformity, and loss of function.

 Take Your ID to the MD

An athlete with a deviated septum may be referred to the ear, nose, and throat (ENT) specialist to have the nose set back to its original position. However, the swelling and obvious deformity may make it difficult for the physician to determine the appearance of original preinjury state. To assist the physician with this task, have the athlete take his or her driver's license or university identification card with him or her. This gives the physician a reference point when alleviating the nasal deformity.

DENTAL INJURIES

Dental injuries can largely be prevented by the use of a mouth guard. Injuries can take place due to collisions with opponents or contact with equipment. The front teeth in the upper jaw are the most commonly injured in sport activity. Children are at risk for dental injuries and 25% of all dental injuries in children take place during physical activity or sport.[15] The anatomy of the tooth consists of 4 types of tissue: pulp, enamel, dentin, and cementum (Figure 8-10). The pulp consists of nerve and blood vessels that supply the tooth. The enamel is the outer covering of the crown of the tooth. It is inorganic in nature and thus has a white covering. It is between 1 to 2 mm thick. The dentin lies between the enamel and the pulp chamber. The dentin is organic in nature and has a more yellow color when compared to the enamel. The cementum is the outer covering of the root of the tooth. This is where the periodontal ligament attaches to hold the tooth in place.

Common dental injuries include contusions, luxations, avulsions, and fractures. A contusion is a direct blow to the tooth that can cause irritation to the underlying nerve. Contusions require regular follow-up to insure that the nerve does not become inflamed and cause further pain or damage. A luxation is a tooth that has come loose or has been forced to an abnormal position following a blow. An avulsion is a tooth that has been knocked completely out of the socket. Actual fractures to the teeth are classified based on the

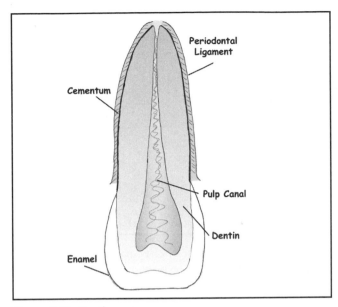

Figure 8-10. Tooth anatomy.

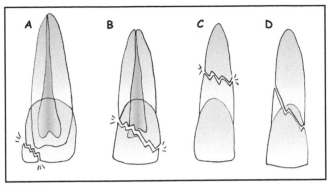

Figure 8-11. Types of tooth fractures. (A) Uncomplicated crown fracture "chip." (B) Complicated crown fracture with nerve exposed. (C) Crown-root fracture with the root involved. (D) Root fracture with crown intact.

specific tissue affected. Some fractures may involve only the surface or enamel of the tooth (ie, a chip) while more severe fractures may involve the root or expose the inner pulp of the tooth (Figure 8-11). A comprehensive sports medicine team should have access to a dentist who is familiar with sport and recreational activities. All of the above injuries warrant a full evaluation by a dentist.

An athlete should see a dentist immediately if he or she has a broken tooth, a tooth that is knocked from the socket, or a tooth that is loose and bleeding as a result of a blow. If a tooth has been completely knocked out, it should be kept and transported to the dentist. The tooth must be kept in an appropriate medium such as saliva, sterile water, or cold milk. Time is of the essence because the prognosis for replacement of the tooth worsens with every passing hour following injury.

INJURIES TO THE EYE

 ## Removing a Foreign Object From the Eye

Most of us have had the following experience: something lands in our eye and the natural response is to rub it, which is probably the worst thing we can do. A foreign object in the eye can cause a corneal abrasion. In addition, the object could become lodged in the tissue, making it even more difficult to remove. If there is a foreign object in the eye, the athletic trainer should do the following:

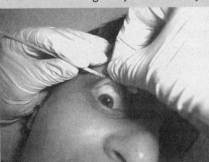

- Grasp the lower eyelid and gently pull it away from the eye. If the object can be seen, use a piece of sterile gauze to gently remove it.
- If the object is under the upper lid, the end of a cotton-tipped applicator can be used to help roll the eyelid up to allow for visualization of the area under the upper lid.
- Flushing the eye with a sterile eye irrigation wash may also help dislodge the object.
- If you cannot remove the object, the eye should be patched and the patient referred to the physician.

Figure 8-12. Anatomy of the eye.

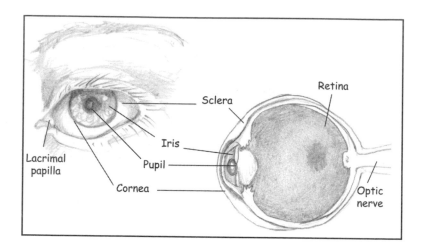

The eye rests in the skull within a bony protective socket created by the surrounding bone. A blow to this region of the face from an object larger than the eye (ie, a ball or fist) can cause injuries to the eye itself, the surrounding bone, or the adjacent soft tissue. Objects that are smaller than the orbital rim (ie, fingers or pointed objects) pose a greater threat to the eye since the orbital rim or surrounding bone can offer no protection from their impact. Serious injuries to the eye can threaten the vision of a patient. Eye injuries must be managed with care and promptly referred to an ophthalmologist.

Any of the following eye conditions are indications for immediate referral to an ophthalmologist[11,15]:

✓ Severe eye pain

✓ Double vision (diplopia)

✓ Blurred vision (loss of acuity)

✓ Decrease in the field of vision (tunnel vision, changes in field of view)

✓ Blood or blurring at the pupil or iris

✓ Presence of a hyphema

✓ Changes in pupil shape

✓ Penetrating injury

✓ Decreased ability to move the eye

One of the most common eye injuries is the corneal abrasion. A corneal abrasion is a scratch to the clear central part of the eye covering the iris. The anatomy of the eye is provided in Figure 8-12. The most common MOI is a foreign object, scratch, or irritation from a contact lens. Signs and symptoms include a scratching or gritty feeling in the eye with sensitivity to bright light or photophobia. Treatment for a corneal abrasion includes antibiotic ointments or eye drops, rest, and an eye patch to decrease photosensitivity. Athletes with a history of abrasions may wish to consider protective eyewear.

Another common condition seen in physically active populations includes inflammation of the con-

junctiva. Conjunctivitis is the inflammation of the tissue that lines the eyelid and covers the eyeball. Bacteria or irritants like dust, smoke, or allergens can cause the tissue to become inflamed. The condition may also be associated with the common cold or upper respiratory infections.[11] Signs and symptoms include redness in the eye, swelling of the eyelid, possible drainage, with burning or itching of the eyes. Some forms of conjunctivitis are quite contagious. Patients should use care in sharing towels and linens. Initial care includes referral to a physician.

Two more serious eye injuries include hyphema and retinal detachment. A hyphema is a collection of blood in the anterior chamber of the eye. A blunt blow to the eye can cause a hyphema. A reddish yellow tint of fluid in the anterior chamber is a common sign concurrent with a logical MOI. Failure to wear protective eyewear while playing racquetball or squash increases the risk for such an injury. The presence of a hyphema should be treated as an emergency. Long-term care consists of compressing dressing and bed rest with the head held at 35 to 45 degrees for several days. Medications may also be used to decrease the pressure in the eye. While a hyphema often heals without complications, secondary glaucoma or blood staining of the cornea may ultimately impair vision.[15] Retinal detachment can occur as a result to a blow to the eye. Patients with a retinal detachment often get the sense of a "curtain" falling over their field of vision. Any patient with changes in the field of vision or limitations in vision following a blow should be referred for evaluation.

COMMON INJURIES TO THE SPINE

Injuries to the spine present a challenge for the athletic trainer in terms of evaluating and recognizing problems and then developing appropriate long-term treatment programs to address them. The spinal column is a complex arrangement of articulations, discs, and nerves covered by layers of muscle tissue that is dependent upon a balance of strength, stability, and flexibility to function properly. The injuries that can occur in this region range from simple contusions or strains to potentially life-threatening injuries. As always, the athletic trainer is responsible for understanding the relationship between the anatomy, MOI, and possible injuries that may occur in order to provide proper initial management and long-term care.

INJURIES TO THE CERVICAL SPINE

Fractures, Instability, and Sprains

The 7 vertebrae of the cervical spine serve to support the skull, protect the spinal cord, and allow for movement. While injuries to the cervical spine represent a small percentage of athletic injuries, they have the potential to be the most devastating. As we evolved to upright walking, our need for mobility in the cervical spine increased. This allows us to turn our head, look around, and see where we want to go. Anatomical structure always dictates function. Our cervical spine allows for mobility at the expense of stability. The cervical vertebrae are less stable than their thoracic or lumbar counterparts. Thus, the opportunity for a cervical vertebrae subluxation or dislocation is possible. Any subluxation or dislocation of a vertebra has the potential to cause damage to the spinal cord. The common MOI for a subluxation or dislocation includes a forced flexion and rotation movement. Signs of a dislocation may be similar to those of a fracture and include pain, point tenderness, cervical muscle spasm, radiating pain, weakness, or paralysis in the extremities. An injury at or above the level of the third cervical vertebrae may cause the patient to experience respiratory distress or failure. Proper first aid is required while immobilizing and transporting this patient. A dislocation may result in the head being tilted in the direction of the dislocation.[11] Suspicion of a cervical vertebrae dislocation is cause to activate your emergency response plan, perform a primary survey, and stabilize the patient until he or she can be transported.

Paralysis or death is a possible complication secondary to a cervical fracture. The athletic trainer must be prepared to identify a possible cervical fracture and activate the emergency response plan if needed. The most common MOI for a fracture is an axial load (force to the top of the head) combined with flexion of the cervical spine. When the cervical spine is flexed,

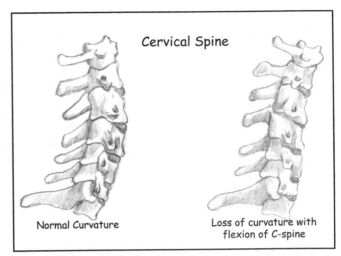

Figure 8-13. Cervical spine in flexion. Note the loss of curvature.

it loses some of its normal curvature (Figure 8-13). A blow to the top of the head will reproduce this mechanism. It is for this reason that hitting with the top of the helmet is illegal in football. An athlete with a cervical spine fracture may have pain, point tenderness, loss of sensation in the extremities, or paralysis. If the patient is not lucid and cannot respond to questions, the clinician must assume the worst and immobilize and transport accordingly.

A sprain to the ligamentous structures that support the cervical spine can take place when the cervical spine is rapidly extended then flexed. The most common mechanism for a sprain is whiplash. Though typically associated with motor vehicle accidents, this mechanism can be seen in physical activity as well. Signs of a sprain injury include persistent pain, spasm of cervical musculature, difficulty with motion, and point tenderness. Initial care involves use of a soft cervical collar to relieve the muscle spasm and referral to a physician to rule out fracture or possible disk injury.

Muscle Strain Injury

Muscle strains to the muscles that control the movements of the cervical spine can be seen when the muscles are either stretched or absorb an abnormal force associated with the movements of the cervical spine. Pain and loss of movement in flexion, extension, or rotation are common indicators of muscle injury. The patient may also have a muscle spasm or hold the neck in a protective position. Initial care should include PRICE and use of a soft cervical collar to alleviate the stress of supporting the head.

Nerve-Related Injuries

Cervical disc injuries can occur when the cervical disc has degenerated and caused a protrusion that

Appropriate Care of Spinal Injuries

The NATA Inter-Association Task Force for Appropriate Care of the Spine-Injured Athlete was formed to develop guidelines for management of catastrophic spine injuries. The task force was composed of professionals from 29 various organizations and professional societies. Athletic trainers, physicians, emergency medical services groups, and various allied health personnel contributed to the final guidelines and recommendations regarding on-the-field management and immediate care of these catastrophic injuries. Below are highlights of the task force-recommended guidelines for appropriate care of the spine-injured athlete.

General Guidelines

- Any athlete suspected of having a spinal injury should not be moved and should be managed as though a spinal injury exists.
- The athlete's airway, breathing, circulation, neurological status, and level of consciousness should be assessed.
- The athlete should not be moved unless absolutely essential to maintain airway, breathing, and circulation.
- If the athlete must be moved to maintain airway, breathing and circulation, the athlete should be placed in a supine position while maintaining spinal immobilization.
- When moving a suspected spine-injured athlete, the head and trunk should be moved as a unit. One accepted technique is to manually splint the head to the trunk.
- The emergency medical system (EMS) should be activated

Face Mask Removal

- The face mask should be removed prior to transportation regardless of respiratory status.
- Those involved in the prehospital care of injured football players should have the tools for face mask removal readily available.

Football Helmet Removal

The athletic helmet and chin strap should only be removed if:

- The helmet and chin strap do not hold the head securely, such that immobilization of the helmet does not also immobilize the head.
- The design of the helmet and chin strap is such that, even after removal of the face mask, the airway cannot be controlled nor ventilation provided.
- The face mask cannot be removed after a reasonable period of time.
- The helmet prevents immobilization for transportation in an appropriate position.

Helmet Removal

Spinal immobilization must be maintained while removing the helmet.

- Helmet removal should be frequently practiced under proper supervision.
- Specific guidelines for helmet removal need to be developed.
- In most circumstances, it may be helpful to remove cheek padding and/or deflate air prior to helmet removal.

Equipment

Appropriate spinal alignment must be maintained.

- There needs to be a realization that the helmet and shoulder pads elevate an athlete's trunk when in a supine position.
- Should either the helmet or shoulder pads be removed—or if only one of these is present—appropriate spinal alignment must be maintained.
- The front of the shoulder pads can be opened to allow access for CPR and defibrillation.

(continued)

Appropriate Care of Spinal Injuries (continued)

Additional Guidelines

- The task force encourages the development of a local emergency care plan regarding the prehospital care of an athlete with a suspected spinal injury. This plan should include communication with the institution's administration and those directly involved with the assessment and transportation of the injured athlete.

- All providers of prehospital care should practice and be competent in all of the skills identified in these guidelines before they are needed in an emergency situation.

Adapted with permission from Kleiner DM, Almquist JL, Bailes J, et al. *Prehospital Care of the Spine-Injured Athlete: A Document from the Inter-Association Task Force for the Appropriate Care of the Spine-Injured Athlete.* Dallas, TX: National Athletic Trainers' Association; 2001.

puts pressure on a nerve root as it leaves the spinal cord and travels to the upper extremity. Disc injuries can cause pain, radiating numbness or tingling into the upper extremity, weakness in the muscles of the upper extremity, and pain that increases when bending the neck forward (flexion). Referral to a physician for a full evaluation is essential if a disc injury is suspected.

An injury to the cervical nerve roots that arise in sport and physical activity is the brachial plexus stretch injury. The common name for this injury is the burner or stinger. The injury is so named due to the painful electric shock-like burning sensation that shoots down the upper extremity when the injury occurs. The mechanism for a brachial plexus stretch injury is shoulder abduction, often depressed, and the head laterally flexed to the opposite side. The brachial plexus is the group of nerves that leave the cervical vertebrae (C5-T1) and innervate sensation and motor function in the upper extremity. The signs and symptoms include a logical mechanism, tingling, pain, and weakness in the upper extremity. A burning sensation is felt that shoots out the upper extremity. An athlete with a burner will often leave the field of play with his or her arm hanging limp by his or her side. Change in sensation and muscle weakness may be present for a few minutes or several days. In some cases, damage to the nerve plexus can cause permanent disability.

No athlete who has sustained a brachial plexus injury should be allowed to return to activity until all symptoms are resolved, full strength is present, and a physician has cleared him or her.

Ice is sometimes used in the initial care to help alleviate pain. Referral to the physician is needed to document available strength and sensation in the upper extremity. Radiographs should be taken to rule out bony changes in the vertebrae that can cause additional pressure on the nerve roots. Repetitive

injuries to the brachial plexus may result in long-term deficits.

INJURIES TO THE LUMBAR SPINE

Fractures

Much like acute fractures of the cervical vertebrae, fractures to the lumbar vertebrae have the potential to cause damage to the underlying spinal cord. The most common fractures to these structures are the compression fracture and fractures to the spinous and transverse processes. Compression fractures are caused by hyperflexion, falls, or high velocity accidents, while direct blows to the lumbar region most often cause fractures to the transverse and spinous processes. Isolated dislocations without an associated fracture are rare in this region of the spine.[15]

A stress reaction fracture is commonly found in the lumbar vertebrae at the neural arch. This fracture is called a spondylolysis (Figure 8-14). A spondylolisthesis is a spondylolysis that has completely fractured, causing the vertebrae to slide forward. Patients with a "spondy" will have pain that increases when the back is extended. This injury is common in adolescents and young adults who participate in activities that require forced extension such as diving, gymnastics, and some swimming strokes. Treatment consists of alleviating discomfort (ice, heat, etc) and performing therapeutic exercises to help strengthen the core muscles and thus stabilize the trunk. In addition, avoiding forced extension exercises is encouraged.

Sprains

Awkward bending and rotation movements may lead to sprains to the ligaments that support the lumbar spine. This may be a one-time event (acute injury) or the result of repetitive movements that cause increasing discomfort. Some back injuries are

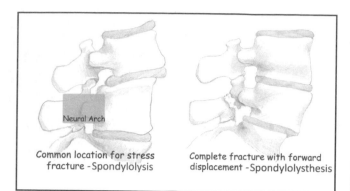

Common location for stress
fracture - Spondylolysis

Complete fracture with forward
displacement - Spondylolysthesis

Neural Arch

Figure 8-14. Spondylolysis.

 Is There Kryptonite in Here?

My athletes used to ask me the obvious question following injuries, "Do you think it is broken?" My standard wise guy response was always, "There must be a lot of kryptonite in here because my x-ray vision is out of whack." Many injuries to the skull and spine can have serious consequences if an injury is not properly identified. The only way to confirm the absence of fracture is to get a radiograph. Spine injuries, possible fractures to the facial bones, and injuries to the skull cannot be left to chance. The athletic trainer must know the signs and symptoms of possible fractures and readily refer to the physician to assist his or her patients in securing the proper diagnostic testing. If you are not sure, you must refer! Do not trust your x-ray vision.

associated with increased pain when you move in a given direction (ie, spondys hurt in extension) but sprain injuries may be uncomfortable in all planes of movement. Patients with back pain must be evaluated thoroughly to insure they do not have an underlying disc or bone problem. The athlete with a sprain injury should receive PRICE to improve pain, referral to a physician to rule out serious injury, and begin a course of rehabilitation to regain pain-free motion and improve core strength.

Muscle Strains and Contusions

Muscle strain injury is a common occurrence associated with low back pain. Muscles will often assume a position of spasm as a protective mechanism if there is an underlying problem with the bone or a disc. Often the muscle can be injured in isolation. Rapid movements, awkward positioning, and long-term poor posture can contribute to muscle strain injury. Once again, patients with muscle pain in the lumbar region must be evaluated thoroughly to insure they do not have an underlying disc or bone problem. The athlete with a muscle strain injury should receive PRICE to improve pain, referral to a physician to rule out serious injury, and begin a course of rehabilitation to regain pain-free motion and improve core strength.

The lumbar region is often exposed to direct blows in many activities and thus exposed to contusions. The potential for contusions or lacerations to internal organs is a concern (see Chapter 9) as are contusions to the spinous processes. The athletic trainer must be aware of the possibility of fracture and readily refer any patient with pain directly to the spinous process for a radiograph.

Nerve-Related Injuries

The intervertebral discs that sit between the lumbar vertebrae can degenerate and cause the middle portion of the disc to protrude or bulge outward and put pressure on nerve roots (Figure 8-15). The most common herniated disc lies between the 4th

and 5th lumbar vertebrae. Athletes may experience disc problems associated with heavy lifting as well as rapid rotation and bending movements. The signs and symptoms of a disc rupture include pain that is central to the lumbar region and radiating down one of the lower extremities. Changes in sensation and muscle weakness will be associated with the location innervated by the affected nerve root. Reflexes in the lower extremity may be diminished. Patients with disc pain will have increased discomfort or pain with flexion. The movement of trunk flexion forces the disc toward the nerve root. Coughing and holding your breath may increase the signs and symptoms. Treatment includes assistance with pain and avoiding positions that increase symptoms (flexion). Extension positions and exercise may provide relief. Long-term rehabilitation includes developing core strength and a balance of flexibility and stability. Surgery may be required if the pressure on the nerve root is persistent and conservative (nonoperative) treatment fails.

The sacral plexus exits below the sacrum on each side and forms the large sciatic nerve, which travels down the back of the lower extremity and branches into several major nerves that serve the lower extremity. Sciatica is a term that is sometimes used to describe pain that travels down the leg from the back. However, it is best to determine the underlying cause of that pain. Is it the result of a disc putting pressure on a lumbar nerve root, or is it caused by irritation to the sciatic nerve? A unilateral straight leg raise will often reproduce pain in the same leg when the sciatic nerve is irritated. One cause of this irritation or inflammation is tightness of the piriformis muscle group as it passes over the sciatic nerve. This tightness is called piriformis syndrome (Figure 8-16).

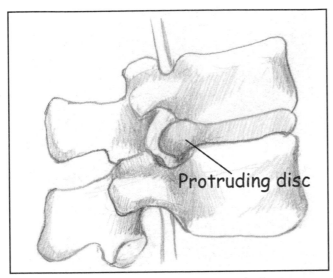

Figure 8-15. Disc injury causing pressure on the lumbar nerve root.

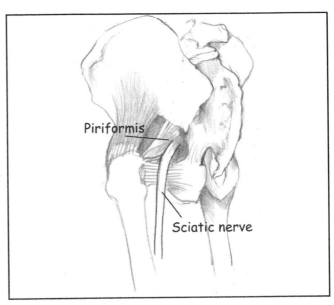

Figure 8-16. Sciatic nerve.

INJURIES TO THE SACROILIAC JOINT

A variety of injuries to the pelvis and hip are discussed in Chapter 6. Injuries to the SI joint are worth discussing in this chapter because of the common association between SI joint irritation and low back pain. Irritation at the lumbosacral junction is a common cause of discomfort. Often referred to with the generalized term of *SI dysfunction*, chronic pain in the SI joint can be a result of rotation of one of the innominate bones of the pelvis (one side of the pelvis). This may be characterized by an uneven alignment of the ASIS or the posterior superior iliac spine (PSIS) and possibly a functional leg length discrepancy. Correction of this problem requires evaluation and treatment by a skilled practitioner who can prescribe specific strengthening and stretching maneuvers in combination with mobilization of the SI joint. Sprain injuries to the SI joint can also occur with a variety of forceful twisting motions. Patients with an SI joint sprain may experience tenderness with palpation over the SI joint. They may also report generalized low back discomfort. They may have some tightness or guarding in the muscles. Pain may be increased with standing on one leg or with rotation of one side of the pelvis (eg, pulling a knee toward the chest or extension of the hip). Patients may also experience pain as they move from a seated to a standing position.[15] These sprain injuries are treated with therapeutic interventions for pain, mobilization exercises to address asymmetries, and strengthening exercises for improved stability.

SUMMARY

The skull and spine provide a wide range of challenges for the athletic trainer. These bony structures protect the very essence of our being, our CNS. The athletic trainer must develop superior evaluation skills, recognize life-threatening or potentially catastrophic situations, and understand the complex relationship between the neuroanatomy and other tissue structures to properly recognize and manage injuries to the head and spine.

REFERENCES

1. Thurman JD, Branche C, Sniezek JE. The epidemiology of sports-related traumatic brain injuries in the United States: recent developments. *J Head Trauma Rehabil.* 1998;13:1-8.
2. Guskiewicz KM, McCrea M, Marshall SW, et al. Cumulative effects of recurrent concussion in collegiate football players: the NCAA Concussion Study. *JAMA.* 2003;290:2549-2555.
3. Walking Tall: PBS Evolution Series. WGBH Educational Foundation and Clear Blue Sky Productions; 2001.
4. Nachemson A, Waddell G, Norlund A. Epidemiology of neck and back pain. In: Nachemson A FJ, ed. *Neck and Back Pain: The Scientific Evidence of Causes, Diagnosis, and Treatment.* Philadelphia, PA: Lippincott, Williams & Wilkins; 2000:165-188.
5. Consumer Product Safety Commission. National electronic injury surveillance system. Available at www.cpsc.gov/LIBRARY/neiss.html. Accessed July 25, 2008.
6. Oliario S, Anderson S, Hooker D. Management of cerebral concussion in sports: the athletic trainer's perspective. *Journal of Athletic Training.* 2001;36:257-262.
7. Congress of Neurologic Surgeons. Glossary of head injury including some definitions of injury to the cervical spine. *Clin Neurosurg.* 1966;14:424-445.

8. Guskiewicz KM, Bruce SL, Cantu RC, et al. National Athletic Trainers' Association position statement: management of sport-related concussion. *Journal of Athletic Training*. 2004;39(3):280-297.

9. Aubry M, Cantu R, Dvorak J, et al. Summary and agreement statement of the First International Conference on Concussion in Sport, Vienna 2001: recommendations for the improvement of safety and health of athletes who may suffer concussive injuries. *Br J Sports Med*. 2002;36:6-10.

10. Guskiewicz KM, Weaver N, Padua DA, Garrett WE. Epidemiology of concussion in collegiate and high school football players. *Am J Sports Med*. 2000;28:643-650.

11. Prentice WE. *Arnheim's Principles of Athletic Training*. 13th ed. New York: McGraw-Hill Higher Education; 2009.

12. Guskiewicz KM, Riemann BL, Perrin DH, Nashner LM. Alternative approaches to the assessment of mild head injury in athletes. *Med Sci Sports Exerc*. 1997;29(7 supp.):S213.

13. McCrea KM, Kelly JP, Randolph C, et al. Standardized assessment of concussion (SAC): on-site mental status evaluation of the athlete. *J Head Trauma Rehabil*. 1998;13:27-35.

14. Cantu RC, Voy R. The second impact syndrome: a risk in any contact sport. *Physician and Sports Medicine*. 1995;23:27-34.

15. Peterson L, Renstrom, P. *Sports Injuries: Their Prevention and Treatment*. 3rd ed. Champaign, IL: Human Kinetics; 2001.

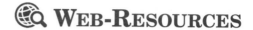 # WEB-RESOURCES

Brain Injury Association of America
www.biausa.org
The mission of the Brain Injury Association of America is to create a better future through brain injury prevention, research, education, and advocacy.

Centers for Disease Control and Prevention
www.cdc.gov
A helpful government site sponsored by the US Department of Heath and Human Services. Information regarding injuries and specific information available regarding TBI is given.

 ## Management of Sport-Related Concussion

The following recommendations are derived from the most recent scientific and clinic-based literature on sport-related concussion. Readers are encouraged to read the entire journal article, which is available at www.nata.org/jat/readers/archives/39.3/i1062-6050-39-3-280.pdf.

Recommendations
Defining and Recognizing Concussion

1. The athletic trainer should develop a high sensitivity for the various mechanisms and presentations of traumatic brain injury (TBI), including mild, moderate, and severe cerebral concussion, as well as the more severe, but less common, head injuries that can cause damage to the brainstem and other vital centers of the brain.

2. The colloquial term *ding* should not be used to describe a sport-related concussion. This stunned confusional state is a concussion most often reflected by the athlete's initial confusion, which may disappear within minutes, leaving no outwardly observable signs and symptoms. Use of the term *ding* generally carries a connotation that diminishes the seriousness of the injury. If an athlete shows concussion-like signs and reports symptoms after a contact to the head, the athlete has, at the very least, sustained a mild concussion and should be treated for a concussion.

3. To detect deteriorating signs and symptoms that may indicate a more serious head injury, the athletic trainer should be able to recognize both the obvious signs (eg, fluctuating levels of consciousness, balance problems, and memory and concentration difficulties) and the more common, self-reported symptoms (eg, headache, ringing in the ears, and nausea).

4. The athletic trainer should play an active role in educating athletes, coaches, and parents about the signs and symptoms associated with concussion, as well as the potential risks of playing while still symptomatic.

5. The athletic trainer should document all pertinent information surrounding the concussive injury, including but not limited to (1) mechanism of injury; (2) initial signs and symptoms; (3) state of consciousness; (4) findings on serial testing of symptoms and neuropsychological function and postural-stability tests (noting any deficits compared with baseline); (5) instructions given to the athlete and/or parent; (6) recommendations provided by the physician; (7) date and time of the athlete's return to participation; and (8) relevant information on the player's history of prior concussion and associated recovery pattern(s).

(continued)

Management of Sport-Related Concussion (continued)

Evaluating and Making the Return-to-Play Decision

6. Working together, ATCs and team physicians should agree on a philosophy for managing sport-related concussion before the start of the athletic season. Currently 3 approaches are commonly used: (1) grading the concussion at the time of the injury, (2) deferring final grading until all symptoms have resolved, or (3) not using a grading scale but rather focusing attention on the athlete's recovery via symptoms, neurocognitive testing, and postural-stability testing. After deciding on an approach, the athletic trainer-physician team should be consistent in its use regardless of the athlete, sport, or circumstances surrounding the injury.

7. For athletes playing sports with a high risk of concussion, baseline cognitive and postural-stability testing should be considered. In addition to the concussion injury assessment, the evaluation should also include an assessment of the cervical spine and cranial nerves to identify any cervical spine or vascular intracerebral injuries.

8. The athletic trainer should record the time of the initial injury and document serial assessments of the injured athlete, noting the presence or absence of signs and symptoms of injury.

The athletic trainer should monitor vital signs and level of consciousness every 5 minutes after a concussion until the athlete's condition improves. The athlete should also be monitored over the next few days after the injury for the presence of delayed signs and symptoms and to assess recovery.

9. Concussion severity should be determined by paying close attention to the severity and persistence of all signs and symptoms, including the presence of amnesia (retrograde and anterograde) and LOC, as well as headache, concentration problems, dizziness, blurred vision, and so on. It is recommended that ATCs and physicians consistently use a symptom checklist.

10. In addition to a thorough clinical evaluation, formal cognitive and postural-stability testing is recommended to assist in objectively determining injury severity and readiness to return to play (RTP). No one test should be used solely to determine recovery or RTP, as concussion presents in many different ways.

11. Once symptom free, the athlete should be reassessed to establish that cognition and postural stability have returned to normal for that player, preferably by comparison with preinjury baseline test results. The RTP decision should be made after an incremental increase in activity with an initial cardiovascular challenge, followed by sport-specific activities that do not place the athlete at risk for concussion. The athlete can be released to full participation as long as no recurrent signs or symptoms are present.

Concussion Assessment Tools

12. Baseline testing on concussion assessment measures is recommended to establish the individual athlete's "normal" preinjury performance and to provide the most reliable benchmark against which to measure postinjury recovery. Baseline testing also controls for extraneous variables (eg,, attention deficit disorder, learning disabilities, age, and education) and for the effects of earlier concussion while also evaluating the possible cumulative effects of recurrent concussions.

13. The use of objective concussion assessment tools will help ATCs more accurately identify deficits caused by injury and postinjury recovery and protect players from the potential risks associated with prematurely returning to competition and sustaining a repeat concussion. The concussion assessment battery should include a combination of tests for cognition, postural stability, and self-reported symptoms known to be affected by concussion.

14. A combination of brief screening tools appropriate for use on the sideline (eg,, Standardized Assessment of Concussion [SAC], Balance Error Scoring System [BESS], symptom checklist) and more extensive measures (eg,, neuropsychological testing, computerized balance testing) to more precisely evaluate recovery later after injury is recommended.

15. Before instituting a concussion neuropsychological testing battery, the athletic trainer should understand the test's user requirements, copyright restrictions, and standardized instructions for administration and scoring. All evaluators should be appropriately trained in the standardized instructions for test administration and scoring before embarking on testing or adopting an instrument for clinical use. Ideally, the sports medicine team should include a neuropsychologist, but in reality, many ATCs may not have access to a neuropsychologist for interpretation and consultation, nor the financial resources to support a neuropsychological testing program. In this case, it is recommended that the athletic trainer use screening instruments (eg,, SAC, BESS, symptom checklist) that have been developed specifically for use by sports medicine clinicians without extensive training in psychometric or standardized testing and that do not require a special license to administer or interpret.   (continued)

Management of Sport-Related Concussion (continued)

16. Athletic trainers should adopt for clinical use only those neuropsychological and postural stability measures with population-specific normative data, test-retest reliability, clinical validity, and sufficient sensitivity and specificity established in the peer-reviewed literature. These standards provide the basis for how well the test can distinguish between those with and without cerebral dysfunction in order to reduce the possibility of false-positive and false-negative errors, which could lead to clinical decision-making errors.

17. As is the case with all clinical instruments, results from assessment measures to evaluate concussion should be integrated with all aspects of the injury evaluation (eg., physical examination, neurologic evaluation, neuroimaging, and player's history) for the most effective approach to injury management and RTP decision making. Decisions about an athlete's RTP should never be based solely on the use of any one test.

When to Refer an Athlete to a Physician After Concussion

18. The athletic trainer or team physician should monitor an athlete with a concussion at 5-minute intervals from the time of the injury until the athlete's condition completely clears or the athlete is referred for further care. Coaches should be informed that in situations when a concussion is suspected but an athletic trainer or physician is not available; their primary role is to ensure that the athlete is immediately seen by an athletic trainer or physician.

19. An athlete with a concussion should be referred to a physician on the day of injury if he or she lost consciousness, experienced amnesia lasting longer than 15 minutes.

20. A team approach to the assessment of concussion should be taken and include a variety of medical specialists. In addition to family practice or general medicine physician referrals, the athletic trainer should secure other specialist referral sources within the community. For example, neurologists are trained to assist in the management of patients experiencing persistent signs and symptoms, including sleep disturbances. Similarly, a neuropsychologist should be identified as part of the sports medicine team for assisting athletes who require more extensive neuropsychological testing and for interpreting the results of neuropsychological tests.

21. A team approach should be used in making RTP decisions after concussion. This approach should involve input from the athletic trainer, physician, athlete, and any referral sources. The assessment of all information, including the physical examination, imaging studies, objective tests, and exertional tests, should be considered prior to making an RTP decision.

When to Disqualify an Athlete

22. Athletes who are symptomatic at rest and after exertion for at least 20 minutes should be disqualified from returning to participation on the day of the injury. Exertional exercises should include sideline jogging followed by sprinting, sit-ups, push-ups, and any sport-specific, non-contact activities (or positions or stances) the athlete might need to perform on returning to participation. Athletes who return on the same day because symptoms resolved quickly (<20 minutes) should be monitored closely after they return to play. They should be repeatedly reevaluated on the sideline after the practice or game and again at 24 and 48 hours postinjury to identify any delayed onset of symptoms.

23. Athletes who experience LOC or amnesia should be disqualified from participating on the day of the injury.

24. The decision to disqualify from further participation on the day of a concussion should be based on a comprehensive physical examination; assessment of self-reported postconcussion signs and symptoms; functional impairments, and the athlete's past history of concussions. If assessment tools such as the SAC, BESS, neuropsychological test battery, and symptom checklist are not used, a 7-day symptom-free waiting period before returning to participation is recommended. Some circumstances, however, will warrant even more conservative treatment (see recommendation 25).

25. Athletic trainers should be more conservative with athletes who have a history of concussion. Athletes with a history of concussion are at increased risk for sustaining subsequent injuries as well as for slowed recovery of self-reported postconcussion signs and symptoms, cognitive dysfunction, and postural instability after subsequent injuries. In athletes with a history of 3 or more concussions and experiencing slowed recovery, temporary or permanent disqualification from contact sports may be indicated.

(continued)

Management of Sport-Related Concussion (continued)

Special Considerations for the Young Athlete

26. Athletic trainers working with younger (pediatric) athletes should be aware that recovery may take longer than in older athletes. Additionally, these younger athletes are maturing at a relatively fast rate and will likely require more frequent updates of baseline measures compared with older athletes.

27. Many young athletes experience sport-related concussion. Athletic trainers should play an active role in helping to educate young athletes, their parents, and coaches about the dangers of repeated concussions. Continued research into the epidemiology of sport-elated concussion in young athletes and prospective investigations to determine the acute and long-term effects of recurrent concussions in younger athletes are warranted.

28. Because damage to the maturing brain of a young athlete can be catastrophic (ie,, almost all reported cases of second-impact syndrome are in young athletes), athletes under age 18 years should be managed more conservatively, using stricter RTP guidelines than those used to manage concussion in the more mature athlete.

Home Care

29. An athlete with a concussion should be instructed to avoid taking medications except acetaminophen after the injury. Acetaminophen and other medications should be given only at the recommendation of a physician. Additionally, the athlete should be instructed to avoid ingesting alcohol, illicit drugs, or other substances that might interfere with cognitive function and neurologic recovery.

30. Any athlete with a concussion should be instructed to rest, but complete bed rest is not recommended. The athlete should resume normal activities of daily living as tolerated while avoiding activities that potentially increase symptoms. Once he or she is symptom free, the athlete may resume a graded program of physical and mental exertion, without contact or risk of concussion, up to the point at which postconcussion signs and symptoms recur. If symptoms appear, the exertion level should be scaled back to allow maximal activity without triggering symptoms.

31. An athlete with a concussion should be instructed to eat a well-balanced diet that is nutritious in both quality and quantity.

32. An athlete should be awakened during the night to check on deteriorating signs and symptoms only if he or she experienced LOC, had prolonged periods of amnesia, or was still experiencing significant symptoms at bedtime. The purpose of the wake-ups is to check for deteriorating signs and symptoms, such as decreased levels of consciousness or increasing headache, which could indicate a more serious head injury or a late-onset complication, such as an intracranial bleed.

33. Oral and written instructions for home care should be given to the athlete and to a responsible adult (eg,, parent or roommate) who will observe and supervise the athlete during the acute phase of the concussion while at home or in the dormitory. The athletic trainer and physician should agree on a standard concussion home-instruction form and it should be used consistently for all concussions.

Equipment Issues

34. The athletic trainer should enforce the standard use of helmets for protecting against catastrophic head injuries and reducing the severity of cerebral concussions. In sports that require helmet protection (football, lacrosse, ice hockey, baseball/ softball, etc), the athletic trainer should ensure that all equipment meets either the National Operating Committee on Standards for Athletic Equipment (NOCSAE) or American Society for Testing and Materials (ASTM) standards.

35. The athletic trainer should enforce the standard use of mouth guards for protection against dental injuries; however, there is no scientific evidence supporting their use for reducing concussive injury.

36. At this time, the athletic trainer should neither endorse nor discourage the use of soccer headgear for protecting against concussion or the consequences of cumulative, subconcussive impacts to the head. Currently no scientific evidence supports the use of headgear in soccer for reducing concussive injury to the head.

Reprinted in part with permission from Guskiewicz KM, Bruce SL, Cantu RC, et al. National Athletic Trainers' Association position statement: management of sport-related concussion. *Journal of Athletic Training*. 2004;39(3):280-297.

Career Spotlight: Clinical Athletic Trainer

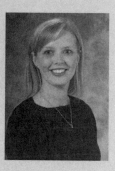

Beth Chorlton, MA, LAT

Licensed Athletic Trainer

UW Health Sports Rehabilitation Clinic

My Position

As a clinical licensed athletic trainer (LAT), my primary responsibilities include evaluation, manual treatment, rehabilitation, and education of athletes/patients. I work in Wisconsin where the practice act allows LATs to carry their own clinical caseload, which includes initial evaluation and overall coordination of patient care. My role requires a close working relationship with various internal health care personnel, including members of the sports rehabilitation staff, physicians, nurses, fitness center staff, exercise physiology staff, radiology staff, and clerical staff. External health care personnel/contacts include physicians, outreach athletic trainers, patient and/or family members, coaches, athletic directors, insurance representatives, and equipment vendors. I also assist in providing a clinical athletic training internship each summer for one or two students who have completed their athletic training education program (ATEP) undergraduate coursework.

Unique or Desired Qualifications

Our clinic requires an athletic trainer to have a master's degree. Although not required, a clinically focused experience during graduate studies can be very helpful in developing the skill set required for attaining a clinic position. These skills include an emphasis on the understanding of repetitive loads and tissue stress as well as pathomechanics associated with overuse injuries.

Favorite Aspect of My Job

I enjoy the clinical setting because I am able to see a wide variety of patients with acute and chronic injuries. Contrary to traditional athletic training settings, I do not have the opportunity to see the injury occur on the field or see the athlete immediately after injury. This often results in the challenge of determining the underlying dysfunctional movement patterns that may have developed since the injury occurred. I also enjoy the opportunity to work with the variety of postsurgical patients/athletes that we see in our clinic. The opportunity to educate and assist my patients in their return to sport/activity is the most fulfilling aspect of my job. In addition, the clinical schedule allows me to have the work and personal life balance that I desire.

Advice

Try to experience as many different athletic training environments as you can to determine your career path focus.

CHAPTER 9

COMMON INJURIES TO THE ABDOMEN AND THORAX AND GENERAL MEDICAL CONDITIONS

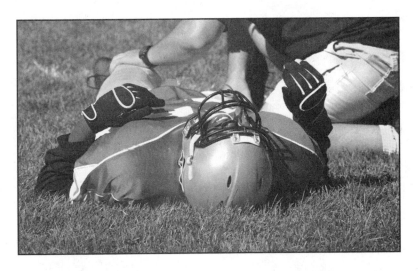

First do no harm. Don't be afraid to take on a task or skill that you understand and know. Be hesitant to get in over your head until you have the specific knowledge and training. Remember, you are dealing with human lives.

Ronnie P. Barnes, MS, ATC
Head Athletic Trainer, Vice President for Medical Services
National Football League–New York Giants

In the past decade, the educational programming for athletic training has continued to evolve beyond the scope of just orthopedic injuries and conditions to include a broader base of general medicine knowledge and skills. While a significant portion of this text is dedicated to describing some of the specific orthopedic conditions encountered in the sports medicine setting, athletic trainers must be equally comfortable in the general medicine realm. Prevention, recognition, evaluation, management, and treatment of illnesses and medical conditions are well within the range of duties the athletic trainer performs. Furthermore, specific attention to psychosocial issues is emphasized in athletic training education programs.

Athletic training falls under the larger umbrella of sports medicine. Sports medicine is defined by the American College of Sports Medicine as being multidisciplinary, including the physiological, biochemical, psychological, and pathological phenomena associated with exercise in sport.[1] The clinical application of

---

Table 9-1

Cardiac Issues and the Preparticipation Examination

Crucial Questions for the Cardiac History

Athletes should be asked if they have the following:

- History of chest pain or discomfort
- History of syncope (fainting) or near syncope
- History of excessive, unexplained, and unexpected shortness of breath or fatigue with exercise
- Past detection of a heart murmur or increased systolic blood pressure
- Family history of premature death (sudden or otherwise) or significant disability from cardiovascular disease in close relatives younger than 50 years old
- Any knowledge of occurrence within their family of any cardiac-related conditions (eg, Marfan, arrhythmia, cardiomyopathies)

Answering yes to any of these questions in the cardiac history warrants further diagnostic testing and referral to a cardiologist.

Adapted from Landry GL, Bernhardt DT. *Essentials of Primary Care Sports Medicine.* Champaign, IL: Human Kinetics; 2003.

---

these disciplines is performed to improve and maintain functional capacities and includes the prevention and treatment of diseases as well as injuries related to exercise and sport.

Pathological, psychological, and prevention and treatment of diseases are included for good reason, and each reaches far beyond just the treatment of injury. Athletic training as a component of sports medicine must address all of these issues. Athletic training students must commit themselves to looking beyond just the orthopedic components of athletic training and strive to learn as much as possible about the illnesses and conditions frequently seen among the populations we serve.

Upon completion of this chapter, the student will be able to:

- ✓ List the benefits and limitations of the preparticipation examination (PPE)
- ✓ Explain the benefits and drawbacks of station-based and office-based PPEs
- ✓ Identify the issues surrounding detection of risk factors for sudden cardiac death (SCD) in young athletes
- ✓ Describe medical conditions commonly seen among physically active populations
- ✓ Identify common injuries of the abdomen that require immediate referral
- ✓ Explain the quadrant system and its use in evaluation of abdominal injuries
- ✓ Describe common medical conditions and injuries of the thorax
- ✓ Discuss the athletic trainer's role in recognizing and properly referring patients with medical conditions

- ✓ Identify the 3 most common skins conditions seen in physically active populations
- ✓ Describe the concerns surrounding community-associated methicillin-resistant *Staphylococcus aureus* (CA-MRSA)
- ✓ List precautionary measures used to prevent CA-MRSA outbreaks

PREPARTICIPATION EXAMINATIONS

Prior to exploring some of the common general medical conditions with which the athletic trainer must be familiar, it is beneficial to discuss a key event that must take place prior to athletic competition. The PPE is designed to protect the safety of participants. Interscholastic and intercollegiate governing bodies mandate that competitors undergo PPEs prior to competition. These may be an annual event or may consist of a comprehensive physical exam followed by annual updates and medical reviews. While disqualification from competition is rare, it is important to try to identify participants who may be at risk for sudden death. Unfortunately, even a complete well-reviewed history and physical exam may not detect a risk factor for sudden death. While this is a key limitation of the PPE, it is still a worthwhile event to review on-going problems, treatment plans (eg, exercise-induced asthma [EIA]), and athlete concerns.[2] Table 9-1 presents guidelines for an appropriate cardiac history and issues surrounding sudden cardiac arrest and the PPE.

Sudden Cardiac Death

Athletes and family members often hope that the PPE can identify all risk factors related to SCD. In reality this is not the case. SCD is defined as nontraumatic, nonviolent, unexpected natural death of cardiac origin occurring within 1 hour of the onset of symptoms in a person who does not have a previously recognized cardiovascular condition that would appear fatal. SCD may occur during or immediately after the exercise or competition.

When SCD occurs in a high-profile athlete, the media attention may lead people to believe that this is a common occurrence. The actual incidence of SCD in athletic activity is low (1 case per 200,000 to 2.3 cases per 100,000 are annual incidence rates that have been reported). It is predisposing cardiovascular conditions (undetected) that make the athlete susceptible to the SCD, and vigorous physical activity may be the trigger.

The common causes of SCD in athletes below 35 years of age are as follows:

- Structural cardiac abnormalities
  - Cardiomyopathies
  - Coronary artery abnormalities
- Cardiac diseases
  - Marfans syndrome
  - Valvular heart disease
  - Premature coronary artery diseases
- A smaller percentage of SCDs are likely related to ionic-channel disorders such as congenital long QT syndrome, and rhythmic disturbances

Prevention of SCD is challenging. It may not be feasible to evaluate all athletic participants with a full cardiac work-up given the number of athletes evaluated for sport annually, and lack of agreement on what screening tests should be used. In addition, the cost may be prohibitive given the low incidence of occurrence. It is clear that an appropriate PPE must include relevant family history, complete medical history, and brachial artery blood pressure screening as a minimum. While less than 30% of SCD victims have symptoms prior to the catastrophic event, any athlete with symptoms (eg, exertional syncope, heart palpitations, shortness of breath, chest pain) must be held from activity and referred immediately for further evaluation. Access to CPR-trained professionals and availability of AEDs are essential for all participants and the efficacy of this prompt response warrants further study. However, it may not be enough to save those with previously undetected cardiac conditions. The possibility of SCD is frightening for any health care provider. All providers who work with active people must continue to educate themselves on the nature of these problems and improvements in screening and pre-participation procedures.

Adapted from:

Maron BJ, Epstein SE, Roberts WC. Causes of sudden death in competitive athletes. *J Am Coll Cardiol.* 1986;7:204-214.

Maron BJ, Shirani J, Polia LC, et al. Sudden death in young competitive athletes: clinical, demographic, and pathological profiles. *JAMA.* 1996;276:199-204.

Pigozzi F, Rizzo M. Sudden death in competitive athletes. *Clin Sports Med.* 2008;27:153-181.

The nature and style of administering the PPE will strongly influence its value. For some athletes, the PPE may be their only involvement with the health care system. For this reason, it should be as comprehensive as is reasonable. The PPE may provide an opportunity for care providers to educate and identify risk factors, for psychosocial problems involving sexuality, substance abuse, violence, or other emotional or psychological factors.[2] A well-constructed PPE is more likely to identify these types of problems in adolescents more so than those in danger of cardiac problems that can lead to sudden death.[2] For example, in a study reviewing 158 SCDs between 1985 and 1995, 48 were due to hypertrophic cardiomyopathy and only 20% of these showed any clues through history or physical exam.[3] The same is true for coronary artery anomalies, which cannot be detected on physical exam. That is why any adherence to the questions outlined in Table 9-1 is of such importance and why parents and athletes should be aware that the PPE cannot eliminate the risk of potentially lethal cardiovascular events.[4]

PPEs should be done 6 weeks before the start of a sport season. This allows any problems that may exist to be addressed. The exams are usually done in

Table 9-2

Example of Appropriate Preparticipation Examination

Exam	Comment
Medical history	Review family history, previous injury or illness, and immunizations
Blood pressure	Consideration must be made for the patient's age, height, and sex when evaluating blood pressure
General appearance	Look for signs of Marfan syndrome
Eyes	Evaluate vision
Cardiovascular	Assess for murmur, suggestions of hypertrophy
Respiratory	Evaluate for normal lung sounds and evidence of wheezing
Abdominal	Assess for liver or spleen enlargement
Genitourinary	Hernia check for male athletes
Musculoskeletal	Complete orthopedic history and examination of any previous injuries
Skin	Exam for evidence of skin infections that may prohibit participation

Adapted from Kurkoswki K, Chandran S. The pre-participation athletic evaluation. Available at www.afp.org. Accessed July 25, 2008.

either an office-based exam or a station-based exam. Assembly line exams performed by one practitioner are neither practical nor comprehensive enough to meet the goals of the PPE. Station-based exams allow large numbers of people to be evaluated at one time. It also allows more specialists to be used for various portions of the exam and therefore increases the odds of detecting problems. The drawback to this exam is that the providers may not have any previous connection to the patients. The office-based exam allows providers to discuss key issues with patients whom they have a previous health care relationship. This is particularly helpful in creating a trusting environment to discuss some of the psychosocial issues outlined previously. Table 9-2 outlines an example of an appropriate PPE.

 ## Preparticipation Physical Examinations

Athletes who participate in athletics in both secondary school and collegiate settings are required to have PPE. The National Federation of State High School Associations (NFHS) stipulates that a student may not practice for or participate in interscholastic athletics until the school has written evidence of permission to participate and evidence that he or she has been deemed fit to participate in sports as determined by a physician or advanced practice nurse prescriber (APNP). Intercollegiate athletes are required to have a PPE upon entrance into college. This initial evaluation should include a comprehensive health history; immunization history ad defined by current Centers of Disease Control and Prevention guidelines; and a relevant physical exam with strong emphasis on the cardiovascular, neurologic, and musculoskeletal evaluation. Subsequent to the initial medical evaluation, an updated history should be performed annually.

The primary goal of the PPE is to detect any conditions that may limit an athlete's participation and predispose the athlete or others to injuries or illness during competition. Secondary goals are to determine the general health of the individual, assess fitness level, and counsel the athlete on health-related issues. The PPE is often the only involvement many student athletes have with the health care system, so it is important that examiners make this encounter as comprehensive as possible. An important function of the exam is to identify athletes who are not only at risk for general medicine and orthopedic conditions but also for psychosocial problems involving sexuality, substance abuse, violence, or any other emotional or psychological factors.

(continued)

Preparticipation Physical Examinations (continued)

Exam Type

There are 2 primary styles of PPE that can be arranged: the office-based examination and the station-based examination. In the high school setting, many athletes will see their personal physician for their PPE. However, given the range of insurance coverage and economic needs of many students, it is equally common for local high schools or sports medicine clinics to sponsor station-based exams as a community service. The station-based exam is common in the intercollegiate setting given the number of athletes reviewed annually. The station-based examination is used to examine a large number of people in a fairly short period of time. In station-based exams, athletes move from station to station (in separate rooms for the sake of privacy) to complete the exam. The station exam is cost-effective and efficient and allows for more access, improved communications, and the use of specialized physicians. The disadvantages of the station-based exam include possible noise and confusion, possible compromised care, and lack of privacy.

The office-based examination allows the athlete to see his or her personal physician in the privacy of the physician's office. This is advantageous since the physician is familiar with the patient and has more time to address sensitive issues. Identifying adolescent stressors surrounding peer relationships, drugs and alcohol, sex, safety, and family can more easily be done in the office-based PPE. This private setting will allow for greater attention to anticipatory guidance such as identifying overbearing parents, providing fitness and nutritional counseling, and spending time discussing injury prevention.

Medical History and Exam Content

Collecting a complete medical history in advance of the PPE is one of the most important organizational tasks in the athletic health care setting. A complete and accurate medical history is the cornerstone of the PPE. The history should give special focus to cardiovascular and musculoskeletal anomalies since these 2 areas are most likely to result in disqualification or require patient follow-up prior to clearance to participate. An orthopedic history is of particular importance as well. Of particular importance are previous injuries that limit the athlete's ability to participate in sports and any injury associated with chronic discomfort, swelling, weakness, or that causes the athlete to compensate by changing his or her mechanics, position of the field, duration of intensity of play.

The physical exam should include the following:

- Documentation of height, weight, and vital signs
- Examination of eyes (vision assessment), ears, nose, and throat
- Heart auscultation
- Some intercollegiate groups may perform echocardiograms
- Pulmonary auscultation
- Abdominal palpation
- Genitalia/hernia assessment
- Skin evaluation
- Musculoskeletal assessment
- Neurologic examination
- Lab testing if warranted by history or physical exam

GENERAL MEDICAL CONDITIONS

The scope of this introductory text does not allow for an in-depth presentation of all the possible medical conditions the athletic trainer may encounter. The following sections are highlights of some of the more common conditions. A student completing an accredited athletic training education program will be exposed to a wide variety of educational competencies related to general medical conditions and a number of clinical proficiencies directly related to the care of medical conditions (Table 9-3).

UPPER RESPIRATORY INFECTIONS

The respiratory tract is defined as all the mucosal-covered surfaces located above the level of the vocal cords. These surfaces are subject to a variety of infections caused by viruses and bacteria. The lining of

Table 9-3

Examples of Athletic Training Clinical Proficiencies for General Medical Conditions

Students must be able to:

- Obtain a basic medical history
- Ascertain body temperature
- Ascertain vital signs
- Palpate the 4 abdominal quadrants for pain, guarding, and rigidity
- Use a stethoscope to identify normal breath, heart, and bowel sounds
- Identify pathological breathing patterns to make a differential assessment of respiratory conditions
- Demonstrate proficiency in the use of an otoscope to examine the nose, outer ear, and middle ear
- Measure urine values using chemical dipsticks

In addition, students in an athletic training education program must learn to recognize the signs, symptoms, and predisposing conditions associated with the following:

- Skin
- Eyes, ears, nose, and throat
- Respiratory system
- Cardiovascular system
- Endocrine system
- Gastrointestinal system
- Eating disorders
- Sexually transmitted diseases/diseases transmitted by body fluid
- Genitourinary tract and organs
- Gynecological disorders
- Viral syndromes
- Neurological disorders
- Systemic disease

Adapted from National Athletic Trainers' Association. *Athletic Training Educational Competencies*. 4th ed. Dallas, TX: Author; 2006.

 Shots Up to Date?

The NCAA recommends that student-athletes participating in athletics be immunized for the following:

- Measles, mumps, and rubella
- Hepatitis B
- Diptheria and tetanus (including boosters)

Any athlete with an abrasion or laceration should have his or her tetanus status determined. If a patient is uncertain about having received the last dose of a primary series or booster within the last 10 years, tetanus immunization is recommended. Given the close quarters commonly found in dormitories and apartment complexes, it is also advised that college-age students receive a vaccination for meningitis. College-age students are at an elevated risk for contracting meningitis.

Bibliography

American College Health Association. Recommendations for institutional prematriculation immunizations. Available at www.acha.org/info_resources/RIPIstatement.pdf. Accessed July 25, 2008.

Centers for Disease Control and Prevention. Meningococcal disease. Available at www.cdc.gov/meningitis/bacterial/faqs.htm. Accessed July 25, 2008.

NCAA Committee on Competitive Safeguards and Medical Aspects of Sports. Blood-borne pathogens and intercollegiate athletics. *2006-2007 NCAA Sports Medicine Handbook*. Indianapolis, IN: NCAA; 2006-2007;54-60.

the upper respiratory tract is covered with cells that produce mucus. The mucus serves a necessary function in lubricating the tissue and trapping particles. In addition, these cells contain cilia. Cilia are tiny "hair-like" structures that move back and forth to move mucus and clear it from the lungs and sinuses. Smoke and viral infections can irritate the lining of the tract and affect the cilia. When the cilia are unable to move mucus, a build up can occur. This is why upper respiratory infections (URI) have many common signs and symptoms: stuffy or runny nose, fullness in the head, irritation to the throat, etc. The athletic trainer should be aware of the signs and symptoms of common illnesses that affect the upper respiratory structures because they will be the most common illnesses seen in the sports medicine environment. The illnesses described next represent some of the more common URIs.

 ## Who Is Dr. Ignaz Semmelweis?

Come on! You do not know? Next time you wash your hands for dinner, you will think of the good Dr. Semmelweis! In 1847, Dr. Ignaz Semmelweis's close friend, Jakob Kolletschka, cut his finger while he was performing an autopsy. Kolletschka soon died. He had symptoms similar to puerperal fever. Semmelweis's attention was aroused since this fever was usually associated with childbirth and killed about 13% of the women who gave birth in his hospital. This death rate was too high for Dr. Semmelweis to accept. He noticed that a nearby hospital run by midwives lost only 2% of its patients to fever.

At this point in history, no one had connected germs with disease yet. This infection would prove to be caused by bacteria. The first hint of that connection would come from England 6 years later. Lister would not show us how to kill germs for another 18 years. Semmelweis was a Hungarian doctor teaching medicine in Vienna. He noticed that students moved between the dissection room and the delivery room without washing their hands. On a hunch, he set up a policy. Doctors had to wash their hands in a chlorine solution when they left the cadavers. Mortality from puerperal fever promptly dropped to 2%.

Instead of reporting his success, Semmelweis kept this information to himself. Yet, by the time a friend published 2 papers on the method, Semmelweis had started washing medical instruments as well as his hands. However, the situation in Vienna was not good. He was criticized and accused of undermining the hospital's leadership with his methods.

In frustration, he went back to Budapest. There he brought his methods to a far more primitive hospital. He cut death by puerperal fever to less than 1%. He systematically isolated causes of death, autopsied victims, set up control groups, and studied statistics. In 1861, he wrote a book on his methods. The establishment gave it poor reviews. Semmelweis grew angry. He hurt his own cause with rage and frustration. In 1865, he suffered a mental breakdown and friends committed him to a mental institution. There, in a cruel twist of fate, he cut his finger. In days, he died at the age of 47 from the very infection that killed his friend Kolletschka and from which he had saved thousands of mothers.

That same year, Joseph Lister began using a carbolic acid solution during surgery to kill germs. In the end, it is Lister who gave our unhappy hero his due. He said, "Without Semmelweis, my achievements would be nothing."

Even in today's modern times, health care providers consider hand washing the single most effective way to prevent the transmission of disease. The value of hand washing in the larger public health picture is well accepted. Despite this acceptance, in our busy world we need to remind ourselves of the most basic defense in infection control: WASH YOUR HANDS.

Athletic training environments must be as clean as possible. The athletic trainer is like any health care worker who must adhere to a stringent policy of cleanliness. Dr. Semmelweis would be proud of you!

Adapted with permission from John H. Lienhard. Engines of Our Ingenuity Episode #622. www.uh.edu/engines/. 1988-1997.

Common Cold

The common cold is caused by a variety of viruses. Colds tend to appear during the winter season. Despite myth and folklore, it is not the cold that causes the spread of rhinoviruses (cold viruses). It is the tendency for people to be inside more and in close contact. Contaminated respiratory secretions spread colds from person to person, either by the inhalation of airborne particles or direct contact with virus-laden surfaces. When you are under stress, your immune system is weakened and you are more susceptible to "catching a cold." When you are under stress, do the things your grandma told you to do: do not go outside without a hat, do not dry your hair, etc. These will not cause a cold, but if you are under stress, you are at greater risk to catch one.

Signs and symptoms of the common cold include the following:

✓ Runny/stuffy nose (dysfunction of the cilia)

✓ Sneezing

✓ Low-grade fever

✓ Sore throat

   o Postnasal drip (worse in morning after sleeping)

✓ Cough

   o Often occurs 2 or 3 days into illness as cough is needed to clear mucus

   o Asthma patients may have a worse cough due to viral illness

The common cold usually lasts about 1 week. The cough may linger for a couple of weeks beyond that. Cold symptoms can affect other aspects of the respiratory tract, including the ears, sinuses, and lungs. There is currently no cure for the common cold. Treatment includes supportive care such as rest, use of a cool mist humidifier, and medication to treat symptoms. Patients with the common cold may be susceptible to secondary bacterial infections. The athletic trainer should refer the patient to a physician if cold symptoms linger.

 Is It a Cold or the Flu?

	Common Cold	Influenza (Flu)
Illness	Respiratory illness caused by viruses	Respiratory illness caused by influenza virus
Treatment	Treat symptoms Does not respond to antibiotics	Antiviral flu medications started in the first 2 days of illness can reduce the severity and duration of influenza illness
Vaccine	None	Annual flu shots can reduce your risk of getting the flu
Transmission	Easily spread from person to person when an infected person touches someone else, sneezes, or coughs	Easily spread from person to person when an infected person sneezes or coughs
Symptoms		
Fever at or above 100°F	Uncommon in adults and older children	Usual and can last 3 to 4 days
Headache	Usual	Usual with sudden onset and can be severe
Muscle aches	Mild	Usual and often severe
Tiredness and exhaustion	Mild	Usual with sudden onset; can be severe and last 2 or more weeks
Runny nose	Usual	Usual
Cough	Usual	Usual
Chest discomfort	Uncommon	Uncommon
Vomiting	Uncommon	Uncommon in adults but more likely in very young children

Adapted from Centers for Disease Control and Prevention. Cold versus flu. Available at http://www.cdc.gov/flu/about/qa/coldflu.htm. Accessed February 26, 2009.

Influenza

Influenza is also a common winter problem caused by a specific type of influenza virus. Unlike the common cold, using a vaccine prior to the winter flu season can often prevent influenza. Influenza is spread by respiratory droplets and contact with contaminated objects. Patients with influenza will be much more ill than those with the common cold. Signs and symptoms of influenza include the following:

✓ Fever and chills (>101°F) (much higher than the low-grade fever sometimes seen with a cold)

✓ Headache

✓ Muscle aches

✓ Runny nose

✓ Sore throat

✓ Cough

Effective pharmacological treatments for the flu must be initiated within the first 24 to 48 hours of the illness, and these medications will only decrease the duration of the flu by a couple of days. The most common care includes supportive care and the treatment of symptoms. The severity of the influenza may warrant the patient being examined by a physician. Any patient with a high fever should be evaluated to rule out other potential illnesses.

Sinusitis

As evidenced by the suffix -itis, sinusitis is an inflammation of the nasal sinus membranes. A range of different bacteria can cause sinusitis. It can also be brought on by dysfunction of the cilia, persistent congestion, and changes in the anatomy of the sinus. The swelling of the membranes and presence of excess mucus causes blockage and pressure in the sinuses. Patients with sinusitis will experience nasal discharge, pressure in the sinuses, and often an associated headache. Sinusitis may also present similar to a cold only with symptoms that are more severe than usual such as higher fever, headache, tooth pain, and facial pain. Treatment options for sinusitis include antibiotics, symptomatic care with over-the-counter medications, saline nasal washes, and steam treatments.

Asthma and Exercise-Induced Asthma

Asthma is a lung disease that affects millions of people. If left untreated, complications from asthma can be fatal. Asthma has the following characteristics: bronchospasm (airway obstruction) that is reversible (though not completely in some patients) spontaneously or with treatment, airway inflammation, and increased responsiveness to a variety of stimuli or stressors. Stressors may include respiratory tract infection, emotional stress, allergens, cold air, dry air, hyperventilation, and irritants like smoke and smog. Asthma results in a decreased ability for oxygen to be exchanged due to increased mucus production and spasm causing the narrowing of the airways. Signs and symptoms of an asthma attack include the following[5]:

✓ Intense, labored breathing

✓ Spasmodic coughing

✓ Chest pain and tightness

✓ Wheezing

✓ High pulse

✓ Increased respiratory rate

✓ Retraction of the neck muscles on inhalation

✓ Restlessness and agitation

✓ Possible syncope

✓ An upright hands-on-knees hunched over position is common

✓ The absence of wheezing may indicate that air is not being moved and the attack is severe

Care for an asthma attack should include the following[6]:

✓ Attempt to relax and reassure the athlete

✓ Use a previously specified medication (if cleared by the physician)

✓ Encourage the athlete to drink water

✓ Have the athlete perform controlled breathing and relaxation exercises

✓ If an environmental factor is triggering the attack, remove it or the athlete from the area

✓ Be prepared to activate an emergency plan if the attack appears severe.

EIA and exercise-induced bronchospasm (EIB) are airway diseases in which exercise or physical activity acts as a trigger to asthma symptoms. EIA can occur in athletes who have no previous history of asthma. Signs and symptoms include repetitive cough and/or slight wheezing either during intense exercise or after activity.[5] The athletic trainer must be mindful to refer the athlete with suspected EIA to the physician for a complete evaluation. Treatment may involve the use of a prescribed bronchodilator using a metered dose inhaler. Treatment may also involve gradual warm up and (if possible) avoiding environments that trigger the reactions. Proper consistent patient compliance is essential to successful care. Some asthma medications have been banned from competition. The athlete and physician must work together to select medications that are allowed during competition.

What Value Good Health?

Alcohol. Tobacco. High-fat diets. Think about it. Do we really still have questions about these particular health issues? Despite the available knowledge of health dangers, it is amazing how people will push the limits. As athletic trainers find themselves in a range of professional practice settings, they will observe many patients who seem unwilling to move beyond their poor health behaviors. They all seem to know someone who has lived to a ripe old age despite these poor behaviors. They run to a place of skepticism to defend their poor choices. For them, the answers are not true.

Everyone knows that tobacco is an addictive drug yet many young people take up smoking. Low-fat, plant-based diets can help reduce heart disease yet our food choices are creating a nation of obese citizens. Alcohol is destructive on so many levels yet we accept the damage of alcohol abuse.

Caring for illnesses takes 27% of the federal budget and creates an amazing drain on the economy. If we could simply focus on tobacco, alcohol, obesity, and lack of exercise, it would have a dramatic effect on our nation's health and economy. Maybe we are all part of the problem. Many a stock portfolio gains profit from these unhealthy behaviors. Television advocates exercise while turning us into couch potatoes.

Yet many of our patients will still be skeptical. We know, without a doubt, the many causes of obesity and heart disease, that tobacco kills more Americans in a year and a half than the total deaths in all the wars this country has ever fought, that much of our alcohol use is physically and mentally destructive, and that lack of exercise opens the door to illness.

By accepting these truths and making a few changes, we could all but eliminate heart disease, adult-onset diabetes, emphysema, and more than half the cancers. Simply acknowledging the obvious could solve the health care problem in America before it bankrupts us. It could save countless loved ones from suffering illness and death.

The fact that folks will not always take advice on healthy behavior is not a new concept. Plato wrote over 2400 years ago:

> To stand in need of the medical art through sloth and intemperate diet...
> do you not think this is abominable?

If this seems off topic for athletic trainers, we need to think again. As the profession continues to expand into a range of health care settings, these problems—and patients who do not want to face them—will be front and center.

Adapted with permission from Leinhard JH. Engines of Our Ingenuity. Episode #1194: Self-Deception. [transcript]. Available at www.uh.edu/engines/epi1194.htm. Accessed April 10, 2007.

Pharyngitis

Pharyngitis is a sore throat associated with nasal symptoms or a sore throat as a result of a primary infection. Both viruses and bacteria cause sore throats. Sore throats can be seen with mononucleosis, influenza, common colds, and other illnesses. Bacterial sore throats are caused by the streptococci bacteria. An athlete with a case of strep throat may present with a fever, redness in the throat, possible pus on the tonsils, headache, and nausea. The signs and symptoms of strep throat may overlap with mononucleosis; in fact, both conditions can coexist. Treatment for a bacterial infection like strep includes a course of oral antibiotics. However, viruses cause most pharyngitis and care should be taken not to use antibiotics because they will not be effective.

COMMON INFECTIONS TO THE EAR

Otitis Externa

Otitis externa is also known as swimmer's ear and refers to general inflammation and infection of the ear canal. Swimmer's ear is caused by exposure to water that can contain various organisms (especially hot tubs). Patients with swimmer's ear complain of ear pain and an itching sensation. A gentle tug on the ear can produce pain and examination of the ear canal can reveal redness or pus in the ear canal. Treatment of swimmer's ear can include topical antibiotics or anti-inflammatory drops. If the infection has spread beyond the ear canal, it may require oral antibiotics. Those who are repeatedly exposed to water (like swimmers) should take preventative measures to keep the ear canal dry using a drop solution of vinegar, alcohol, and saline (1:1:1). An athlete showing persistent signs of otitis externa should be referred for a complete evaluation.

Otitis Media

Otitis media is an infection to the middle ear. Middle ear infections result in a collection of fluid behind the tympanic membrane (ear drum). Individuals with otitis media will present with ear pain and may have difficulty hearing. Other signs and symptoms can include headache, fever, and nausea. The patient must be referred to a physician for a thorough evaluation of the tympanic membrane. Both viruses and bacteria cause middle ear infections and this can make treatment choices difficult. Treatment options include symptomatic treatment and time, pain control, and antibiotics.

MONONUCLEOSIS

Mononucleosis is an acute infection that is caused by the Epstein-Barr virus. The virus is carried in the throat and transmitted in the saliva, thus its reputation as the "kissing disease." Adolescents and young adults who live in close quarters and share utensils are commonly at risk. An athletic trainer working in a setting with high school and college athletes will need to be familiar with the recognition and care of patients with mononucleosis.

A patient with mononucleosis may present initially with a fever, sore throat, loss of energy, and muscle aches. The lethargy and fatigue associated with the illness can last a number of weeks. It is this malaise that makes "mono" problematic for the competitive athlete. In addition, mononucleosis can produce an enlargement of the spleen (splenomegaly), thus creating a risk of splenic rupture. Patients with mononucleosis can often return to activities 4 weeks following the onset of the illness if there is no concern about the enlargement of the spleen.[7] Specific time to return to competition will vary by sport requirements and the demands of the activity. Further diagnostic tests may be used (CT scan and ultrasound) to determine the size of the spleen. Treatment of mononucleosis requires rest and treatment of symptoms.

 ## Diabetes: Guidelines for Diabetic Athletes

There approximately 21 million people living with diabetes in the United States, and many athletes are among that population. The NATA has produced a position statement, *Management of the Athlete With Type 1 Diabetes Mellitus*. This statement provides relevant information on type 1 diabetes mellitus and offers specific recommendations for athletic trainers who work with diabetic athletes. Type 1 diabetes is a chronic (lifelong) disease that occurs when the pancreas does not produce enough insulin to properly control blood sugar levels. Type 1 diabetes is often called juvenile or insulin-dependent diabetes. In this type of diabetes, cells of the pancreas produce little or no insulin, the hormone that allows glucose to enter body cells.

The position statement from the NATA outlines several guidelines that can help athletes and their parents, coaches, and health care professionals effectively manage diabetes. The primary goal of diabetes management is to maintain blood-glucose levels consistently in a normal or near-normal range. Strategies to recognize, treat, and prevent hypoglycemia (low blood glucose) typically include blood-glucose monitoring, carbohydrate supplementation, and insulin adjustments.

Recommendation for Diabetes Management

Athletes with type 1 diabetes can benefit from a well-organized plan that allows them to compete on equal ground with their teammates and competitors. This plan should include the following 7 elements:

1. Blood glucose monitoring guidelines: These should address the frequency of monitoring as well as pre-exercise blood glucose levels where beginning exercise could be unsafe.
2. Insulin therapy guidelines: These should include the type of insulin used, dosages, and adjustment strategies for planned activities types, as well as insulin correction dosages for high blood glucose levels.
3. List of other medications: Make sure to include medicines used to assist with blood glucose control and/or to treat other diabetes-related conditions.
4. Guidelines for low blood glucose (hypoglycemia) recognition and treatment: These guidelines include prevention, signs, symptoms, and treatment of hypoglycemia, including instructions on the use of the hormone glucagon to metabolize carbohydrates.   (continued)

> ### ⓘ　Diabetes: Guidelines for Diabetic Athletes (continued)
>
> 5. Guidelines for high blood glucose (hyperglycemia) recognition and treatment: These guidelines include prevention, signs, symptoms, and treatment of hyperglycemia and diabetic ketoacidosis, a condition in which insufficient levels of insulin lead to hyperglycemia and the build-up of ketones (by-products of fat metabolism that can reach toxic levels) in the blood. Diabetic ketoacidosis can be life threatening.
> 6. Emergency contact information: Include parents' and/or other family member's telephone numbers, physician's telephone number, and consent for medical treatment (for minors).
> 7. Medic alert: Athletes with diabetes should have a medic alert tag with them at all times.
>
> Since travel is also often a part of life for those on sports teams, athletes with diabetes are also advised to carry prepackaged meals and snacks in case food availability is interrupted. If travel occurs over several time zones, insulin therapy may need to be adjusted to coordinate with changes in eating and activity patterns.
>
> Carolyn C. Jimenez, PhD, ATC and lead author of NATA's position statement commented, "Athletic trainers play a critical role in the prevention, recognition and immediate care of athlete with diabetes." She added, "We are there to provide perspectives on proper exercise and nutrition, counsel them on proper hydration and help them keep track of the intensity of exercise sessions, so they can adjust glucose and insulin levels accordingly."
>
> ### Bibliography
> Jimenez CC, Corcoran MH, Crawley JT, et al. National Athletic Trainers' Association position statement: management of the athlete with type 1 diabetes mellitus. *J Athl Train*. 2007;42(4):536-545.
> NATA Press Release. Journal of Athletic Training *offers care plan to manage diabetes in athletes*. December 2007.

MENINGITIS

Meningitis is an infection of the covering of the brain and the spinal cord. It can be caused by the bacteria *meningococcus* as well as a number of viruses. The infection can present similar to cold symptoms and may resemble the flu. However, it can progress to meningococcemia (infection of the blood) or full-blown meningitis very rapidly. These infections can be fatal. College-age students living in close quarters like dormitories are considered a high-risk group for meningococcal infections and should be vaccinated. Meningitis is spread by droplets or direct contact with infected persons. The symptoms to look for include the following:

- ✓ High fever
- ✓ Nausea or vomiting
- ✓ Severe headache
- ✓ Stiffness and pains in the neck
- ✓ Skin rash of small purple/red spots on the skin

The symptoms can occur within 2 to 10 days (usually 3 to 4) after the person has been exposed. The symptoms can occur suddenly.

A physician should evaluate a patient with a high fever and neck pain!

Remember, meningitis can be fatal. The athletic trainer must know the signs and symptoms of this illness and be quick to refer the patient. In addition, the athletic trainer will often be called upon to educate teammates and roommates of those infected. The Centers for Disease Control and Prevention (CDC) recommends preventative treatment under the following conditions[8]:

- ✓ Somebody living in the same house.
- ✓ A person who has come in contact with the patient's mouth or nose secretions, such as through kissing or by sharing cigarettes, or using the same eating and drinking utensils, glasses, and plates.
- ✓ A person who has done medical treatments like giving mouth-to-mouth resuscitation on the patient or intubating the patient.
- ✓ Children sharing toys, such as in group day care centers, family child care homes, or in nurseries.

SKIN INFECTIONS

Skin infections are a common occurrence with athletes and physically active individuals. Many sport activities require lots of equipment that can become dirty and easily contaminated. In addition, the close contact required of some sports (wrestling, boxing, etc) makes athletes more susceptible to skin-related problems. Early identification and treatment of skin infections is essential to patient comfort and containing the infection. If left unchecked, some skin problems can

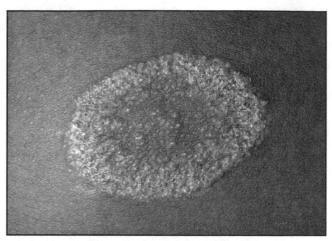

Figure 9-1. Tinea corporis. (Courtesy of Dr. Gary Williams, University of Wisconsin–Madison School of Medicine and Public Health.)

spread through an entire team. Personal cleanliness combined with proper cleaning of equipment and

facilities are key strategies to addressing skin infection issues. The most common skin infections that the athletic trainer will encounter are caused by bacteria, fungi, and viruses.

Note: Skin infections are often associated with specific skin wounds. A complete discussion of wounds and proper wound care is found in Chapter 14.

Fungal

Fungal infections are very common in athletic and sport environments. Tinea is a group of fungi commonly associated with ringworm. Ringworm is named for the red ring that appears when the fungus is present on the body. Fungal conditions are named (usually in Latin) based on the location of the fungus. Common fungal infections include the following:

✓ Tinea corporis—Tinea of the body or ringworm (Figure 9-1)

✓ Tinea pedis—Tinea on the feet or athlete's foot

✓ Tinea capitis—Tinea of the scalp

Skin Infections in Wrestling: Special Considerations

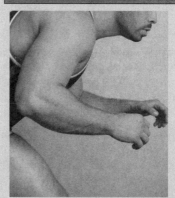

Data from the NCAA Injury Surveillance System (ISS) indicate that skin infections are associated with at least 10% of the time-loss injuries in wrestling. It is recommended that qualified personnel, including a knowledgeable, experienced physician, examine the skin of all wrestlers before any participation.

Open wounds and infectious skin conditions that cannot be adequately protected should be considered cause for medical disqualification from practice or competition. The term *adequately protected* means that the wound or skin condition has been deemed noninfectious and adequately medicated and is able to be covered by a securely attached bandage made of nonpermeable material that will withstand the rigors of competition.

Wrestlers who are undergoing treatment for a communicable skin disease at the time of a competition are required to provide written documentation to that effect from a physician. This documentation should include the wrestler's diagnosis, culture results (if possible), date and time therapy began, and the exact names of medication for treatment. The *NCAA Sports Medicine Handbook* provides specific guidelines for the disposition of a range of skin infections. Athletic trainers caring for wrestling teams must work closely with team physicians to insure proper guidelines are followed.

Skin infections may be transmitted by both direct (person to person) and indirect (person to inanimate surface to person) contact. Infection control measures, or measures that seek to prevent the spread of disease, should be utilized to reduce the risks of disease transmission. Efforts should be made to improve wrestler hygiene practices, to utilize recommended procedures for cleaning and disinfection of surfaces, and to handle blood and other bodily fluids appropriately. Suggested measures include promoting hand hygiene practices; educating athletes not to pick, squeeze, or scratch skin lesions; encouraging athletes to shower after activity; educating athletes not to share protective gear, towels, razors, or water bottles; ensuring recommended procedures for cleaning and disinfection of wrestling mats, all athletic equipment, locker rooms, and whirlpool tubs are closely followed; and verifying clean up of blood and other potentially infectious materials is done, according to the OSHA Blood-Borne Pathogens Standard #29 CFR 1910.1030.

Adapted from the National Collegiate Athletic Association. *NCAA Sports Medicine Handbook.* Indianapolis, IN: Author; 2006.

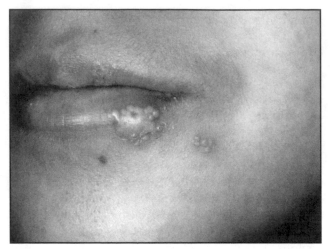

Figure 9-2. Herpes simplex. (Courtesy of Dr. Gary Williams UW Madison School of Medicine and Public Health.)

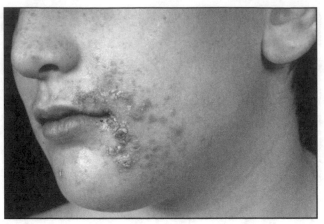

Figure 9-3. Impetigo. (Courtesy of Dr. Gary Williams UW Madison School of Medicine and Public Health.)

✓ Tinea cruris—Tinea of the groin region or jock itch

✓ Tinea unguium—Tinea of the nail bed (most often the toes)

Fungus needs a wet, dark, warm environment to grow. A key component of this treatment will involve changing this environment. Itching and redness are common. However, persistent scratching can lead to an open wound environment and a secondary infection. Over-the-counter antifungal medications (powders and sprays) combined with improved drying to the infected area are the appropriate initial care. Fungal infections that do not respond to treatment or any infection that is not isolated (ie, is spreading) should be referred to a physician.

Viral

A virus is an opportunistic organism that must live in a host cell. Once a virus is present, it may cause a condition that appears rapidly or it may live in a cell for an extended period. The most common viral skin infections seen in athletic populations are the herpes group of viruses.

✓ Herpes simplex type 1—Responsible for cold sores and fever blisters (Figure 9-2)

✓ Herpes simplex type 2—Responsible for genital herpes

Herpes simplex that appears on the shoulders and back is referred to as herpes gladiatorum (named after the gladiators on whom it often appeared) and is common in wrestlers. These viruses are opportunistic and can appear during times of stress (final exams or competitions) or when the host is fatigued or ill. Given the contagious nature of the problem, herpes outbreaks must be treated aggressively and covered to prevent spreading. In NCAA wrestling, any infected area that cannot be covered adequately is considered cause for disqualification.

Herpes outbreaks result in a tingling sensation followed by an outbreak of fluid-filled vesicles. The lesion may be painful. Since the virus can live dormant in the host cells, herpes outbreaks tend to reoccur in the same place. While medications can be used to treat the outbreak and lessen their severity, the virus will not be killed and can return. Over-the-counter topical creams and oral antiviral medications can be used. Herpes virus can spread with contact and thus universal precautions must be practiced at all times.

Bacterial

Bacterial infections can also be seen among physically active individuals. Collectively, bacterial infections are known as pyoderma. These are pus-producing infections of the superficial layer of the skin and include the following:

✓ Impetigo contagiosa (Figure 9-3)

✓ Folliculitis—Inflammation and inflection of hair follicles

✓ Furuncles—Commonly called a boil

The most common culprits to bacterial infections are streptococci and staphylococcus bacteria often secondary to a wound that has not received proper care. Impetigo contagiosa warrants specific discussion since it is highly contagious and is frequently seen in children or athletes that have close skin-to-skin contact (eg, wrestlers). The infection presents as a group of skin erosions with honey-colored crusts on them. This crusting is a characteristic of impetigo infections. Other bacterial infections may be characterized by redness, warmth, and swelling. Pus formation is not uncommon. Treatment requires use of a topical antibacterial agent or the use of a systemic antibiotic.

Methicillin-Resistant Staphylococcus aureus

Methicillin-resistant *Staphylococcus aureus* (MRSA) is a type of "staph" infection that has proven to be resistant to several common antibiotics.[9] The seriousness of this potentially fatal infection is gaining greater public awareness. A recent case of the death of a high school wrestler from complications secondary to a staph infection was reported in *USA Today*.[10] It is believed the boy acquired the infection at a summer wrestling camp. MRSA was traditionally viewed as a hospital pathogen; however, it is more commonly found in other community settings and is now described as either hospital-associated MRSA (HA-MRSA) or community-associated MRSA (CA-MRSA).[9,11] Because of the crowded and close contact environments inherent to athletic practice and competition, team sports have become a target population for CA-MRSA.[12] Infections are facilitated by turf burn abrasions, chafing, shaving, prolonged physical contact, and also by the sharing of towels and equipment. Outbreaks have been reported in several team sports. One case study of a professional football team reported that players with turf burns were 7 times more likely to develop CA-MRSA than those without turf burns.[13]

The significance of the MRSA infection lies in the unfortunate combination that it is resistant to some antibiotics but it is also virulent. Clinically, CA-MRSA presents with skin and soft tissue lesions in an estimated 70% to 80% of the infections.[12] Most of these infections are in the mild form of common skin lesions (folliculitis, furuncles or boils, impetigo, or small abscesses that can be incised and drained). Cases of necrotizing fasciitis (tissue death) and necrotizing soft tissue abscesses requiring surgical resection are being reported with increased frequency.[14] Fully invasive CA-MRSA is not common but it can cause significant mortality and disabling outcomes. Death from septic shock syndrome can occur. Management is determined by the clinical presentation and may involve drainage of abscesses or treatment with oral antibiotics. Severe cases can require hospitalization.

Athletic trainers working in team environments should consult with team physicians regarding any potential skin infections. The NATA has put out an official statement on CA-MRSA that outlines good hygiene practices and guidelines for prevention of CA-MRSA outbreaks.

 ## Official Statement from the National Athletic Trainers' Association on Community-Acquired MRSA Infections

In an effort to educate the public about the potential risks of the emergence of community-acquired methicillin-resistant staphylococcus infection (CA-MRSA), the NATA recommends that health care personnel and physically active participants take appropriate precautions with suspicious lesions and talk with a physician.

According to the Centers for Disease Control and Prevention (CDC), approximately 25% to 30% of the population is colonized in the nose with *Staphylococcus aureus*, often referred to as "staph" and approximately 1% of the population is colonized with MRSA.[1]

Cases have developed from person-to-person contact, shared towels and soaps, improperly treated whirlpools, and equipment (mats, pads, surfaces, etc). Staph or CA-MRSA infections usually manifest as skin infections, such as pimples, pustules, and boils that present as red, swollen, painful, or have pus or other drainage. Without proper referral and care, more serious infections may cause pneumonia, bloodstream infections, or surgical wound infections.

Maintaining good hygiene and avoiding contact with drainage from skin lesions are the best methods for prevention.

Proper prevention and management recommendations may include, but are not limited to, the following:

- Keep hands clean by washing thoroughly with soap and warm water or using an alcohol-based hand sanitizer routinely.
- Encourage immediate showering following activity.
- Avoid whirlpools or common tubs if you have an open wound, scrape, or scratch.
- Avoid sharing towels, razors, and daily athletic gear.
- Properly wash athletic gear and towels after each use.
- Maintain clean facilities and equipment.

(continued)

ⓘ Official Statement from the National Athletic Trainers' Association on Community-Acquired MRSA Infections (continued)

- Inform or refer to appropriate health care personnel for all active skin lesions and lesions that do not respond to initial therapy.
- Administer or seek proper first aid.
- Encourage health care personnel to seek bacterial cultures to establish a diagnosis.
- Care for and cover skin lesions appropriately before participation.

Reference

1. Centers for Disease Control and Prevention. CA-MRSA information for the public. Available on-line at: http://www.cdc.gov/ncidod/hip/aresist/ca_mrsa_public.htm. Accessed July 25, 2008.

Official Statement; National Athletic Trainers' Association March 1, 200. Reprinted with permission of NATA.

THE FEMALE ATHLETE TRIAD

The female athlete triad is a syndrome that occurs in physically active girls and women. The triad consists of the inter-related components of disordered eating, menstrual irregularities, and bone health (osteoporosis).[1] Disordered eating represents a spectrum of behaviors that need not meet the full diagnostic criteria for anorexia or bulimia. These disordered behaviors may include caloric restriction, binging and purging, use of pills or laxatives, and induced vomiting.

The second component of the triad is menstrual irregularity. Studies indicate that the prevalence of menstrual irregularities among active women can vary greatly. Menstrual irregularities may include absence of onset of menses (primary amenorrhea) or absence of menses for 3 consecutive months following onset of menses (secondary amenorrhea). Menstrual irregularity is more common in athletes than the general population.[15] The highest frequency of irregularity is seen among ballet dancers and runners. Amenorrhea may be triggered by changes in the endocrine system through exercise or secondary to an eating disorder. It is important for the athletic trainer to be aware that an athlete with menstrual irregularity should be referred for a complete evaluation. The evaluation may indicate an eating-related problem, female athlete triad, or a stand-alone menstrual dysfunction.

The final component of the triad is bone health. Specifically, bone loss or osteoporosis. Within the context of the female athlete triad, changes in bone health may include premature bone loss, inadequate bone, or possibly both. These changes are due to inadequate levels of available estrogen. Athletes with the female athlete triad will experience deterioration in the normal bone architecture due to increased skeletal fragility. Due to these changes, these athletes are at risk for stress fractures.

ⓘ Common Risk Factors and Sports-Related Triggers for Disordered Eating

Risk Factors	Sports-Related Triggers
Chronic dieting	Inappropriate idea that low weight will improve performance
Low self-esteem	Pressure to lose weight from coaches, parents, and peers
Family dysfunction	Drive to win at any cost
Physical or sexual abuse	Self-identity as athlete only
Biologic factors	Over-trained and undernourished
Perfectionism	Traumatic event (injury, grief, loss of coach)
Lack of nutritional knowledge	Vulnerable times of life (growth spurt, adolescence, entering college)

Adolescents and women training for activities that stress appearance or low body weight are at greatest risk for the female athlete triad.[1] Alone or in combination, female athlete triad disorders can decrease performance and in extreme cases have catastrophic consequences. The athletic trainer and all individuals who work with physically active girls and women should be educated about the triad and develop plans to prevent, recognize, treat, and reduce risks.[1]

PSYCHOLOGICAL CONSIDERATIONS

Athletes and physically active individuals (like anyone) may find themselves facing a specific psychosocial crisis. The athletic trainer must be able to facilitate the referral or guidance for psychosocial crisis by implementing intervention strategies to meet the needs of the patient.[16] These psychosocial issues may stem from a variety of sources, such as stress, family issues, depression, sexual identity issues, conflict resolution difficulties, and a host of other possibilities. The athletic trainer has an obligation to understand the problems common to the population with which he or she works and have skills in the appropriate referral techniques. Athletic trainers will often work closely with the resources available on their campus or in the community to establish a plan for assisting patients with psychosocial issues.

INJURIES AND CONDITIONS OF THE ABDOMEN

Layers of muscle and soft tissue protect the abdomen. The nature of this anatomical arrangement makes the region susceptible to muscular strain injuries as well as contusions. While most contusions and strain injuries to the abdomen are minor, trauma to the region can result in injury to the internal organs. Both solid and hollow organs are contained in the abdomen. Hollow organs include the stomach, large and small intestine, ureters, and bladder. Solid organs include the liver, spleen, pancreas, and kidneys. Solid organs have rich blood supply and are of particular concern. Internal bleeding secondary to injury, if left undetected, can become life threatening. This requires the athletic trainer to be aware of such injuries and to evaluate the athlete with care. Immediate referral for a full medical evaluation is in order if there are any signs of acute abdominal injury.

The abdomen can be divided into 4 quadrants (Figures 9-4 and 9-5). This allows the athletic trainer to orient him- or herself to the location of specific organs. Acute abdominal injuries may include splenic rupture, kidney contusion, and contusion/laceration of the liver. A common illness that can cause abdominal pain is the acute appendix.

Recommendations and Strategies for the Female Athlete Triad

- Exercise and sports participation should be promoted in girls and adolescents for health benefit and enjoyment.

- Preparticipation histories and evaluations should review dietary practices; exercise intensity, duration, and frequency; and menstrual history.

- Amenorrhea should be considered a normal response to exercise. A complete evaluation is required for any adolescent with primary or secondary amenorrhea.

- Disordered eating should be considered in adolescents with amenorrhea. Treatment of disordered eating may require a team of health care professionals that includes a physician, nutritionist, and mental health professional. All should have experience in the treatment of eating disorders. Cooperation of coaches, parents, and teammates is an essential component of treatment.

- Education and counseling should be provided to athletes, parents, and coaches regarding the female athlete triad and the need for adequate energy (calorie) and nutrient intake to meet energy expenditure and maintain normal growth and development.

- Weight should not be considered an accurate estimate of fatness or fitness. A body composition measure that suggests a range of values rather than specific values is preferable. It is difficult and potentially dangerous to define an ideal level of weight and/or body fat for each sport or individual participant.

- Adolescents with menstrual dysfunction attributed to exercise should be encouraged to increase their energy (caloric) intake and modify exercise activity. If the athlete's weight is too low, she may be required to gain weight before resuming athletic activity.

- Estrogen-progesterone supplementation may be considered in the mature amenorrheic athlete.

- Measurement of bone mineral density may be considered as a tool when making treatment decisions for the amenorrheic athlete.

Adapted from AAP Committee on Fitness and Sports Medicine. Medical concerns in the female athlete. *Pediatrics*. 2000;106:610-613.

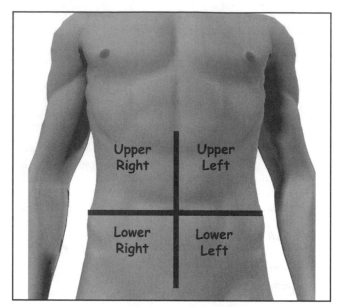

Figure 9-4. The abdomen can be divided into 4 quadrants intersecting at the umbilicus.

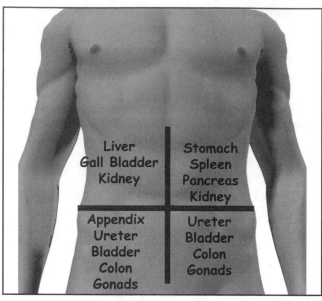

Figure 9-5. The solid organs of the abdomen can be identified through palpation by knowing the quadrant system.

Splenic Rupture

The spleen is the most commonly injured abdominal organ due to sports-related trauma. The spleen is located in the upper left quadrant and is protected by the lower ribs. The spleen stores red blood cells and is responsible for producing antibodies and white blood cells during illness. Some illnesses, like mononucleosis, can cause the spleen to be enlarged and more susceptible to trauma. The mechanism for an injury to the spleen includes a direct blow to the upper left quadrant. Other mechanisms can include a fall or landing on an object over the upper left quadrant. Signs and symptoms of a splenic injury include the following[5]:

✓ Upper left quadrant pain

✓ Nausea and vomiting may be present

✓ Signs of shock

  ○ Decreasing blood pressure

  ○ Cold, clammy skin

  ○ Pale color

  ○ Weak rapid pulse

✓ Signs of abdominal bleeding

  ○ Abdominal rigidity (with palpation)

  ○ Tenderness (especially rebound tenderness [ie, tenderness when the hand is removed from the abdomen])

✓ Kehr's sign

  ○ Radiating pain to the left shoulder or arm

If an athlete displays any of the above signs, he or she should be referred immediately for care. A splenic rupture is a medical emergency (see Chapter 11 for a discussion of emergency plans). Splenic injuries can present in a delayed fashion. Any athlete who has sustained blunt trauma to the abdomen should be evaluated and the signs and symptoms of delayed hemorrhage should be discussed.[5] It is the risk of splenic rupture that requires patients with mononucleosis to avoid contact and vigorous activity until the spleen has returned to normal size.

 Splenic Rupture and Removal: An NFL Case Study

In September 2006 in a game with the Carolina Panthers, Tampa Bay quarterback Chris Simms took several hard hits behind the line of scrimmage. He felt a bit dehydrated and labored due to some sore ribs sustained late in the game but played on in a 26-24 losing effort. Hours after the game, he was recovering in a hospital following a splenectomy to remove his ruptured spleen. It was reported he lost up to 5 pints of blood prior to his emergency surgery.

This case serves as a reminder that not all spleen injuries will present with the "classic" symptoms. It also brings to light the need for follow-up evaluation of athletes who have had abdominal or thoracic region trauma. The sideline or courtside evaluation is only a "snapshot," and some signs and symptoms of more serious injury do not present readily. The potential for delayed hemorrhage is an all too real possibility.

Simms spent 2007 on injured reserve and is still pursuing a NFL career.

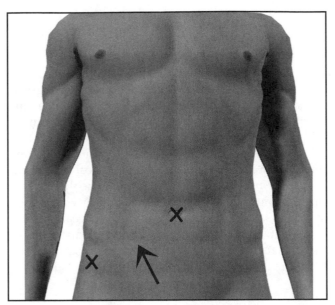

Figure 9-6. McBurney's point is located halfway between the umbilicus and the ASIS. It is the location of tenderness with acute appendix.

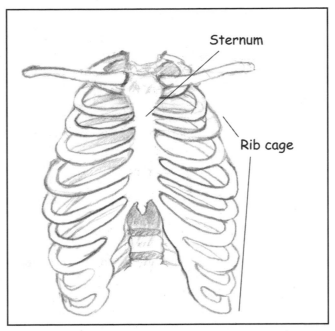

Figure 9-7. The rib cage and sternum serve to protect the internal organs of the thorax.

Contusion to the Kidney

The kidney is susceptible to contusions as a result of direct trauma from sports such as boxing and football. The MOI involves a direct blow or blunt trauma. The athlete may report a deep ache in the lower back, and muscle guarding and hematuria (blood in the urine) may be present. Severe injury can result in signs of shock, nausea, vomiting, and severe hematuria.[5] Hematuria is not always visible and may need to be confirmed by urinalysis. An athlete with a suspected kidney contusion should be referred immediately for a full evaluation. Care of the contused kidney may involve hospitalization for observation and gradual increase in fluid intake. If the bleeding is severe, surgical intervention may be needed.[6]

Contusion/Laceration of the Liver

Injuries to the liver are rare. The MOI involves direct trauma to the right side of the rib cage. The liver may become contused or lacerated. Liver injuries may take place secondary to injuries to the ribs. The primary concern is bleeding into the abdominal cavity. If the liver is enlarged secondary to hepatitis, it may be more susceptible to injury. A patient with a liver injury will have pain and tenderness in the upper right quadrant. However, pain may refer to the chest and shoulders. Suspected liver injuries require immediate referral.

Acute Appendix

Acute appendix is a common illness that affects the abdominal region. It is common in younger adults and presents with pain in the lower right quadrant, low-grade fever, nausea, vomiting, and pain that increases with walking or coughing. Palpation over McBurney's point (Figure 9-6) mid way between the navel and the ASIS may reveal point tenderness or rebound tenderness. The inflamed appendix can rupture if it is not treated. A rupture can cause infection to the entire abdominal cavity. As with any abdominal pain, prompt referral to the physician is in order.

THORACIC INJURIES

The organs of the thoracic cavity are well protected by the skeletal arrangement of the rib cage (Figure 9-7). However, injuries to the internal organs can take place and injuries to the musculoskeletal structures that protect those organs are commonplace. In sport and physical activities, direct blows, falls, or contact with an implement like a ball or bat can cause injuries to the ribs, supporting structures, or internal organs. Since the heart and lungs are contained in the thoracic cavity, injuries to this area can be life threatening. Possible serious internal injuries in this area include a pneumothorax and cardiac contusion. Common musculoskeletal injuries include contusions, sprains, and fractures to the ribs and sternum.

Pneumothorax

A pneumothorax occurs when air is allowed to enter the pleural sac that surrounds the lungs. The entrance of air into this cavity will cause the lungs to collapse and pull away from the chest wall. This reduces the lungs' ability to inflate and deflate properly. While this injury is not common in sport, it can occur. It may be caused by trauma (spontaneous collapse) or penetration secondary to a rib injury. The signs and symptoms associated with pneumothorax include pain in the chest region, dyspnea (difficulty breathing), deviation of the trachea, and light-headedness. A full evaluation including listening to lung sounds is required. A severe pneumothorax may cause the patient to take on a blue or cyanotic appearance.[5] Any patient with a suspected pneumothorax injury should be referred immediately by activating an emergency action plan.

Lung collapse may progress to a tension pneumothorax. A tension pneumothorax occurs when air trapped in the pleural cavity places tension on the heart and other lung. This increased pressure can compromise function of these vital organs. A tension pneumothorax can cause fatal loss of oxygen due to circulatory and respiratory system collapse. Any suspected respiratory trauma warrants activation of the emergency plan.

Cardiac Contusion

Cardiac contusions can occur secondary to blunt trauma to the chest. Being struck by a hockey puck or baseball is a common MOI. The contusion is caused by compression of the heart between the sternum and the rib cage. Damage to the heart can take place and can be life threatening. Signs and symptoms may include chest pain, signs of shock, changes in heart rhythm, and possible respiratory distress. Blunt trauma to the chest should always cause the health care provider to suspect internal injuries and evaluate with care. Immediate referral is the appropriate action.

Another condition known as cardiac concussion (commotio cordis) can also occur following blunt trauma. The condition presents with immediate cardiac arrest and sudden death following the injury. The injury need not be severe enough to damage musculoskeletal tissue to result in a fatality. Such conditions again reinforce the need for emergency action plans and the availability of trained personnel at venues where such injuries may occur.

SUMMARY

Injuries to the abdomen and thorax can range from simple muscle strains to medical emergencies. The skilled athletic trainer must be able to recognize, manage, and make appropriate referrals when dealing with abdominal and thoracic injuries. The domains of athletic training extend beyond just the care of athletic injuries. The ability to provide recognition, care, and referral for illnesses and general medical conditions round out an approach to sports medicine that is more inclusive and holistic. The athletic trainer who understands the need for this global view and can become proficient in both the musculoskeletal and general medical realm will be well prepared to serve his or her patients.

REFERENCES

1. American College of Sports Medicine. ACSM position stand on the female athlete triad. *Med Sci Sports Exerc*. 1997;29:i-ix.
2. Landry GL, Bernhardt DT. *Essentials of Primary Care Sports Medicine*. Champaign, IL: Human Kinetics; 2003.
3. Marion BJ, Shirani J, Poliac LC, Mathenge R, Roberts WC, Mueller FO. Sudden death in young competitive athletes: clinical, demographic and pathological profiles. *JAMA*. 1996;276:199-204.
4. Mick TM, Dimeff RJ. What kind of physical examination does a young athlete need before participating in sports? *Cleve Clin J Med*. 2004;71(7):587-597.
5. Shultz SJ, Houglum PA, Perrin DH. *Assessment of Athletic Injuries*. 2nd ed. Champaign, IL: Human Kinetics; 2005.
6. Prentice WE. *Arnheims's Principles of Athletic Training*. 13th ed. New York: McGraw-Hill Higher Education; 2009.
7. Sullivan AJ, Anderson SJ. *Care of the Young Athlete*. Oklahoma City, OK: American Academy of Orthopaedic Surgeons & American Academy of Pediatrics; 2000.
8. CDC. Meningococcal disease. Center for Disease Control: frequently asked questions. Available at www.cdc.gov/meningitis/bacterial/faqs.htm. Accessed July 2008.
9. MedlinePlus. MRSA. Available at www.nlm.nih.gov/medlineplus.print.mrsa.html. Accessed August 2008.
10. USA Today. Mother says son died from complications of staph infection. Available at www.usatoday.com/sports/preps/2008-07-25-staph-infection_N.htm. Accessed April 20, 2009.
11. Rihn JA, Marian GM, Harner CD. Community-acquired methicillin-resistant *Staphylococcus aureus*. *Am J Sports Med*. 2005;33(12):1924-1929.
12. Lu D, Holtom P. Community-acquired methicillin-resistant *Staphylococcus aureus*: a new player in sports medicine. *Curr Sports Med Rep*. 2005;4(5):265-270.
13. Kazakova S, Hageman J, Matava M, et al. A clone of methicillin-resistant *Staphylococcus aureus* among professional football players. *N Engl J Med*. 2005;352:468-475.
14. Miller LG, Perdreau-Remington F, Rieg G, et al. Necrotizing fasciitis caused by *Staphylococcus aureus* in Los Angeles. *N Engl J Med*. 2005;352:1445-1453.

15. American Academy of Pediatrics Committee on Sports Medicine and Fitness. Medical concerns in the female athlete. *Pediatrics.* 2000;106:610-613.
16. Board of Certification Inc. *Role Delineation Study.* 5th ed. Omaha, NE: NATA Board of Certification, Inc; 2004.

🌐 WEB RESOURCES

Centers for Disease Control and Prevention
www.cdc.gov
A helpful government site sponsored by the US Department of Health and Human Services. Information regarding infectious disease, information for travelers, health bulletins on various topics, and current funding and research projects are provided.

American Academy of Pediatrics
www.aap.org
The Web site for the AAP provides information regarding many aspects of providing care for children and adolescents. Professional publications section allows for searches of current position statements and reports.

American College of Sports Medicine
www.acsm.org
Position stands and general health and fitness information are available from the Web site.

American Academy of Allergy, Asthma, and Immunology
www.aaaai.org
This Web site provides information for consumers, patients, and professionals regarding asthma, allergies, and immunology issues.

Career Spotlight: Director of Performing Arts Rehabilitation

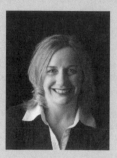

Julie O'Connell, PT, ATC

Director of Performing Arts Rehabilitation

AthletiCo at East Bank Club, Chicago, IL

My Position

I am a clinical physical therapist and athletic trainer and the Director of Performing Arts Rehabilitation. I spend my day treating patients in a clinical environment and providing on-site services backstage with professional dance companies and Broadway shows. I also work as an administrator to create relationships with current affiliations and to foster opportunities with new companies in need of on-site services.

Unique or Desired Qualifications

A performing arts clinician exhibits a unique balance of dance-, music-, and art-specific knowledge with a strong manual therapy background. It is important to speak the language of the performers in order to assist them with assessment and treatment of their injuries. Within the backstage environment, the clinician needs to be flexible and creative in determining an appropriate treatment space as there are not allocated health care locations in the theaters. Performing arts medicine is a great new field for clinicians that have had previous experience in dance and music and want to share their medical knowledge with these professionals.

Favorite Aspect of My Job

The favorite aspect of my job is the opportunity to see performers return to the stage in a healthy environment following an injury. There is so much creativity that goes into taping, bracing, and padding the injuries of these performers in order for them to maintain the integrity of their costuming without compromising their health.

Advice

I would encourage students with dance and music expertise to give back to the arts community as a health care provider. These athletes/artists could really benefit from clinicians with the passion to return them to the stage injury free.

SECTION III

PLANNING, PREVENTION, AND CARE

CHAPTER 10

BLOOD-BORNE PATHOGENS AND UNIVERSAL PRECAUTIONS

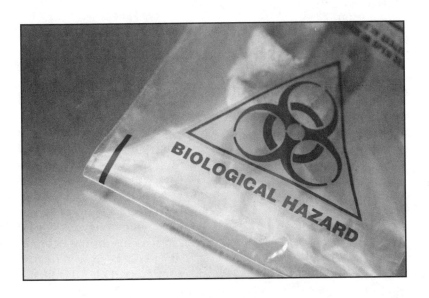

To be a good athletic trainer requires an odd mix of interpersonal skills, science-based knowledge/skill, and personal empathy.

Chad Starkey, PhD, ATC, FNATA
Associate Professor
Ohio University

Blood-borne pathogens (BBP) continue to be a major world health concern. Hepatitis B virus (HBV), hepatitis C virus (HCV), and human immunodeficiency virus (HIV) are the most common BBP. According to the World Health Organization (WHO),[1] there are over 350 million people worldwide infected with HBV. The CDC reports an estimate of 1.25 million people in the United States with the HBV infection.[2] It is estimated that 180 million people worldwide are infected with HCV with an estimate of 130 million being chronic carriers. In the United States, 1.8% of the population is infected with HCV, with 3.8 million exposed and 2.7 million chronically affected.[1] HBV and HCV are major causes of acute hepatitis and chronic liver

disease, including primary hepatocellular carcinoma (liver cancer) and cirrhosis, which eventually leads to liver failure. Liver cancer and cirrhosis kill more than 1 million people annually.[1] At the end of 2003, an estimated 1,039,000 to 1,185,000 persons in the United States were living with HIV/acquired immunodeficiency syndrome (AIDS), with 24% to 27% undiagnosed and unaware of their HIV infection. HIV/AIDS refers to cases of HIV infection, regardless of whether they have progressed to AIDS. The HIV virus infection is a progressive disease leading to immune suppression and the development of AIDS.

Blood-borne infections like HIV, HBV, and HCV are transmitted through unprotected sexual contact, exposure to blood and blood components through use of needles, contamination of open wounds or mucous membranes by infected blood, and perinatally from an infected mother to fetus or infant.[3] Due to potential exposure from patients infected with BBP, health care providers are considered an at-risk group. Dealing with wounds and potential needle sticks are common exposure mechanisms in health care settings. Given this risk, understanding the nature of these viruses and the need for adherence to universal precautions is imperative for practicing athletic trainers.

Upon completion of this chapter, the student will be able to:

✓ Identify the nature of BBP, including HIV, HBV, and HCV

✓ Describe common high-risk activities associated with the transmission of BBP

✓ Explain the risks of transmission during sporting activities

✓ Evaluate the common position statements regarding BBP in the athletic setting

✓ List appropriate vaccination strategies for health care providers

✓ Apply universal precautions

✓ Discuss the role of the athletic trainer in minimizing the risk of exposure to BBP in an athletic environment

BLOOD-BORNE PATHOGENS

BBP are disease-causing micro-organisms that can be potentially transmitted through contact with blood. These pathogens can cause serious or fatal infections. The most serious include HIV, HBV, and HCV. BBP are transmitted through unprotected sexual contact, direct contact with infected blood or blood components, and perinatally from mother to baby.[4] Activities like unprotected sexual contact, intravenous (IV) drug use, and the sharing of needles are known forms of transmitting BBP. Behaviors such as body piercing and tattoos cause exposure to blood and therefore must be considered an increased risk for contracting HBV, HIV, or HCV.[4] It is these off-field behaviors, not sports participation, that place the athlete at the greatest risk of contracting a BBP infection.[3]

HUMAN IMMUNODEFICIENCY VIRUS

HIV infection is a progressive disease leading to immune suppression and the development of AIDS. AIDS is characterized by the development of opportunistic infections and malignancies that ultimately lead to the death of the patient. It is associated with Kaposi's sarcoma, a cancer of the soft tissues that causes highly visible purplish lesions and is extremely rare among those with normal immunity. Upon infection, HIV infects the lymph nodes, which may enlarge in a similar fashion to a mononucleosis infection. About 2 to 6 weeks after exposure, 50% of all newly infected people experience fever, chills, headache, and sore throat similar to flu-like symptoms. Half of all newly infected people experience no symptoms. Both groups will enter an asymptomatic stage that may be protracted (months to several years). This period of time may present issues for health care providers regarding a patient's involvement in athletics. HIV specifically targets a type of white blood cell called a T lymphocyte, or simply T cell. There are several types of T cells; the CD 4 cells are targeted by HIV.[5] T lymphocytes are responsible for the cell-mediated immunity that is critical for fighting viral infections, fungal infections, and certain bacteria. CD 4 cells are essential to normal function because of the immunity they provide.[5] In the AIDS stage of the disease, the immune system is severely compromised and the body loses its ability to fight disease.

Patients who have developed full-blown AIDS may notice fatigue and weight loss. Pneumonia may be the first sign of immunodeficiency. Patients with HIV infection may develop pneumonia that is often caused by infectious agents that do not normally cause pneumonia. Pneumonocystis carinii was previously only seen in patients immunocompromised by chemotherapy. It had not been seen in any other group before the discovery of AIDS. All infections are difficult to treat because of the weakened immune response.

HEPATITIS B VIRUS

There are estimated to be over 1 million carriers of HBV in the United States. HBV causes infection of the liver and can make individuals very ill will fever, chills, loss of appetite, nausea, abdominal pain, jaundice, or any combination of these signs and symptoms. One third of patients will experience severe hepatitis, which will cause death in 1% of those.[2] Of the 3 viruses discussed in this chapter, HBV is the most contagious but it is not the most virulent.[5] Infected individuals may have no symptoms or only experience mild symptoms similar to influenza (flu). About half of all infected patients have subclinical HBV, which means the infection does not make them ill. There are 2 major problems associated with HBV infections[5]:

1. In about 6% to 10% of infected adults, the virus remains in the liver and bloodstream because the immune system cannot kill the virus. These individuals become carriers of the virus. Their

A Few Words About Gloving

Prior to donning a pair of gloves, the athletic trainer should take a look at his or her hands. Are there cuts? Scrapes? Hangnails?

Covering broken skin areas with a dressing before gloving will provide you with some increased protection. Wearing rings, especially those with large stones, or having long fingernails may cause small perforations in the gloves, thereby decreasing their protective value. Long fingernails can harbor significant amounts of bacteria and may contribute to infection.

Just wearing your gloves to protect yourself and your patient is not enough. You must remove them in the proper fashion. Gloves should be removed in a manner that prohibits contact with the contaminated surface of the glove. This means that your hands should never come in contact with the outer, dirty surfaces of the gloves. This can be accomplished by following these steps:

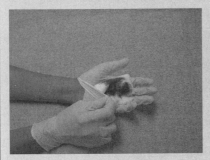 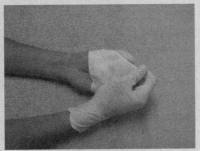 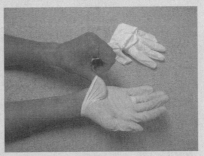

| Grab the first glove on the outer surface at the wrist. | Pull the glove back onto itself so that when it is completely removed it will be inside out. | Remove the other glove by slipping your bare fingers inside the glove, and pulling it off so that it is also inside out when completely removed. |

bodily fluids can infect other people at any time. There are an estimated 400 million carriers of HBV.

2. About 5% of infected individuals develop chronic liver infection, and another 20% eventually die from cirrhosis or liver cancer, which tends to develop several decades after the original infection.

HEPATITIS C VIRUS

Prior to its discovery in 1989 and effective testing methods to detect the virus in blood products, millions of people were infected with HCV. Tainted blood transfusions or blood products accounted for millions of infections. Today, developed countries screen for such infections and this is no longer a risk for infection. Most of the currently HCV+ patients in the United States contracted the disease prior to 1990. There are fewer than 30,000 new cases of infection in the United States annually. However, it may take decades for liver symptoms to manifest. In the United States, 8000 to 10,000 deaths and approximately 1000 liver transplants are attributed to HCV.

Initial symptoms of HCV include diminished appetite, fever, muscle aches, fatigue, and sometimes jaundice. A large majority of people (~75%) have subclinical cases at first, meaning they experience no symptoms.[5] Eighty percent to 85% of cases are chronically infected for the rest of their lives. Approximately 6 to 12 develop cirrhosis of the liver within about 20 years, and as many as 12 per 100 develop cirrhosis within 40 years of the infection. HCV is spread through blood transfusions and needle sharing among IV drug users. Estimates of the percentage of cases acquired through sexual activity range from 6% to 35%. The odds of acquiring the virus through sexual activity seem in proportion to the number of sexual partners and the presence of a secondary infection (eg, genital herpes or HIV).[5] Like all BBP, avoidance of high-risk behaviors is the first line of defense.

RISK OF BLOOD-BORNE INFECTIONS IN SPORT

While the risk of HIV transmission in sports is not considered to be zero, it is so sufficiently small that it cannot be accurately quantified. Transmission of HIV in sports has not been documented.[6] Despite this low risk, some sports such as boxing, wrestling, and

Universal Precautions

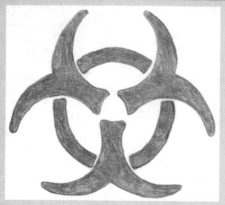

OSHA is a division of the US Department of Labor. OSHA in conjunction with other federal agencies publishes the *Blood-Borne Pathogens Standard*, a federal directive that dictates how employers must protect workers and the public with regards to BBP. The concept of universal precautions grew from a series of documents published in the 1980s by the CDC that instructed how blood and bodily fluids should be handled in hospital settings. That original document evolved to the *Universal Blood and Bodily Fluid Precautions* published in 1987. These guidelines are now simply known as universal precautions.

- Barrier protection should be used at all times to prevent skin and mucous membrane contamination with blood, body fluids containing visible blood, or other body fluids (cerebrospinal, synovial, pleural, peritoneal, pericardial, and amniotic fluids, semen and vaginal secretions). Barrier protection should be used with ALL tissues. The type of barrier protection used should be appropriate for the type of procedures being performed and the type of exposure anticipated. Examples of barrier protection include disposable lab coats, gloves, and eye and face protection.

- Gloves are to be worn when there is potential for hand or skin contact with blood, other potentially infectious material, or items and surfaces contaminated with these materials.

- Wear face protection (face shield) during procedures that are likely to generate droplets of blood or body fluid to prevent exposure to mucous membranes of the mouth, nose, and eyes.

- Wear protective body clothing (disposable laboratory coats) when there is a potential for splashing of blood or body fluids.

- Wash hands or other skin surfaces thoroughly and immediately if contaminated with blood, body fluids containing visible blood, or other body fluids to which universal precautions apply.

- Wash hands immediately after gloves are removed.

- Avoid accidental injuries that can be caused by needles, scalpel blades, laboratory instruments, etc when performing procedures, cleaning instruments, handling sharp instruments, and disposing of used needles, pipettes, etc.

- Used needles, disposable syringes, scalpel blades, pipettes, and other sharp items are to be placed in puncture-resistant containers (Figure 10-1) marked with a biohazard symbol for disposal (shown above).

Adapted from Occupational Safety & Health Administration. Revision to OSHA's Bloodborne Pathogens Standard: Technical Background and Summary; 2001 and National Institute of Environmental Health Sciences. Biological Safety—Universal Precautions. 2001.

contact sports where bleeding is a possibility require vigilant use of universal precautions. HIV cannot be transmitted through normal body contact such as touching and sharing of sports equipment (though equipment sharing should be discouraged) or using facilities such as locker rooms or bathrooms.

The risk of transmission of HBV in sports is also considered quite low; however, it may be assumed to be higher than HIV given the number of potential carriers. There is one documented case of transmission in an athletic setting among sumo wrestlers in Japan. There is also evidence that household contact with HBV carriers may result in infection without participation in risk behaviors. These are rare and likely occur through unrecognized wound or mucous membrane exposure.[7] HBV is resistant to drying,

ambient temperatures, simple detergents, and alcohol and can be stable on environmental surfaces for at least 7 days. Hence transmission can occur via environmental surfaces. This is another reason that the theoretical risk is higher than HIV. However, like HIV, the risk is greatest for individuals who participate in high-risk behaviors.[7] A comparison of HBV and HIV viruses is provided in Table 10-1. Table 10-2 compares sport playability and risk of transmission issues for HBV and HIV.

HCV transmission is not as contagious as HBV and not as virulent as HIV. While it is a serious threat, it is not likely to be seen among participants on sports teams in developed nations. Again, the practice of universal precautions and avoidance of high-risk activities is the cornerstone to all prevention programs.

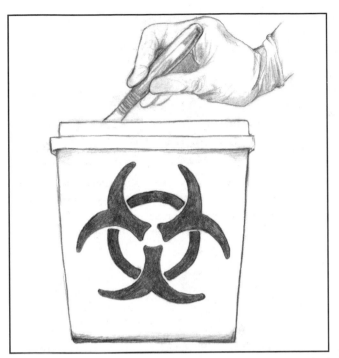

Figure 10-1. Biohazard receptacles for the proper disposal of needles, syringes, and scalpel blades are essential for adherence to universal precautions.

Doping and Drug Abuse

Blood-borne infections can be transmitted through blood doping and there is a significant risk of infection from sharing needles that may be associated with drug abuse in sports. Three separate cases of HIV infection among bodybuilders sharing needles for steroid use have been cited in the literature; two in the United States and one in France.[8] In one of these cases, there was a simultaneous infection of HBV. A case study of a weightlifter with HCV has also presented secondary to needle sharing. A 1993 study estimated that there were 1 million people in the United States who were either current or past users of anabolic steroids.[9] Of these, 50% were intramuscular drug users (they injected steroids), and about 25% admitted to sharing of syringes. Therefore, the risk of infection among this population is clearly elevated.

Travel and Risk Behaviors

BBP can be transmitted through sexual activity. Having unprotected homosexual sex with men and multiple sex partners are the most significant risk factors for these types of infections. However, the most common method of transmission of HBV during adulthood is heterosexual contact with an infected individual, followed by injected drug use, and then homosexual contact.[3] There are limits in the literature as to whether the transmission of infections among athletes through sexual activity is more common than

in the general population. Some literature suggests male athletes may participate in high-risk behaviors specific to the number of sexual partners and less adherence to safe sex practices when compared to nonathletes.[10,11] There appears to be some evidence that sexual activity and having multiple partners is less common among female athletes.[12] Athletic trainers must be prepared to provide sound advice and serve in an educational role when fielding questions regarding these practices. Communication with team physicians and a trusting nonjudgmental approach will be helpful.

PREVENTION OF BLOOD-BORNE INFECTIONS

Education

The main methods of transmission of BBP are not through athletic activity. Potential infections for athletes are similar to those in the general population. Educational efforts should focus on these high-risk activities that are unrelated to sport. In certain environments, the athletic trainer will be called on to serve as an educator. Athletic trainers can create

Table 10-2

Participation by Student Athletes With Hepatitis B Virus or Human Immunodeficiency Virus

	HIV	HBV
Individual health considerations	• Participation decisions should be based on the health status of the individual • Must be asymptomatic with no evidence of immunologic deficiencies • Presence of infection alone does not mandate removal from play • Physician with knowledge of HIV management is critical. • Open patient and care provider communication	• Playability is determined by clinical signs and symptoms (eg, fatigue and fever) • No evidence suggesting competitive training is problematic for HBV carrier • Simple infection presence does not mandate removal from play
Risk of transmission	• Concerns focus on exposure to contaminated blood through open wounds or mucous membranes • Precise risk is impossible to calculate, but evidence suggests that it is extremely low • No validated reports of HIV transmission in the athletics setting and currently no recommended restriction • One state court has upheld exclusion of HIV+ athlete from combative sports (karate)	• Athletes with either acute or chronic HBV infection present limited risk for disease transmission in most sports • HBV risk is greater than HIV in sports with higher potential for blood exposure and sustained close contact (eg, wrestling) • It is prudent to consider removal of the individual with acute HBV illness (acute or chronic) from combative, sustained close-contact sports

Adapted from: NCAA Committee on Competitive Safeguards and Medical Aspects of Sports. Blood-borne pathogens and intercollegiate athletics. *2006-2007 NCAA Sports Medicine Handbook*. Indianapolis, IN: NCAA; 2006-2007:54-60.

 ## Safe Sex Is Also a Universal Precaution

OK, let us be candid. While practicing universal precautions is an essential component to duties as a health care provider, your duties as a citizen of the planet extend a bit further. If you choose to be sexually active, practicing safe sex is the responsible choice you must make. Make safe sex a universal precaution.

The only 100% sure way to protect yourself is to not have sex. If you are going to be sexually active, you should make condom use a habit. Using a condom is still considered the best way to protect yourself from HIV and many other sexually transmitted diseases, but it is by no means foolproof. Human error can decrease the effectiveness in the real world. In order to stay completely protected, make sure you use a condom every time and make sure to put the condom on before any sexual contact.

Always avoid sexual activity when using drugs or alcohol because they can impair your judgment and your ability to use the condom correctly. As health care providers in training, it is important to model specific healthy behaviors and to be comfortable discussing sensitive issues.

More information about universal precautions and safe sex practices can be found at the National Library of Medicine National Institutes of Health public information site at www.nlm.nih.gov.

and distribute information to athletes and patients, co-workers, families, and communities concerning the risk of blood-borne infections, availability of HIV testing, HBV testing and vaccine, and other questions that may arise in their employment setting.[4] These educational efforts must rely on a team approach and utilize physicians, coaches, community health resources, and others to insure their effectiveness and appropriate scope. There are often fears and misconceptions about blood-borne diseases. The athletic trainer can play an important role by serving as an educational resource to allay fears and provide appropriate information.

Dealing with patients infected with blood-borne diseases requires special attention to medical confidentiality. The identity of individuals infected must remain confidential. Only those persons in whom the patient chooses to confide have the right to know about those medical issues. Medical confidentiality is essential to maintain the patient-provider relationship. This level of confidentiality and security of records should always be afforded patients with any illness or injury.

 ## Vaccination and Blood-Borne Pathogens

An effective vaccine to prevent HBV is available, and the CDC recommends that all health care workers be vaccinated for HBV. In addition, the American College Health Association recommends all college students be vaccinated. Based on these 2 recommendations, it is important that athletic training students make efforts to protect themselves, beyond adherence to universal precautions, and get vaccinated. HBV vaccination may be a requirement to meet the health requirements and technical standards of an athletic training education program.

Prevention and Management: Care Provider Roles

The Committee on Sports Medicine and Fitness of the AAP in 1999 released recommendations titled *Human Immunodeficiency Virus and Other Blood-Borne Pathogens in the Athletic Setting.* This document has served as the template for numerous other organizational statements, including the NCAA and NATA. Because athletes and athletic program staff members can be exposed to blood during athletic activity, they have a small risk of infection from HIV, HBV, or HCV. The AAP position statement discusses sports participation for athletes infected with these pathogens and precautions that should be taken to lower the risk of infection to other persons in the athletic setting.

The following is a summary of the AAP committee recommendations[6]:

✓ Athletes with HIV, HBV, or HCV infection should be allowed to participate in all competitive sports.

✓ The infection status of patients should be kept confidential. Confidentiality about an athlete's infection with a BBP is necessary to prevent exclusion of the athlete from sports because of inappropriate fear among others in the program.

✓ Athletes should not be tested for BBP simply because they are sports participants. Physicians should counsel athletes who are infected with HIV, HBV, and HCV that they have a very small risk of infecting other athletes. These athletes can then consider choosing a sport with a low risk of virus transmission. This will not only protect other participants from infection but also will protect the infected athletes themselves by reducing their possible exposure to BBP other than the one(s) with which they are infected. Wrestling and boxing, a sport opposed by the AAP, probably have the greatest potential for contamination of injured skin by blood.

✓ Athletic programs should inform athletes and their families that they have a very small risk of infection, but that the infection status of other players will remain confidential.

✓ Physicians and athletic program staff should aggressively promote HBV immunization of all persons who may be exposed to athletes' blood. If possible, all athletes should receive HBV immunization. More than 95% of persons who receive this immunization will be protected against infection.

✓ Coaches and athletic trainers should receive training in first aid and emergency care and in the prevention of transmission of pathogens in the athletic setting.

✓ Coaches and health care team members should teach athletes about the precautions listed above and about high-risk activities that may cause transmission of BBP. Sexual activity and needle sharing during the use of illicit drugs, including anabolic steroids, carry a high risk of viral transmission. Athletes should be told not to share personal items, such as razors, toothbrushes, and nail clippers, which might be contaminated with blood.

✓ In some states, depending on state law, schools may be required to comply with OSHA regulations for the prevention of transmission of BBP. The rules that apply must be determined by each athletic program. Compliance with OSHA regulations is a reasonable and recommended precaution, even if it is not required by the state.

The AAP committee also recommends that the following precautions be taken in sports with direct body contact and sports in which an athlete's blood or other bodily fluids may contaminate the skin or mucous membranes of other participants or staff members of the athletic program[6]:

✓ Athletes should cover existing cuts, abrasions, wounds, or other areas of broken skin with an occlusive dressing before and during participation. Caregivers must also cover their own damaged skin to prevent transmission of infection to or from an injured athlete.

✓ Disposable, water-impervious vinyl or latex gloves should be worn to avoid contact with blood or other bodily fluids visibly tinged with blood and any object contaminated with these fluids. Hands should be cleaned with soap and water or an alcohol-based antiseptic hand wash as soon as gloves are removed.

✓ Athletes with active bleeding should be removed from competition immediately and bleeding should be stopped. Wounds should be cleaned with soap and water or skin antiseptics. Wounds should be covered with an occlusive dressing that remains intact during further play before athletes return to competition.

✓ Athletes should be told to report injuries and wounds in a timely fashion before or during competition.

✓ Minor cuts or abrasions that are not bleeding do not require interruption of play but can be cleaned and covered during scheduled breaks. During breaks, if an athlete's equipment or uniform is wet with blood, the equipment should be cleaned and disinfected and the uniform should be replaced.

✓ Equipment and playing areas contaminated with blood should be cleaned and disinfected with an appropriate germicide. The decontaminated equipment or area should be in contact with the germicide for at least 30 seconds. The area may be wiped with a disposable cloth after the minimum contact time or be allowed to air dry.

✓ Emergency care should not be delayed because gloves or other protective equipment are not available. If the caregiver does not have appropriate protective equipment, a towel may be used to cover the wound until a location off the playing field is reached and gloves can be obtained.

✓ Breathing bags and oral airways should be available for giving resuscitation. Mouth-to-mouth resuscitation is recommended only if this equipment is not available.

✓ Equipment handlers, laundry personnel, and janitorial staff should be trained in the proper procedures for handling washable or disposable materials contaminated with blood.

As first-line care providers, the athletic trainer must be prepared to address the issue of BBP from many perspectives. As a health care provider, the athletic trainer must be aware of the risk of transmission of BBP and utilize universal precautions at all times. In addition, the athletic trainers must be aware of the federal regulations and standards that govern specific health care settings and know how to respond should they be exposed to a potential BBP. Table 10-3 outlines recommendations for care of athletes and environmental surfaces. These recommendations for athletic trainers and other caregivers are outlined in the most recent *NCAA Sports Medicine Handbook*. These recommendations are drawn from the original AAP items listed previously with some modifications.

Testing

Mandatory testing or widespread screening of athletes for blood-borne diseases is not recommended. These tests could not be effectively used for prevention measures, the cost would be excessive, and there are legal and ethical issues surrounding such an invasive program.[3] However, in combative sports such as international wrestling and boxing, governing bodies can dictate that AIDS detection testing is mandatory for participants in their sanctioned events. The International Amateur Boxing Association has recommended that HIV testing be part of the preparticipation screening process.[3]

Voluntary testing should be encouraged for all individuals who participate in high-risk behaviors (athletes and nonathletes). Those who have multiple sexual partners, inject drugs (of any kind), or have sexual contact with persons at risk should be tested.[3]

Testing alone is not effective without educational intervention to try to change behaviors.

EXPOSURE AND REPORTING PROTOCOLS

Athletic training students must know the proper procedures to follow if they feel they have had a potential BBP exposure incident. An exposure means a specific eye, mucous membrane, nonintact skin, or

Table 10-3

Care of Environmental Surfaces

Individuals responsible for cleaning and disinfecting blood spills must be properly trained on procedures and the use of universal precautions.

- Cleaning supplies should be assembled and stored for easy access and should include the following:
  - Barrier protections—goggles, mask, and fluid-resistant gown if chance of splatter
  - Supply of absorbent paper towels or disposable cloths
  - Red plastic bag with biohazard symbol to collect waste or another appropriate receptacle in accordance with facility protocols
  - Properly diluted germicide disinfectant or freshly prepared diluted bleach solution (1:10 bleach/water)
- Clean up procedure:
  - Gloves should be donned prior to clean up
  - Remove visible organic material by covering with paper towels or disposable cloths
  - Place soiled materials in red bag or proper biohazard receptacle
  - Spray the surface with properly diluted chemical germicide used according to manufacturer's label specifications
  - Place soiled towels in waste biohazard receptacle
  - Spray the surface with either a properly diluted germicide disinfectant or freshly prepared diluted bleach solution (1:10 bleach/water) and place towels in receptacle
  - Remove gloves and wash hands thoroughly
  - Dispose of waste according to facility protocol
- Restock supplies

Adapted from NCAA Committee on Competitive Safeguards and Medical Aspects of Sports. Blood-borne pathogens and intercollegiate athletics. *2006-2007 NCAA Sports Medicine Handbook.* Indianapolis, IN: NCAA; 2006-2007:54-60.

parenteral (not by mouth) contact with blood or potentially infected material. While blood is the most likely source in an athletic training environment, infections materials also include semen, vaginal secretions, CSF, synovial fluid, pleural fluid, pericardial fluid, amniotic fluid, saliva in dental procedures, and any body fluid visibly contaminated with blood.

As part of an accredited athletic training education program, students must be instructed in the reporting protocol for the various clinical settings in which they will be learning. Individuals will be designated to gather information and provide instructions for follow-up care should a student have a potential exposure incident. While notification and procedures will vary by institution, the outline below provides common steps to follow if there is a potential exposure incident.

- ✓ Needlestick or other sharp object injury:
  - Immediately wash the affected area with disinfectant soap and water.
  - Gently squeeze the injured area to induce bleeding, if possible.
  - Notify your clinical supervisor or designated site coordinator.
  - Immediately follow-up with your physician or designated university health care provider.

- ✓ Splash of blood or body fluids to mucosa of eyes, nose, or mouth:
  - Immediately flush the affected area with water or saline.
  - Notify your clinical supervisor or designated site coordinator.
  - Follow-up with your physician or designated university health care provider.

- ✓ Splash of blood or body fluids onto nonintact skin:
  - Immediately wash the affected area with disinfectant soap and water.
  - Notify your clinical supervisor or designated site coordinator.
  - Follow-up with your physician or designated university health care provider.

- ✓ Splash of blood or body fluids onto intact skin:
  - Immediately wash the affected area with disinfectant soap and water.
  - Notify your clinical supervisor or designated site coordinator.
  - Follow-up with your physician or designated university health care provider if instructed.

General Wound Care

Health care providers must take the proper steps to provide wound care while adhering to universal precautions and sterile technique. Sterile technique is used to prevent a wound from being infected while it is being managed. The steps below outline proper wound care:

- Control bleeding with the use of direct pressure while adhering to universal precautions.

- Irrigate the wound with a sterile water solution for several minutes (if not available, clean running tap water is acceptable). All wounds should be considered contaminated and thus cleaned appropriately. Irrigation can be performed using a large syringe (500 mL) and a sterile saline solution. This solution may be diluted with 3% hydrogen peroxide.

- Clean the area around the wound with a mild antibacterial soap and water.

- Adhesive strips are often used to bring the edges of a wound together and allow for greater healing. They also can help close a wound until a physician can evaluate it. Adhesive may be used only to the edges of the wound. Once the adhesive is sticky and dry, the strips should be secured on one side of the wound. The strips should be pulled in one direction and secured on the opposite side.

- Dressings and ointments. The moisture content of a healing wound is always changing. Maintaining this moisture and using a dressing that allows the wound to be protected during healing may increase the rate of healing. Clean, moist dressings are associated with faster healing and less discomfort for patients than dry dressings. If available, a moist dressing such as a hydrocolloid or polyurethane semipermeable film should be used to cover the wound.

A more complete discussion of minor and major wounds is presented in Chapter 13.

SUMMARY

Skin injuries and the potential for exposure to BBP are a common occurrence in the sports medicine setting. This chapter provides an overview of BBP and the use of universal precautions. As a health care provider who is often the first responder to injury, the athletic trainer must set the example for proper use of universal precautions and serve as an educator to dispel myths and provide factual information concerning BBP.

REFERENCES

1. World Health Organization. WHO and HIV/AIDS. Available at www.who.int/hiv/en. Accessed July 25, 2008.
2. Centers for Disease Control and Prevention. Blood borne infectious diseases HIV/AIDS, hepatitis B virus, and hepatitis C virus. Available at www.cdc.gov/niosh/topics/bbp. Accessed June 10, 2008.
3. Kordi R, Wallace WA. Blood borne infections in sport: risks of transmission, methods of prevention, and recommendations for hepatitis B vaccination. *Br J Sports Med.* 2004;38:678-684.
4. NCAA Committee on Competitive Safeguards and Medical Aspects of Sports. Blood-borne pathogens and intercollegiate athletics. *2006-2007 NCAA Sports Medicine Handbook.* City, ST: Publisher; 2006-2007:54-60.
5. Landry GL, Bernhardt DT. *Essentials of Primary Care Sports Medicine.* Champaign, IL: Human Kinetics; 2003.
6. American Academy of Pediatrics Committee on Sports Medicine and Fitness. Human immunodeficiency virus and other blood-borne viral pathogens in the athletic setting (RE9821). *Pediatrics.* 1999;104:1400-1403.
7. American Medical Society for Sports Medicine, American Orthopaedic Society for Sports Medicine. Joint position statement human immunodeficiency virus (HIV) and other blood-borne pathogens in sports. Available at http://www.newamssm.org/hiv.html. Accessed February 27, 2009.
8. Sklarek HM, Mantovani RP, Erens E, et al. AIDS in a bodybuilder using anabolic steroids. *N Engl J Med.* 1984;311:1701.
9. Dickenson BP, Mylonakis E, Strong LL, et al. Potential infections related to anabolic steroid injection in young adolescents. *Pediatrics.* 1999;103:694.
10. Nattiv A, Purffer JC, Green GA. Lifestyles and health risks of collegiate athletes: a multi-center study. *Clin J Sports Med.* 1997;7:262-272.
11. Nattiv A, Puffer JC. Lifestyles and health risks of collegiate athletes. *J Fam Pract.* 1991;33:585-590.
12. Pate RR, Trost SG, Levin S, et al. Sports participation and health-related behaviors among US youth. *Arch Pediatr Adolesc Med.* 2000;154:904-911.

WEB RESOURCES

American College Health Association
www.acha.org
The ACHA serves as an advocate and leadership organization for issues surrounding college and university health. Several ACHA guideline reports available on-line and frequently updated.

American Academy of Pediatrics
www.aap.org
The Web site for the AAP provides information regarding many aspects of providing care for children and adolescents. Professional publications sections allow for searches of current position statements and reports.

Centers for Disease Control and Prevention
www.cdc.gov

A helpful government site sponsored by the US Department of Health and Human Services. Information regarding infectious disease, information for travelers, health bulletins on various topics, and current funding and research projects is provided.

Occupational Health & Safety Administration
www.osha.gov

This Web site is dedicated to providing information from OSHA regarding workplace safety. Significant information is available regarding health care work settings and BBP.

 ## Career Spotlight: High School Athletic Trainer

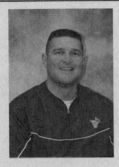

Keith Skinner, MS, ATC

Voorhees High School

Glen Gardner, New Jersey

My Position

I am a full-time athletic trainer at a mid-sized New Jersey high school. I am employed by the school district on a 240-day contract to provide medical coverage to 25 varsity and subvarsity sports. This position requires no teaching responsibilities and is strictly athletic training coverage beginning in the middle of August thru early June.

Unique or Desired Qualifications

Take psychology classes; many times half the battle is dealing with the psychological effects of injury and the return to play. Try to work with as many different sports as possible because they all have their own equipment, rules, etc that factor into injury and recovery.

Favorite Aspect of My Job

I love sports so this job is perfect for a sports fanatic like myself. Although working with young athletes has its own issues, it does help me "feel" young as I enter the mid-life part of my career. Lastly, there is no better feeling than seeing an athlete return to action after helping him or her overcome an injury and battle through the rehabilitation process.

Advice

Treat every athlete, freshman sub to varsity starter, the same. I try to imagine they are one of my own kids and treat them the way I would want my own kids to be treated.

CHAPTER 11

EMERGENCY PLANNING AND INJURY EVALUATION

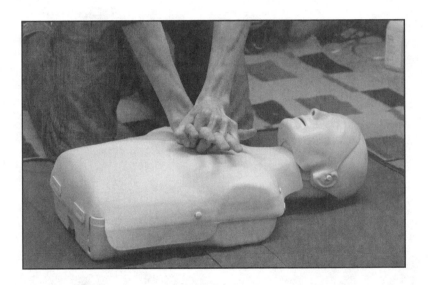

I think students need to understand that they are assisting in the role of health care provider, a student health-care provider, but assisting with patient care nonetheless. They need to follow the instructions of their supervisor and be very willing to ask lots of "why" questions.

Patrick J. Sexton, EdD, ATC/R, CSCS
Director of Athletic Training Education
Minnesota State University–Mankato

The ability of the athletic trainer to determine the severity of a specific injury or condition, outline a course of action (emergency or otherwise), and provide the appropriate care is a vital skill. Significant portions of the athletic training domains are dedicated to these skills. Athletic training students who understand how these skills fit into the professional domains of a certified athletic trainer will be better prepared to make the most of their clinical rotations. The skills outlined in this chapter are presented as an overview. Any student advancing in an athletic training education program will take individual courses (both didactic and clinical) in each area and have significant exposure to the content described below.

Upon completion of this chapter, the student will be able to:

✓ Know the difference between a primary and secondary injury survey

✓ Describe the components of a physical exam

✓ Appreciate the importance and obligation of adequate emergency response plans

✓ Explain the key components to an emergency response plan

✓ Discuss the essential role of the AED in ECC

✓ Differentiate the portions of the SOAP format

✓ Apply the SAMPLE approach to taking a medical history

✓ Identify common diagnostic testing associated with sports injuries

DEFINING EMERGENCIES

EMERGENCY PLANNING

An emergency plan is a comprehensive document that outlines how an emergency situation will be handled. Emergency plans can be thought of as blueprints.[1] Like blueprints that must be drawn before a building is built, the emergency plan must be in place before it is needed. Proper planning will allow the sports medicine team to respond to an emergency smoothly. The ability to properly respond when called upon may make the difference between life and death. In addition to planning, teamwork is the second essential component of a response plan. Everyone involved must know their role, work within their boundaries, and be prepared to act accordingly.

Emergency plans are not one size fits all. The plan must be specific to the sport activity in question and will need to be tailored to specific facilities. Compare the needs of the athletic trainer at a track and field event to one at an equipment-intensive event like a football game. How you immobilize and transport an individual with a suspected cervical injury will require some equipment-specific planning. The most common equipment example is having a plan to remove a football helmet facemask if needed. The 2 main questions that an emergency plan should address are as follows:

1. What are the roles and responsibilities of each member of the sports medicine team as he or she responds to an emergency?
2. What steps will be taken to activate EMS?

Emergency documents should not be written for the sole benefit of the sports medicine team. The plan should be distributed to administrators, coaches, facilities staff, and any personnel that may be impacted by such an event. While plans must be flexible, each should provide information on implementation, personnel, emergency equipment, communication, transportation, venue location, emergency care facilities, and documentation.[1] Table 11-1 outlines the NATA's position statement on emergency planning in athletics.[2]

 Emergency Action Steps—Check, Call, Care

When responding to an emergency, always remember the following steps:

- CHECK the scene and the victim
- CALL 9-1-1- or your local emergency number (or have someone call)
- CARE for the victim

 Emergency Cardiac Care Requirements for the Athletic Trainer

Certified athletic trainers are required to maintain ECC certification. It is identified as ECC because it extends beyond just CPR. Although CE credits are no longer awarded for ECC certification, athletic trainers need to be current with the ECC requirements throughout the CEU reporting period. ECC certification must include the following:

- Adult and pediatric CPR
- AED
- 2nd rescuer CPR
- Airway obstruction
- Barrier devices (eg, pocket mask, valve mask)

Acceptable ECC providers are those adhering to the most current *International Guidelines for Cardiopulmonary Resuscitation and Emergency Cardiac Care*. The 2 most common courses that meet these requirements are:

- CPR/AED for the Professional Rescuer through the American Red Cross
- BLS Healthcare Provider through the American Heart Association

Bibliography

Board of Certification, Inc. Emergency Cardiac Care (ECC) Recertification Requirements 2006-2011. Available at www.bocatc.org. Accessed July 11, 2008.

TYPES OF EVALUATION

Primary Survey

Athletic trainers must be prepared to assess emergent injury situations as well as the more common non-life–threatening injuries. Any on-the-field injury assessment begins with a primary survey. The primary survey involves an assessment of the ABCs

---

Table 11-1

Emergency Planning in Athletics

The recommendations provided below are based on the most current literature and expert review of common practices. Students are encouraged to visit the NATA Web site at www.nata.org to view their position statement on emergency planning.

- Each institution or organization that sponsors athletic activities must have a written emergency plan. The emergency plan should be comprehensive and practical, yet flexible enough to adapt to any situation.

- Emergency plans must be written documents and should be distributed to certified athletic trainers, team and attending physicians, athletic training students, institutional and organizational administrators, and coaches. The emergency plan should be developed in consultation with local emergency medical services personnel.

- An emergency plan for athletics identifies the personnel involved in carrying out the emergency plan and outlines the qualifications of those executing the plan. Sports medicine professionals and coaches should be trained in automatic external defibrillation (AED), cardiopulmonary resuscitation (CPR), first aid, and prevention of disease transmission.

- The emergency plan should specify the equipment needed to carry out the tasks required in the event of an emergency. In addition, the emergency plan should outline the location of the emergency equipment. Further, the equipment available should be appropriate to the level of training of the personnel involved.

- Establishment of a clear mechanism for communication to appropriate emergency care service providers and identification of the mode of transportation for the injured participant are critical elements of an emergency plan.

- The emergency plan should be specific to the activity venue. That is, each activity site should have a defined emergency plan that is derived from the overall institutional or organizational policies on emergency planning.

- Emergency plans should incorporate the emergency care facilities to which the injured individual will be taken. Emergency receiving facilities should be notified in advance of scheduled events and contests. Personnel from the emergency receiving facilities should be included in the development of the emergency plan for the institution or organization.

- The emergency plan specifies the necessary documentation supporting the implementation and evaluation of the emergency plan. This documentation should identify responsibility for documenting actions taken during the emergency, evaluation of the emergency response, and institutional personnel training.

- The emergency plan should be reviewed and rehearsed annually, although more frequent view and rehearsal may be necessary. The results of these reviews and rehearsals should be documented and should indicate whether the emergency plan was modified, with further documentation reflecting how the plan was changed.

- All personnel involved with organization and sponsorship of athletic activities share a professional responsibility to provide for the emergency care of an injured person, including the development and implementation of an emergency plan.

- All personnel involved with the organization and sponsorship of athletic activities share a legal duty to develop, implement, and evaluate an emergency plan for all sponsored athletic activities.

- The emergency plan should be reviewed by the administration and legal counsel of the sponsoring organization or institution.

Adapted with permission of National Athletic Trainers' Association from Anderson JC, Courson RW, Kleiner DM, McLoda TA. National Athletic Trainers' Association position statement: emergency planning in athletics. *Journal of Athletic Training.* 2002;37:99-105.

(ie, airway, breathing, and circulation). The primary survey also requires that you establish the presence of severe bleeding.[1] At anytime during the primary survey, an athletic trainer must be prepared to activate an emergency plan that includes summoning EMS, establishing an open airway, giving CPR, and providing first aid. Emergency care is a series of decisions, and what you find as you assess the ABCs determines what steps must be taken. Figure 11-1 shows a typical decision tree for assessing an emergency.

Athletic training students must be prepared to assist athletic training staff in the event of an emergency. Athletic training students in clinical rotations should hold a current CPR certification and be trained in CPR (including AED), basic care first aid, and the use and maintenance of emergency care equipment and know the location of such equipment. Students may be asked to assist supervising staff in activating an emergency plan. Phoning EMS, assisting with CPR, spine boarding, and patient conveyance are all potential emergency situations for which an athletic training student should be prepared. It is the responsibility of the athletic training education program to insure that students are equipped to handle emergency situations prior to being placed in a clinical situation.

ATCs and EMS—Working Together on Catastrophic Injury

A player down on the field or court with a spinal cord injury marks one of the most severe injuries facing sports medicine teams. The stories of Dennis Byrd's 1992 injury with the New York Jets and more recently Kevin Everett of the Buffalo Bills in 2007 are examples of how proper on-the-field care can contribute to an improved outcome for the most devastating spinal injuries. While innovative treatments (controlled hypothermia of the spine for Everett) and skilled surgeons are central to these stories, it all starts with the on-the-field care.

"The care that I received on the field, the attention to detail and the precision, none of this was a mistake. Procedures, positions, actual practice working with the spine board and neck braces... had been practiced in the summer before the players came into training camp. The only real stroke of fate was my accident." Dennis Byrd, NATA Keynote, 1994

The recovery road for these patients is long. However, their stories do serve as inspiration and hope to victims of spinal injuries and are a testament to the importance of emergency planning and proper prehospital care of spinal injuries.

One key to successful emergency planning and pre-hospital care of the athlete is communication and cooperation between sports medicine teams and EMS personnel. Unfortunately, emergency personnel may not possess the specialized knowledge and skills to respond perfectly to these infrequent but extremely serious sports incidents.

In Dayton, Ohio, they are moving beyond just talking and truly working together.

In 2008, the Wright State University Boonshoft School of Medicine and the Greater Dayton Athletic Trainers Association held an EMS/sports medicine symposium to teach local emergency personnel some ways to assess and treat athletes who become injured while competing.

The symposium focused on spinal injuries to football players and was the first in a series of annual events dedicated to the pre-hospital care of acute athletic emergencies. Dr. Brian L. Springer, sports medicine director for Wright State's department of emergency medicine and the event's organizer, commented, "Some 10% of cervical spine injuries occur in athletes and football has one of the highest incidence rates among all sports. While catastrophic injuries are relatively rare, the risk is still very real, and improving the effectiveness of pre-hospital care can make a tremendous difference."

Bibliography

Byrd, Dennis. 1994 NATA Keynote Address.
Press Release: Local emergency personnel to learn, practice care of spine-injured athletes at Wright State symposium in Kettering. Wright State University Boonshoft School of Medicine. June 2008.

Figure 11-1. A decision tree can be utilized to evaluate on-the-field injuries.

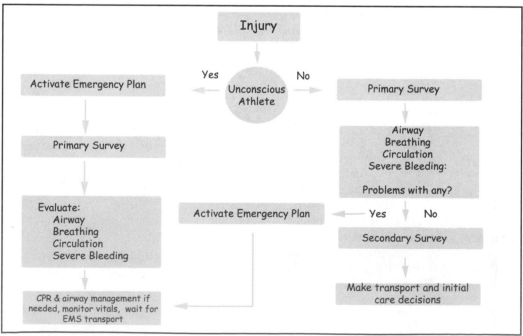

The Emergency Plan in Action: A True Story

During a routine practice in 2007, University of South Florida (USF) softball player Cristi Ecks lay in the infield dirt, lifeless. She had collapsed without warning as she walked to the pitcher's circle at a routine practice. Two days earlier in the same space, the 20-year-old pitcher had struck out 8 and allowed only one hit in a dominating but routine outing against Seton Hall. But on that particular Tuesday afternoon, her heart was still and her breathing absent as an athletic trainer administered CPR. Teammates rushed to nearby fields to call for help. Finally, after about 2 minutes, 45 seconds, a portable defibrillator shocked her heart back into rhythm.

"It seemed like a lifetime," said coach Ken Eriksen, who recounted the scene in detail. "But that's a pretty dang quick response there, from everybody."

The USF's athletic department has a certified trainer at every team's practice, and the athletic facility has 6 portable defibrillators that travel to practices for just such an emergency. When Ecks fell—around 4 pm, 30 min into a light walk-through practice—athletic trainer Kelly Cox was walking back onto the field after working with another player. She immediately remembered her ABCs and after checking those, knew she had to administer CPR, something she had never done outside of her training.

She gave mouth-to-mouth resuscitation and chest compressions until the defibrillator indicated Ecks' heart needed to be shocked. Ecks started breathing again on her own, and Cox felt a great relief. USF associate athletic director Barry Clements said Tuesday's events were an example of proper training and preparation saving a life under difficult circumstances. "We have emergency policies and procedures, so when we go into crisis mode, we do it with a plan," Clements said. "It couldn't have happened any better, or any quicker, which is crucial in those situations. If you'd rehearsed it 100 times, it couldn't have gone better than it went. Preparation is the key to our success. "

This story, though amazing, is far from uncommon. Multiple stories appear in the news every year about people being saved through the conscientious implementation of a well-rehearsed emergency plan. The need for up-to-date ECC training and access to an AED cannot be understated.

Bibliography

Auman G. USF pitcher recovers after heart stopped. *St. Petersburg Times*. April 03, 2008.

National Athletic Trainers' Association Official Statement—Automated External Defibrillators

Official Statement

The National Athletic Trainers' Association (NATA), as a leader in health care for the physically active, strongly believes that the treatment of sudden cardiac arrest is a priority. An AED program should be part of an athletic trainer's emergency action plan. NATA strongly encourages athletic trainers, in every work setting, to have access to an AED. Athletic trainers are encouraged to make an AED part of their standard emergency equipment. In addition, in conjunction and coordination with local EMS, athletic trainers should take a primary role in implementing a comprehensive AED program within their work setting.

Rationale

According to the American Heart Association (AHA), each year, approximately 250,000 Americans die of sudden cardiac arrest (SCA) outside of the hospital.[1] As many as 7000 children die of SCA each year.[2] Evidence suggests that the risk of a cardiac event is higher during or immediately following vigorous exercise. Cardiopulmonary resuscitation (CPR) is critical to maintaining the supply of oxygen to vital organs, but the single most effective treatment for cardiac arrest is defibrillation, a shock delivered to the heart using a small electronic device known as a defibrillator. The AHA recommends defibrillation within 3 to 5 minutes or sooner.[1] Most communities cannot meet these guidelines. As a result, nationwide, survival from SCA is only about 5%. In some communities where shocks from an AED and CPR are provided within 3 to 5 minutes by the first person on the scene, survival rates are as high as 48% to 74%.

References

1. American Heart Association, 2003. Heart Disease and Stroke Statistics – 2003 Update.
2. Berger S, Dhalia A, Freidberg DZ. 1999. Sudden cardiac arrest death in infants, children and adolescents. *Pediatric Clinics of North America*. 1999;46(2):221-34.

THE SECONDARY SURVEY

While the athletic trainer should always be prepared in the event of an emergency, most on-the-field evaluations and decisions are not emergent. In this situation, the athletic trainer must then perform a secondary survey. The secondary survey is a survey for trauma once you have established that the patient is stable. Throughout the secondary survey, the practitioner must always continue to assess the ABCs while checking the patient from head to toe for additional signs of injury or trauma. The secondary survey should help the athletic trainer determine the safest method for removing the athlete from the field of play. A more comprehensive evaluation can be preformed once the athlete is on the sidelines or in the athletic training facility.

A COMPLETE HISTORY AND PHYSICAL EXAM

A Step-by-Step Process

A comprehensive evaluation consists of taking a history and carrying out a physical examination. This type of evaluation is performed when an athlete or patient comes to you with an existing problem or on the sidelines after an acute nonemergent injury. These evaluations will most often follow the SOAP note format. SOAP is a format for evaluation and documentation that stands for Subjective, Objective, Assessment, and Plan.[3] Subjective information is information gathered from the patient (history), while objective information involves visual information and results of tests performed by the athletic trainer and graded in a consistent manner. Assessments are the results of the evaluation. They are an impression of how the injury occurred and the severity of the injury. The plan outlines what management, treatment, or referral actions will be taken to care for the injury.

Athletic training students should only do an evaluation if they have been properly instructed in evaluation techniques and are under the guidance of a supervising athletic trainer. While the SOAP note format for evaluation and documentation guides the evaluation process, the steps in an evaluation are often remembered by the acronym HOPS. This stands for History, Observation, Palpation, and Special tests. The steps below are an overview of the components of an injury evaluation.

History

As the word implies, the history is what has already happened. The athletic trainer must gather information from the patient. This subjective information is critical to establishing a starting point for the athletic trainer to begin his or her "search" for the underlying injury that has brought the athlete to him or her. During a history, the athletic trainer must ask questions to determine:

✓ MOI

✓ History of previous injury

✓ Onset of symptoms

✓ Location of injury

✓ What type of pain is present

✓ Any abnormal sensations

✓ Anything that makes the injury worse or better

✓ What treatment has been done

✓ Taking any medications or supplements

Of all the questions the athletic trainer will ask the patient, the MOI and previous history often are the most informative. The athletic trainer must be equally adept at evaluating illnesses as well as injuries. Refer to More Than Just Injuries on p. 217 for more information on evaluating illnesses.

Observation

The athletic trainer must observe the area of the injury as well as the overall actions of the patient for the following:

✓ Swelling (edema)

✓ Discoloration (ecchymosis)

✓ Deformity

✓ Signs of infection and inflammation

✓ The patient's facial expressions (pain)

✓ Presence of a painful gait (limp)

✓ Smooth and coordinated movement

✓ Bilateral comparison (compare one side to the other)

With practice and experience, the athletic training student will learn to gather observational information while asking questions during the history phase.

Palpation

To palpate means to gather information with your hands. You need to palpate the proper structures to gather information. This brings to light a general assumption of the evaluation process: you must have a strong knowledge of the anatomical structures to gather appropriate information. During a physical examination, you can palpate for the following:

✓ Pain

  ○ Response to touch

✓ Crepitus

  ○ A "crunchy" sensation associated with tendinitis, bursitis, and bone abnormalities

More Than Just Injuries

The evaluation of an illness can differ greatly to that of an injury evaluation. Athletic training students must learn to be comfortable with both types of evaluation situations. Since one point of the evaluation process is to determine appropriate referral, it is essential that the athletic trainer provide the physician with helpful information. The best place to start is with an appropriate history. The history takes on greater importance with illnesses since there are fewer specific tests that the clinician can perform to gather information. An accurate medical history is essential. A technique often used when evaluating ill patients relies on the acronym SAMPLE to obtain thorough information. SAMPLE is used across many health care disciplines and is also used by emergency personnel. Learning this information and using it when evaluating illnesses and general medical conditions will allow for an evaluation that is more specific to the problem at hand.

A "SAMPLE" history includes the following:

- S—Signs and symptoms, including vital signs.
- A—Allergies. Does the patient have any known allergies to medication? Food? Insect bites or stings? Others (ie, respiratory, hay fever)?
- M—Medication. Is the patient taking any medication? Is so, for what condition? Is the medication a prescription or is it over the counter? Is the patient taking any supplements or herbal products?
- P—Past/pertinent medical history. Previous medical conditions? Recent illnesses? Have they been treated? If so, by whom (names of care provider)?
- L—Last meal. When was the last time the patient ate a meal? Did he or she get sick (ie, gastrointestinal distress, nausea, vomiting)? Did anyone with whom he or she ate get sick?
- E—Events leading to episode. What was the patient doing when he or she noticed he or she was ill? What brought him or her in to be evaluated?

✓ Swelling

   o Edema

✓ Deformity

✓ Muscle tone

✓ Changes in temperature

Palpation may be uncomfortable for the patient, therefore the athletic trainer must proceed with caution and palpate areas that he or she suspects will be painful last.

Special Tests

Range of Motion Testing—Functional testing refers to the assessment of active ROM (AROM), passive ROM (PROM), and resisted ROM (RROM). AROM is motion that is initiated and carried out by the patient. The athletic trainer performs PROM with the patient completely relaxed. No active muscle activity is present during PROM. When evaluating active range, the patient must be provided with simple instructions that he or she understands. Asking the athlete to abduct or perform forward flexion may not mean anything to him or her. Therefore, you need to use simple commands like, "Raise your arms over your head." During active motion, any pain with movement, limitation in movement, or asynchronous movement should be noted. Evaluation of AROM and PROM should be done bilaterally to compare extremi-

ties. A goniometer may be used to get a measurement (in degrees of motion) of the available range.

PROM requires the evaluator to "feel" tissues at the end of the available range. The athletic trainer must note any pain with passive movement, limitation in movement, or change in "end-feel." End-feel is the type of tissue resistance that the practitioner feels as the joint is passively moved. For example, if you extend the elbow, the end-feel is hard compared to flexing your knee, which has a soft feel as the tissues of the gastrocnemius contact the thigh. Knowing the expected end-feel allows the athletic trainer to make a comparison to his or her physical exam findings.

Resisted ROM is also known as manual muscle testing (MMT). This portion of the physical examination assesses the strength and muscle function for a specific movement. MMT skills require students to have a working knowledge of the muscles and muscle actions. Manual muscle tests are graded by comparing the strength of a given muscle group to the opposite extremity. Muscle strength is commonly graded on a scale of 5. 5/5 strength would equal 100%, 0/5 would indicate that there is no muscle activity.

Ligament and Special Tests—The athletic trainer utilizes ligamentous tests to apply stress to a joint and determine if specific structures have been injured. The ability to position the patient, place their hands, apply the test, and interpret the results are clinical skills

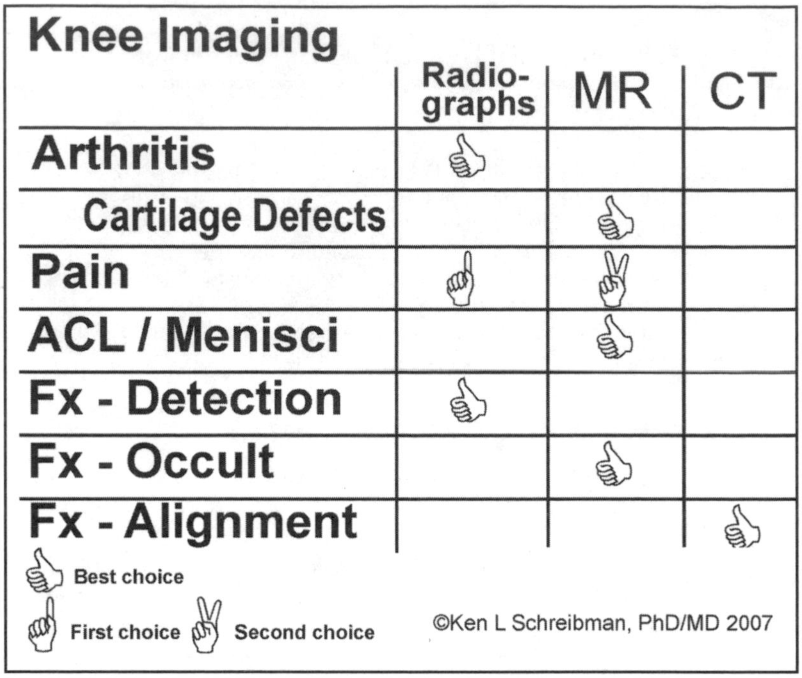

Figure 11-2. A schematic for differentiating decision between radiograph (x-ray), MRI, and CT scans. (© Ken L. Schreibman, PhD, MD, 2007. Used by permission.)

Knee Imaging

	Radiographs	MR	CT
Arthritis	👍 Best choice		
Cartilage Defects		👍 Best choice	
Pain	☝ First choice	✌ Second choice	
ACL / Menisci		👍 Best choice	
Fx - Detection	👍 Best choice		
Fx - Occult		👍 Best choice	
Fx - Alignment			👍 Best choice

👍 Best choice
☝ First choice   ✌ Second choice

©Ken L Schreibman, PhD/MD 2007

required of all athletic trainers. These tests allow the athletic trainer to identify sprain injuries. The amount of laxity, pain, and the quality of the "end-point" of a ligament test are all indicators of injury. Special tests are designed to help identify specific injuries or conditions based on a particular maneuver by the patient or action by the examiner. For instance, an injury to the AC joint of the shoulder may cause the distal clavicle to ride upward and create a deformity. The athletic trainer can perform a special test called a "spring" test, pushing the distal clavicle down to its normal position and observing if it springs back upward when released. This is a special test to determine the severity of an AC sprain. There are several special tests that adequately examine a wide range of injuries and conditions. Special tests are often named after the physician who identified the test (Noble, Ober, Kennedy-Hawkins) or named after the position the patient assumes to perform the test (single leg stance, impingement).

Neurovascular Testing—Several acute and chronic injuries can affect nervous or vascular structures in the body. Nerve injuries may cause changes in sensation, muscle weakness, or loss of function. Athletic trainers evaluate neurological function by assessing dermatomes, myotomes, and deep tendon reflexes. Dermatomes are sensory areas of the skin that are supplied from a specific nerve root. Finding a change in sensation in a specific area may indicate a nerve injury at that level of the spinal nerve root. Myotomes are muscle actions that are related to particular spinal nerve roots. For example, if there is pressure on the 5th cervical nerve root (C5), the patient may demonstrate weakness in his or her deltoid or biceps brachii when it

is evaluated. Deep tendon reflexes can be evaluated in many locations. The patellar tendon, Achilles tendon, biceps brachii tendon, and triceps brachii tendon are common locations for reflex testing. When the patient is properly positioned and the tendon tapped with a reflex hammer, the results can be noted. Some patients display excessive response and are hyper-reflexive, while others may show decreased reflexes. Changes in reflexes can be associated with injury at a specific nerve root level. Athletic trainers must be skilled in assessing the neurological status of an injury for the purpose of initial care and appropriate referral.

It is common practice to check for circulation by checking the pulse distal to the site of a traumatic injury (fracture or dislocation). Vascular structures may be affected by both acute and chronic injury. Taking the pulse and confirming normal circulation should be a part of any physical examination.

DIAGNOSTIC IMAGING

It is common that the patient may need further diagnostic testing following a thorough evaluation. Diagnostic imaging through the use of radiographs, MRI, CT scan, or ultrasound are used in a variety of situations associated with injuries and conditions the athletic trainer will encounter. Other imaging choices are available but outside the scope of this introductory text. The athletic trainer in the physician extender role may take part in the ordering of images at the request of the supervising physician. Athletic trainers must have an understanding of these diagnostic imaging choices and appreciate their application and use under specific conditions. Figure 11-2 is an overview of common knee conditions and the appropriate imaging choices.[4]

Radiographs

The first early radiographs were taken in the 1890s and William Conrad Röntgen is first credited with knowing the potential to harness this "new photographic marvel." X-rays are a form of radiation, much like light or radio waves that can be focused into a beam. Unlike normal light, x-rays can pass through most objects based upon the density of the object. When x-rays strike a piece of photographic film, they produce an image. What is seen on that image depends upon the density of the tissue. Dense tissues such as bones absorb many of the x-rays and appear white on the picture. Less dense tissues such as muscles and organs absorb fewer of the x-rays (more rays pass through) and they appear in shades of gray. If the x-rays pass through the air, they will appear black.[5] Figure 11-3 shows a radiograph of the knee.

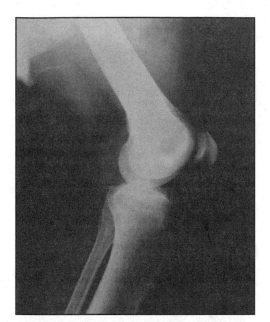

Figure 11-3. Radiograph image of the knee. (Courtesy of Dr. Ken Schreibman, University of Wisconsin–Madison School of Medicine and Public Health.)

 ## Why Do They Call It an X-Ray?

On November 8, 1895, William Conrad Röntgen was working in his lab in Strasburg with a Crookes tube (a type of powerful light). He built a cardboard light seal around it and turned it on. He had meant to illuminate a fluorescent screen with it but found that he was illuminating a nearby bench through the cardboard. In the great tradition of science, he had found something by accident. Also in the great tradition of science, others were working on a similar process in their laboratories. A similar device with the ability to help us see through things had been done in Pennsylvania in 1893, but they did not realize what they had. Röntgen knew exactly what he had. What he did not know was what to call this illumination. He rapidly tried to get a scientific paper out by the following month and titled it, *On a New Kind of X-Rays*.

The discovery brought much hoopla and attention to Röntgen. Three months later, an April copy of *McClure's Magazine* included the article, *The New Marvel in Photography*.

In all the history of scientific discovery [it says] there has never been [so] dramatic an effect wrought on the scientific centers...as has followed, in the past four weeks, upon an announcement [by] William Conrad Röntgen [who] discovered a new kind of light, which penetrated and photographed through everything.

The author of the McClure article went on to suggest that American labs and lecture halls will buzz with a "contagious arousal of interest over a discovery so strange that its importance cannot be measured [or] its utility even prophesied." Röntgen tried to keep his eye on the ball and not get caught up in his press clippings. He did not quite understand the rays or even know if they were a form of electricity. "I am not a prophet," he cried, "I am opposed to prophesying. I pursue my investigations." Others were crazy about the new x-rays. They had already been used to locate foreign objects in ailing bodies and to identify tuberculosis.

Röntgen insisted on the term *x-rays* instead of Röntgen rays. But, in 2004, the new element Röntegenium was named after him. He was also awarded the first physics Nobel Prize for his discovery. He died of cancer at the age of 78, but probably not from his experiments. He was one of the rare x-ray pioneers who shielded himself.

Adapted with permission from Leinhard JH. Engines of Our Ingenuity. Episode #2112: Röntgen in 1896. [transcript]. Available at www.uh.edu/engines/epi2112.htm. Accessed April 10, 2008.

Magnetic Resonance Imaging

MRI uses radiofrequency waves and a strong magnetic field to provide clear and detailed images of internal anatomy. Biologic tissue, when placed within a strong magnet, can be induced to give off a detectable signal immediately following stimulation by a pulse of radio frequency (RF) energy. Different types of tissue (muscle, fat, CSF, etc) each give off measurably different types of "tissue specific" signal following the administration of the same RF pulse. It is these predictable differences between the signals from one tissue versus another tissue type that allows MRI to produce meaningful images.[6]

One Clam, Two Nobel Prizes, and a Dispute!

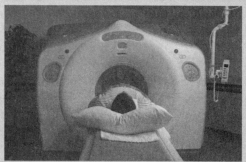

MRI: Magnetic Resonance Imaging

The ability to examine soft tissue structures in the body in a safe, noninvasive fashion is what makes MRI so amazing. Finding a way to scan the body and distinguish healthy tissue from diseased tissue held enormous implications in the field of medicine. From the sports medicine perspective, the advent of MRI has allowed physicians to confirm their clinical suspicions with a scan rather than an invasive procedure prior to surgery. Like so many technological discoveries, the MRI has an interesting and somewhat turbulent history.

In 2003, Paul C. Lauterbur, PhD, an American chemist, and Sir Peter Mansfield, PhD, a British physicist were the winners of the Nobel Prize for Physiology and Medicine for their work in the development of the MRI. Widely recognized as one of the great technological advances of the 20th century, it was a logical choice to be recognized by the Nobel committee. Sir Mansfield was largely recognized for refinements to the use of MRI while Dr. Lauterbur was recognized as a pioneer. In 1973, Dr. Lauterbur submitted the first image of a live subject, a clam, using MRI. This finding was published in the journal *Nature*.

However, there is more to the story. Dr. Lauterbur worked at SUNY Stony Brook. In the late 1960s, a physician named Raymond Damadian worked at SUNY Downstate in Brooklyn. In 1969, he conceived of the idea of a whole body scanner. In 1970, he was able to use MRI to distinguish healthy tissue from cancerous tissue in mice. This confirmed his idea that a whole body scanner may be feasible. His initial results were published in *Science* in 1971. In fact, Dr. Damadian applied for and was granted the first patent for his scanning method. Damadian and his graduate students built their whole body MRI scanner from scratch and in 1977 achieved the first image of the human body. Damadian ultimately left SUNY in 1979 to go into private business to produce MRI scanners.

Here is where it gets tricky. In 1971, Lauterbur observed a graduate student replicate one of Dr. Damadian's experiments. He noted that the imaging method would not produce clear enough images and he proposed a different use of the magnetic fields that employed a second weaker magnetic field that could be controlled to create a magnetic field gradient allowing for better images. It seems that Lauterbur's idea was an extension of Damadian's work. However, he did not clearly cite that work in his 1973 paper in *Nature*. And a feud was born.

Academic egos, competition, patents, and business success—the list goes on and with the potential pitfalls of such an academic rivalry. In time, Dr. Damadian adopted Lauterbur's gradient method for the commercial scanners produced by the FONAR Corporation that he leads. However, the adversarial relationship over the origins of the MRI for human images still rages on. Following the Nobel announcement in 2003 omitting Dr. Damadian, FONAR took out full-page ads in the major newspapers claiming the Nobel committee wronged him. Nobel prizes may be given to 3 individuals for a given discovery and it is curious why Damadian was overlooked. Other precursor discoveries have been noted before. This was not even the first time MRI had been recognized. Physicists and chemists had used MRI for years with the Nobel award for physics in both 1944 and 1952 being tied to this area. It took much longer for MRI to be adapted for medical use.

There is little doubt that Drs. Lauterbur and Mansfield deserve the recognition they have received. However, many question if they would have turned their attention to human applications of this technology without the work of Dr. Damadian. Nobel winners hold an elite spot in history. It is hard to deny Dr. Damadian's goal to have his place recognized. The story is a good reminder. Rarely do technological advances come down to the work of one individual. It also reminds us that adversarial relationships between intelligent, egotistical, driven men can be difficult to mend.

(continued)

ℹ One Clam, Two Nobel Prizes, and a Dispute! (continued)

In 1988, President Ronald Reagan awarded both Dr. Damadian and Dr. Lauterbur the National Medal of Technology for "independent contributions in conceiving and developing the application of medical resonance technology to medical uses including whole-body scanning and diagnostic imaging." It is said that on that day Dr. Lauterbur offered his hand to Dr. Damadian, but Dr. Damadian turned his back on him. I doubt those feelings improved any after the Nobel announcements of 2003.

Next time you view the MRI image of one of your patients, you will know just a little more about the amazing and unfortunate history of this lifesaving technology. A lot of good in the wake of bruised egos and hurt feelings.

Dr. Lauterbur died in 2007. Dr. Damadian returned to SUNY Downstate in 1998 and continues to publish and lecture. His FONAR company has won several patent infringement lawsuits including a multimillion dollar settlement from General Electric in 1997.

Bibliography

Obituaries. *The Week*. April 13, 2007:44.
Powderly KE. 2003 Nobel Prize in Physiology or Medicine…Revisionist History? History News Network. Available at http://hnn.us/articles/1789.html. Accessed February 25, 2009.

Historically, today's term for imaging biologic tissue, *MRI*, stems from the earlier term *nuclear magnetic resonance* (NMR). The acronym NMRI stands for:

- ✓ Nuclear (N): refers to the spin of some nucleus
- ✓ Magnetic (M): refers to an assortment of magnetic fields
- ✓ Resonance (R): refers to the need to match the (radio) frequencies
- ✓ Imaging (I): refers to the ability, flexibility, and sensitivity to produce images

The most common nucleus visualized by MRI is 1H (the atom of hydrogen as it appears in biologic tissue) because it is the predominant element in water. The composition of most biological tissue is dominated by water in some form, and it is the difference in water environments between different tissues that MRI visualizes so effectively (ie, the difference between hydrogen as it appears in complex molecules like fat as opposed to hydrogen as it appears in simple molecules such as H_2O).[6] MRI in athletic training settings is widely used to examine soft tissue structures in the joints (eg, ACL in the knee, cartilage defects in the knee). MRI can also be helpful to look at inflammatory processes in bone thus the use with overuse injuries that do not appear readily on traditional radiographs.[5] MR arthrography is a type of MRI that involves the placement of a contrast dye in the joint prior to the MRI in order to see specific structures in greater detail.[5] Figure 11-4 shows an MRI image of the knee.

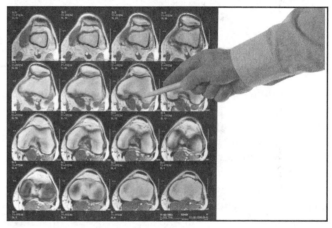

Figure 11-4. MRI of the knee.

Computed Tomography Scan

CT is a procedure that processes information from an x-ray beam that creates a cross sectional 3-dimensional image of the area being scanned. The word tomography is derived from the Greek words *tomos* (slice) and *graphein* (to write). CT is often used to image complex fractures, especially around joints, because of its ability to reconstruct the area of interest in multiple planes. It is particularly useful with fracture alignment (see Figure 11-2).[7] The advantage of the CT scan is the ability to view the anatomical structure from many angles. New multislice CT scans can be reconstructed to allow for visualization of images in 3 dimensions.[5] The anatomical images presented in the Web companion of this text are actual reconstructed CT images from real patients.

Ultrasound

Diagnostic ultrasound or sonography involves using high-frequency sound waves to produce images of anatomical structures. Health care professionals use them to view the heart, blood vessels, kidneys, liver, and other organs. Unlike x-rays, ultrasound does not involve exposure to radiation. Thus, it is commonly used in examining the fetus during pregnancy.[5] Improvements in ultrasound technology have allowed for images to be seen in 3 dimensions. During an ultrasound test, a special technician or doctor moves a device called a transducer over part of the patient's body. The transducer sends out sound waves that bounce off the tissues inside the body. The transducer also captures the waves that bounce back. Images are created from these sound waves. Diagnostic ultrasound is often used to examine the spleen following injury or if it is enlarged from an illness (see Chapter 9). Ultrasound is being used more often to aid in the diagnosis of musculoskeletal problems. Its noninvasive nature and lower costs are appealing. The real-time capture of the images allows for structures to be examined functionally (ie, you can move an extremity and examine an underlying tendon at the same time).

SUMMARY

The athletic trainer must possess the skills to evaluate both emergent and nonemergent injuries to determine an appropriate course of action. Primary and secondary surveys are evaluation schemes that allow the athletic trainer to properly assess the injured individual, render initial care, and make the necessary referral. The primary survey includes the ABCs. The initiation of an emergency response plan is the appropriate action when the athletic trainer identifies an emergency. Institutions and organizations must have well-documented and frequently rehearsed emergency action plans.

The secondary survey is a survey for trauma once the athletic trainer has established that the patient is stable and aids in determining if (and how) the patient will be transported from the field of play. A complete history and physical exam is a step-by-step process that requires an understanding of the underlying anatomy and proper function of the musculoskeletal structures. Athletic trainers must be able to evaluate both injures and illnesses and make appropriate adjustments to the history process.

As athletic trainers find themselves in a wider range of health care settings, they will need to be more familiar with a variety of diagnostic tests. Imaging tests commonly associated with injury evaluation and diagnosis are commonplace in sports medicine settings. The athletic trainer is often called upon to educate the patient regarding the nature of these diagnostic procedures. Athletic trainers must have an understanding of diagnostic imaging choices and appreciate their application and use under specific conditions.

REFERENCES

1. Kleiner DM, Anderson J, Bailes J, et al. *Prehospital Care of the Spine-Injured Athlete: A Document from the Inter-Association Task Force for Appropriate Care of the Spine-Injured Athlete.* Dallas, TX: National Athletic Trainers' Association; 2001:1-31.
2. Anderson JC, Courson RW, Kleiner DM, McLoda TA. National Athletic Trainers' Association position statement: emergency planning in athletics. *Journal of Athletic Training.* 2002;37:99-105.
3. Ginge K. *Writing Soap Notes.* Philadelphia, PA: FA Davis; 1990.
4. Schreibman, K. Imaging of the knee. Athletic Training Lecture Series. Dept. of Kinesiology UW-Madison. April 2008
5. Medlineplus National Library of Medicine. Diagnostic imaging. Available at www.nlm.nih.gov/medlineplus/diagnosticimaging.html. Accessed August 8, 2008.
6. Chan A, Lee R. A brief overview of MRI and NMR. CIBC Web Notes. Available at http://magnet.caltech.edu/mri/mri-overview.php Accessed August 8, 2008.
7. Euclid S. *Computed Tomography: Physical Principles, Clinical Applications, and Quality Control.* 2nd ed. Philadelphia, PA: WB Saunders; 2001.

WEB RESOURCES

National Collegiate Athletics Association
www.ncaa.org/wps/ncaa?ContentID=1446
Links to NCAA Health and Safety page provides copies of position papers, NCAA-sponsored research, and links to the sports medicine handbook.

National Athletic Trainers' Association
www.nata.org
Copies of positions statements regarding emergency planning and pre-hospitalization care of spine-injured athletes can be found at the NATA Web site.

Career Spotlight: Professional Football Athletic Trainer

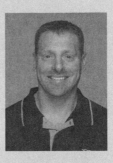

Geoff Kaplan, ATC, LAT, PT, SCS, MA, CSCS

Head Athletic Trainer

Houston Texans

My Position

NFL athletic trainers serve in numerous roles for their respective clubs. The primary role of NFL athletic trainers is to coordinate the medical care of the club's players, coaches, staff, and their families. We are responsible for injury prevention, evaluation, education, treatment, and rehabilitation of all club employees. Communication is essential at this level; all NFL athletic trainers have daily interaction with coaches, players, administration, player personnel, media relations, strength and conditioning, equipment, and football operations.

During the "season," NFL athletic trainers' responsibilities are typical of most athletic trainers—we take care of the players. We are responsible for the players' medical care from the time of injury to their return to the field. NFL athletic trainers work 7 days a week from the first day of training camp to the last day of the season. Our days are spent evaluating, treating, rehabilitating, and educating our players; covering practice; communicating with coaches, administration, and front office personnel; record keeping; and preparing injury reports.

During the "off season," we continue to rehabilitate injured players, evaluate prospective college and professional players, attend the NFL combined physicals, participate in draft meetings, do inventory and order supplies, cover mini-camps and off season conditioning, and attend CE conferences.

Unique or Desired Qualifications

NFL athletic trainers are the only NFL employees that are required to have an advanced certification and at least a baccalaureate degree. The NFL's Collective Bargaining Agreement requires NATA certification of all athletic trainers. Many NFL athletic trainers have additional certifications and advanced degrees. These include master's degrees; degrees in physical therapy; CSCS certification; advanced certifications from NASM, APTA, and NSCA; and EMT certification to name a few. Most NFL athletic trainers completed a NFL athletic training internship prior to being hired full time. Most NFL teams offer summer or seasonal internships. These internships are invaluable ways to learn the role of an NFL athletic trainer.

Favorite Aspect of My Job

There are a few aspects of my job that are very special:

- Working with some of the best athletes in the world
- Being part of a team with a common goal of winning
- Walking out of the tunnel on game day and hearing the roar of the crowd

Advice

The best advice I can give to prospective students is to separate yourself from the pack, make yourself special. This might entail getting an extra degree or certification, doing an internship, or working for a few years in the field. It is important to make yourself as marketable as possible.

CHAPTER 12

ENVIRONMENTAL CONCERNS

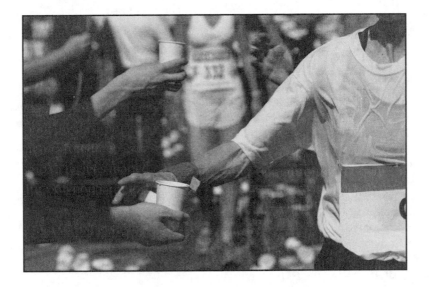

I always knew I wanted to be in a medical field, I liked sciences. When I stumbled upon athletic training in college, I was very excited because here was a medical field that put me in an environment that was exciting and allowed me to work with people who really wanted to get better. That really captured my enthusiasm.

Denise O'Rand, PhD, ATC
Associate Professor and Undergraduate Athletic Training
Program Director
San Diego State University

Exercise and competition in the heat or cold pose special problems for the physically active individual. If handled properly, these situations should be little more than an inconvenience for participants. If not addressed, the consequences could be deadly. Although sport- and exercise-related deaths due to hyperthermia or hypothermia are rare, they can occur. In fact, heat stroke is the third most common cause of exercise-induced death in US high school athletes, following head injuries and cardiac disorders.[1] The athletic trainer must be aware of the environmental conditions that can influence safe participation. Following proper guidelines and educating participants will lessen the risk of a serious heat-related illness or injury.

This chapter addresses the environmental issues of hyperthermia (heat), hypothermia (cold), and lightning safety.

Upon completion of this chapter, the student will be able to:

✓ Describe the metabolic factors that contribute to thermoregulation

✓ Explain the metabolic and environmental factors that contribute to heat loss and heat gain

✓ Identify the signs and symptoms of heat- and cold-related injury and illnesses

✓ List the appropriate prevention strategies to avoid heat- and cold-related conditions

✓ Discuss the importance of monitoring changing weather conditions

✓ List the factors that make up an appropriate lightning safety plan

THERMOREGULATION

Normal body temperature can fluctuate many times throughout the day for the average individual. For instance, body temperatures are lower when we are asleep as compared to the waking hours.[2] However, the slightest changes in temperature due to exercise, heat, or cold will trigger physiologic responses to help maintain homeostasis. The human body can tolerate drops in temperature much easier than an elevation in temperature. However, the extremes in either case can lead to death. The body must maintain a narrow range of core temperature to allow for systems to operate properly. Luckily, your brain is equipped with a built-in thermostat to help you control temperature.

In your brain, the hypothalamus contains a group of specialized neurons that respond to changes in temperature. Any detectable change stimulates a physiologic reaction to either dissipate or to create/conserve heat. The hypothalamus acts within a very narrow range, 37°C±1°C (98.6°F). However, unlike your house or apartment, you cannot turn the heat "off" when it gets too hot. You need to activate mechanisms to dissipate the excess heat. In an exercising athlete, less than 25% of the energy expended during play is transformed into movement—the rest must become heat.[1] The greater the athlete's effort, the greater the amount of heat generated. If you combine this with a warm and humid environment, you can see the stress or "heat load" on the body can be significant.

THERMAL BALANCE: HEAT LOSS AND GAIN

Figure 12-1 shows the constant balance being played out by the thermoregulatory system. The body must constantly adjust to changes in temperature. The resulting core or body temperature is the result of a balance between heat loss and heat gain. Although heat can be gained from the environment, most heat is produced by metabolic activity (work).[3] This balance relies on mechanisms that alter heat transfer from the body's core to the periphery, regulate sweat and evaporative cooling, and vary the body's rate of heat production. If heat production exceeds heat loss, the core temperature can rise quickly. As we will see, this is a dangerous scenario. When heat loss exceeds heat production, the core temperature will fall. If left unchecked, this too is a dangerous scenario.

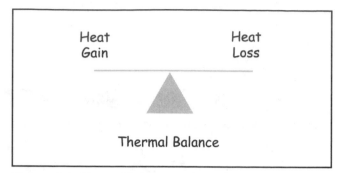

Figure 12-1. Thermal balance is dependent upon both heat gain and heat loss.

Heat regulatory mechanisms can be activated in 2 ways[2]:

1. Thermal receptors in the skin provide peripheral input to the hypothalamus and physiologic responses take place.

2. Temperature changes in the blood perfusing the hypothalamus directly stimulate the hypothalamus.

The hypothalamic-stimulated responses to both heat and cold are presented in Figures 12-2 and 12-3.

Thermoregulation in Heat Stress

During exercise in high heat, the body must be able to cool and dissipate the heat production generated by the large heat loads. There is a constant battle between the metabolic demands of working muscle and the mechanisms that regulate body temperature. The 2 major vehicles for heat dissipation are sweating and increased skin blood flow (SBF). Figure 12-4 illustrates potential avenues of heat exchange during exercise. Heat loss in the body occurs in 4 ways:

1. Radiation
2. Conduction
3. Convection
4. Evaporation

Radiation

All objects emit electromagnetic heat waves. Our body is most often warmer than the objects we encounter in our environment, therefore the net exchange of radiant heat energy occurs from the body through the air to cooler objects in the environment. This form of heat exchange is similar to how the sun warms the earth. It is radiant, therefore it does not require contact. We lose radiant heat during exercise. However, you can imagine if the outside temperature exceeds our own. This may prove ineffective.

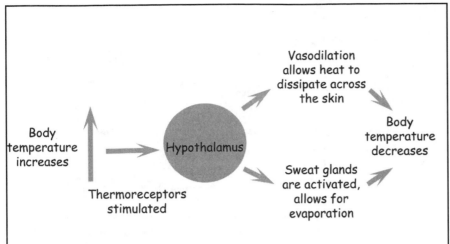

Figure 12-2. Physiologic response to body temperature increases.

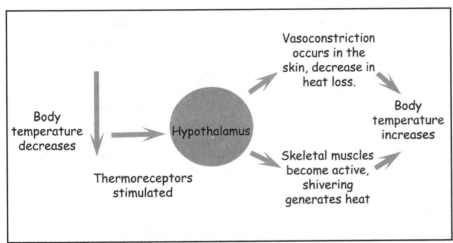

Figure 12-3. Physiologic response to body temperature decreases.

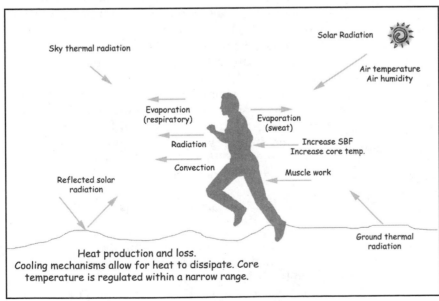

Figure 12-4. Heat production and loss during activity. (Adapted from McArdle WD, Katch FI, Katch VL. *Essentials of Exercise Physiology.* 2nd ed. New York: Lippincott Williams & Wilkins; 2000.)

Conduction

Where radiant heat transmits energy through the air, conduction requires objects to be in contact with one another. Conductive heat loss involves the direct transfer of heat through a liquid, solid, or gas from one molecule to another.[2] The rate of conductive heat loss depends upon the temperature gradient or difference in the temperature of the 2 objects. This is a minor role in heat loss during exercise; however, we will see it is an important aspect of heat gain in the cold.

Convection

The transfer of heat by the circulation of wind or water is known as convection. Convection is also the way that heat is transferred in the blood. If convection is present, a greater amount of heat can be dissipated away from the body. Think of how you feel when a fan blows air on you during a hot day. The heat loss increases because the convective effect of the currents can carry the heat away. Air currents at 4 mph cool twice as effectively as air moving at 1 mph.[2]

Evaporation

Evaporation provides the major physiologic defense against overheating. Evaporation takes place by water evaporation from the respiratory passages and skin surface to the environment. Sweat glands are activated in response to heat stress. The body has 2 to 4 million of these glands available to secrete large quantities of hypotonic saline solution. This sweat is 0.2% to 0.4% NaCl.[1-3] Cooling occurs when the sweat reaches the skin and evaporates. Dripping sweat is of no help; evaporation must take place for cooling to occur. Three factors dictate evaporation of sweat:

1. Surface area exposed
2. Temperature and relative humidity
3. Convective air currents around the body

The cooled skin then cools the blood that has been shunted to the surface. This process takes place all the time. Approximately 350 mL (about a soda can's worth) of water seeps through the skin each day and evaporates to the environment. This insensible perspiration goes unnoticed.[2] Another 350 mL of water evaporates from respiratory passages.

HEAT LOSS: THE EFFECT OF TEMPERATURE AND HUMIDITY

As ambient (air) temperature increases, the effectiveness of heat loss via conduction, convection, and radiation decreases. As the air temperature increases, these 3 methods actually add to the heat gain for the body. There is a constant struggle between heat production and cooling mechanisms (Figure 12-5). When the ambient temperature exceeds body temperature,

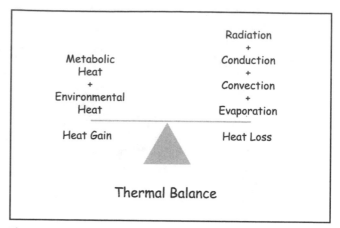

Figure 12-5. Factors contributing to heat loss and heat gain.

only evaporation is left to dissipate heat. As evaporation becomes the only mechanism for cooling, an increase in sweating will increase our fluid requirements. This is true at rest and, as we will see, is accentuated with exercise.

In addition to increases in air temperature, humidity is an important consideration for anyone exercising in the heat. In fact, the relative humidity exerts the greatest impact on the effectiveness of evaporative heat loss. As the relative humidity increases, the ability for sweat to evaporate from the skin is significantly decreased. This clearly illustrates the role of evaporation in cooling: on a humid day you will see an increase in sweat; however, sweat alone does not provide cooling—sweat that is evaporated provides cooling. Thus in the humid environment, fluid requirements are significantly increased. Relatively high ambient temperature can be tolerated provided the relative humidity is low. The combination of high humidity, high temperature, and vigorous exercise can provide a recipe for heat distress unless precautions are taken. It is essential that athletic trainers monitoring athletic events obtain both air temperature and humidity readings at the site of practice or competition. Table 12-1 outlines the physiological responses to exercise in the heat.

WATER LOSS IN THE HEAT

A key prevention strategy for heat-related illness is the availability of water and fluid replacement. Dehydration that is induced by exercise in the heat can reach levels that significantly impair the thermoregulatory system. Figure 12-6 demonstrates the potential water loss per hour for an average adult at moderate activity at various temperatures. The average adult working in the heat can lose 1 L of sweat per square meter of body surface. This may represent a loss of 1.5 to 2.5 L of sweat per hour for an average-sized adult (110 to 155 lbs) and accounts for 2% to 4% of their

Table 12-1

Physiological Responses to Exercise in Elevated Temperatures

Physiological Response	Rationale
Increased heart rate	Increased cardiovascular demand. O_2 delivery to muscles must increase to sustain energy metabolism. Peripheral blood flow to skin must increase to transport metabolic heat from exercise for dissipation; this blood is no longer available for O_2 delivery to muscles.
Decreased energy	As you continue to work to meet the cardiovascular demands, increased amounts of glycogen are being used. Cardiac output and aerobic capacity decrease with exercise in the heat due to changes in blood volume. Fatigue will be achieved sooner.
Increased sweating/decreased blood volume	Exercise in the heat leads to increased sweat production. For an acclimatized individual, fluid losses of more than 3 L of sweat per hour are common during intense exercise. As you lose fluid, your blood also is losing fluid, causing a decrease in blood volume.

Water Loss Per Hour / Moderate Activity

0.4 qt.	0.75 qt	1.0 qt.	1.5 qt.
0.1 gal.	0.186 gal.	0.25 gal.	0.375 gal
0.378 L	0.71 L	0.946 L	1.42 L
80	90	100	110	°F
26.2	32.2	37.8	43.3	°C

Air Temperature

Figure 12-6. Average water loss per hour for a typical adult at various air temperatures. (Adapted from McArdle WD, Katch FI, Katch VL. *Essentials of Exercise Physiology*. 2nd ed. New York: Lippincott, Williams & Wilkins; 2000.)

body weight for each hour of work.[4] Dehydration of greater than 3% of body weight can increase the risk of developing an exertional heat illness (heat cramps, heat exhaustion, or heat stroke). It is easy to see that athletes exercising in warm conditions could exceed this amount with ease. Elite marathon runners can sweat in excess of 5 L of fluid during competition. This represents 6% to 7% of their body weight.[2] There is a positive linear relationship between the volume of fluid lost during exercise and an increase in the relative humidity. When you combine fluid loss, work level, thermal load, and increased difficulty in dissipating heat, the stress on the thermoregulatory system is significant.

THE EFFECTS OF DEHYDRATION

Fluid that is lost and not replaced increases the load on thermoregulation. Any amount of dehydration can stress the thermoregulatory system. Plasma volume decreases with the loss of fluid. As dehydration increases, it will become more difficult to cool the body. Peripheral blood flow (a key cooling mechanism) will diminish and the rate of sweating will diminish. While diminished sweat production may sound desirable, it is problematic because the need to cool the body is still present. The loss of sweating is an important sign for a patient heading for thermoregulatory collapse (see heat stroke). The loss of only 1% of body mass by dehydration has shown significant increases in rectal (core) temperatures when compared to the same exercise in a fully hydrated individual.[2] Compared to a normally hydrated person, the dehydrated athlete will have an increased heart rate (due to plasma volume changes), an elevated core temperature, an increase in his or her perceived exertion, and he or she will fatigue easier and more quickly.

Blood plasma volume is responsible for transporting most of the water lost as sweat. As sweat loss progresses, it is difficult to maintain the appropriate cardiac output. In addition, the loss of blood volume causes an increase in the vascular resistance in the periphery to help maintain blood pressure. The net effect of this loss of volume reduces skin blood flow, compromising a significant heat dissipation source. Dehydration impairs your body's ability to meet the physiologic demands associated with exercise under a thermal load. Proper hydration before, during, and after exercise is a key prevention strategy. The NATA has issued a position statement that provides guidelines for fluid replacement.[5]

Fluid Replacement for Athletes: A Summary of Practical Applications

Background: Dehydration can compromise athletic performance and increase the risk of exertional heat injury.

Recommendations: Educate athletes regarding the risks of dehydration and overhydration on health and physical performance. Work with individual athletes to develop fluid-replacement strategies that optimize hydration status before, during, and after competition.

Consult the Position Statement for a complete description of the following subject areas or to gain better understanding of the scientific literature which supports these recommendations.

Effects of Dehydration

- Dehydration can affect an athlete's performance in less than an hour of exercise—sooner if the athlete begins the session dehydrated
- Dehydration of just 1% to 2% of body weight (only 1.5 to 3 lbs for a 150-lb athlete) can negatively influence performance
- Dehydration of greater than 3% of body weight increases an athlete's risk of heat illness (heat cramps, heat exhaustion, heat stroke)

Warning Signs of Dehydration

Recognize the basic signs of dehydration:

- Thirst
- Irritability
- Headache
- Weakness
- Dizziness
- Cramps
- Nausea
- Decreased performance

What to Drink During Exercise

- Athletes benefit in many situations from drinking a sports drink containing carbohydrate.
- If exercise lasts more than 45 to 50 minutes or is intense, a sports drink should be provided during the session.
- The carbohydrate concentration in the ideal fluid replacement solution should be in the range of 6%-8% (g/100 mL)
- An ingestion rate of 1 g carbohydrate (CHO)/minute during exercise maintains optimal carbohydrate metabolism. For example: 1 L of a 6% carbohydrate sports drink per hour of exercise.
- During events when a high rate of fluid intake is necessary to sustain hydration, sports drinks with less than 7% carbohydrate should be used to optimize fluid delivery.
- Fluids with salt (sodium chloride) are beneficial to increasing thirst and voluntary fluid intake as well as offsetting the amount lost in sweat.
- Cool beverages at temperatures of 50°F to 59°F are recommended.

What NOT to Drink During Exercise

- Fruit juices, carbohydrate gels, sodas and those sports drinks that have CHO levels above 8% are not recommended during exercise as the sole beverage.
- 8% CHO is a warning sign. Replacing fluids with a beverage that has less than 8% carbohydrate would be optimal to assure the fastest rate of fluid absorption.
- Beverages containing caffeine and carbonation are discouraged during activity because they can dehydrate the body by stimulating excess urine production, or voluntary fluid intake.

Hydration Tips

- Drink according to a schedule based on individual fluid needs. By the time you become thirsty, you're already dehydrated.
- Drink before, during, and after practices and games (follow the fluid guidelines listed next to maintain hydration and maximize performance).

(continued)

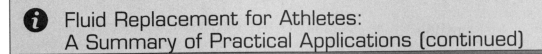

**Fluid Replacement for Athletes:
A Summary of Practical Applications (continued)**

- Avoid soft drinks and juice during play. The high carbohydrates may cause stomach problems.

Fluid Guidelines

Before Exercise

- 2 to 3 hours before exercise drink 17 to 20 oz. of water or a sports drink.
- 10 to 20 minutes before exercise drink another 7 to 10 oz of water or a sports drink.

During Exercise

- Drink Early – Even minimal dehydration compromises performance.
- In general, every 10 to 20 minutes drink at least 7 to 10 oz of water or a sports drink.
- To maintain hydration, remember to drink beyond your thirst. Optimally, drink fluids based on amount of sweat and urine loss.

After Exercise

- Within 2 hours drink enough to replace any weight loss from exercise.
- Drink approximately 20 to 24 oz of a sports drink per pound of weight loss.

Reprinted in part with permission of NATA from Casa DJ, Armstrong LE, Hillman SK, et al. National Athletic Trainers' Association position statement: fluid replacement for athletes. *J Athl Train.* 2000;35(2):212-224.

HYPERTHERMIA/ HEAT-RELATED ILLNESSES

Physiologic stress induced by excess temperature and poor thermoregulation can lead to a spectrum of heat-related illnesses, and the most serious of these can be catastrophic. An athletic trainer must be aware of the signs and symptoms of heat-related illnesses in order to recognize and properly refer patients. Through appropriate monitoring and the implementation of a prevention strategy, serious heat-related illness could be avoided.

HEAT CRAMPS

Heat cramps are strong painful spasms that usually occur in large muscle groups. The gastrocnemius, abdomen, hamstrings, and gluteal groups are commonly affected. Though the mechanism is poorly understood, heat cramps are associated with fluid and electrolyte imbalances caused by profuse sweating. Electrolytes are substances in a solution consisting of various chemicals that can carry electric charges. Electrolytes exist in the blood as acids, bases, and salts (such as sodium, calcium, potassium, magnesium, and bicarbonate). Electrolytes are essential to muscle contraction and even slight imbalances can lead to this problem. Individuals most likely to get

heat cramps are often in good physical condition and simply overexert themselves in the heat.[6] These are extremely painful muscle contractions. Athletes with heat cramps will often not return to activity and may experience subsequent muscle soreness.

The best prevention is adequate fluid and electrolyte intake via nutritional means. Small increases in table salt use, eating foods high in potassium (bananas), and foods high in calcium (dairy) are effective strategies to prevent heat cramps. Salt tablets are not recommended.

Immediate Treatment of Heat Cramps

✓ Fluid intake is essential so drink lots of water

✓ Gentle massage to relax the affected muscle or muscle group

✓ Gentle stretching of the affected muscle group can inhibit the spasm

✓ Ice packs may decrease pain and allow for gentle stretching

HEAT EXHAUSTION

Heat exhaustion is another level of heat illness that is caused by dehydration due to profuse sweating. Heat exhaustion patients have lost the ability to maintain adequate cardiac output, resulting from strenuous exercise and environmental heat stress. The heat exhaustion patient will often collapse or "fall out" of his or her activity. They will present with profuse sweating, often to the point of their skin feeling cool. Dizziness, headache, cool clammy pale skin, an elevation in temperature (can vary from 98.6°F to 104°F), rapid breathing (hyperventilation), mild confusion, decreased blood pressure, decreased urine output, and a rapid weak pulse are indicators of heat exhaustion. This patient may or may not have experienced heat cramps prior to presenting with the above signs and symptoms. Heat exhaustion patients may be nauseous to the point of vomiting, thus exacerbating the onset of dehydration. These patients will often appear disoriented and can be spotted because their performance will begin to falter. Heat exhaustion is more common in patients who are in poor physical condition and overexert themselves in the heat.[6] While heat exhaustion does not lead to physiologic damage, it must be treated aggressively so that the athlete does not progress to a full thermoregulatory collapse or heat stroke.

Immediate Treatment of Heat Exhaustion

✓ Immediate removal from activity, remove clothing and equipment

✓ Remove from heat—Try a shady spot or indoors to cool air

✓ Cooling—Ice packs, fans, cold towels in neck, axilla, and groin regions

✓ Fluid replacement—Oral or IV if unable to drink

✓ Monitor core temperature

✓ If using an electrolyte drink, it must be watered down (3 to 4 times) to allow for faster absorption by the gastrointestinal tract and to avoid an adverse reaction (increased nausea)

✓ If unable to drink, IV fluid (IVF) rehydration may be required

✓ Long-term interventions must include adequate hydration, acclimatization, and physical conditioning

✓ Athletes that do not have a rapid and uneventful recovery should be transported to a medical facility for further testing and observation

HEAT STROKE/EXERTIONAL HEAT STROKE

Heat stroke is the most serious and complex heat-stress malady. It requires immediate medical attention.[2] Heat stroke represents a complete breakdown of the thermoregulatory mechanisms in the body. The body is no longer able to dissipate heat and core temperatures can rise to deadly levels >41°C (106°F). These patients have a low fluid volume and develop dangerously high core temperatures. Core hyperthermia can allow for system and organ failures. Heat stroke is a MEDICAL EMERGENCY. Mortality rates for heat stroke are near 10%. Neurological deficits such as mental impairment are often seen first and may be one of the first signs of organ and system failure.

While classic heat stroke often strikes the elderly and infirm, an exertional heat stroke patient is often a physically fit individual who is not used to exercising in the heat. They may or may not have heat exhaustion symptoms that precede the onset of heat stroke. The exertional heat stroke patient often has been sweating profusely prior to the rapid onset of heat stroke. Abrupt onset or sudden collapse is characteristic of exertional heat stroke. A classic heat stroke patient may have a sudden change in mental status followed by collapse and the skin is hot and red. However, the skin may or may not be damp depending on how much sweating has preceded the collapse (this is one difference from the "typical heat stroke patient"). One key finding is hot, red skin (wet or dry). Patients will have rapid breathing (hyperventilation) and rapid heart rate (tachycardia) and experience a rapid rise in core temperature (rectal temperature >104°F). THIS IS A MEDICAL EMERGENCY. Sudden collapse and LOC are imminent.

The athletic trainer must activate his or her emergency plan (see Chapter 11), take immediate steps to cool the patient, and provide emergency life support. This is essential if the patient is to survive. The magnitude and the duration of the core temperature rise determines the extent of organ damage and mortality. Activation of the emergency plan and rapid cooling cannot be overstated. Table 12-2 outlines the signs and symptoms of heat stroke and heat exhaustion.

Immediate Treatment of Heat Stroke

✓ Activate emergency plan

✓ Heroic efforts must be taken to cool the patient

Table 12-2

Signs and Symptoms: Heat Exhaustion/Heat Stroke

Heat Exhaustion	Heat Stroke
Dizziness	Disoriented or unconscious
Headache	
Profuse sweating	No sweating
Cool, clammy, pale skin	*Hot, dry, reddish skin
Normal, slightly elevated temperature	Significant increase in body temperature
Rapid weak pulse	Rapid, pounding pulse

* Remember, exertional heat stroke patients may have damp skin due to the profuse sweating prior to collapse.

✓ Remove all equipment and clothing, use wet towels combined with fanning to encourage evaporation, and place ice packs at the neck, axilla, and groin

✓ Partial immersion in cold or ice water may be effective; however, the unconscious patient may be difficult to manage, therefore complete submersion must be avoided

✓ Patient must be monitored for ABCs

✓ Transport patient as soon as possible

✓ Monitor for 24 hours for signs of organ system damage

🔑 Strategies for Preventing Heat Illness

- Obtain a complete medical history—Athletes and physically active individuals with a prior history of heat-related illness must be identified. Previous episodes of heat illness are considered a risk factor for future events.

- Gradual acclimatization—Gradual exposure to warm environments combined with good aerobic fitness is an essential prevention strategy. A period of 7 to 10 days is needed to achieve acclimatization.

- Proper clothing and uniforms—Lightweight, lightly colored clothing that helps transfer sweat away from the body is desirable. Avoid dark colors, which absorb solar radiation. If sweating is significant, rest periods that allow for changing from wet to dry clothing are advised. Activities that require lots of protective equipment (ie, football) should slowly acclimate to the full-required equipment. Rubberized clothing that does not transfer sweat away from the body should NEVER be used.

- Monitor environmental conditions—The air temperature and relative humidity must be measured. Wet-bulb, dry-bulb, and globe temperatures can be taken to assess the impact of the humidity, temperature, and solar radiation.

- Fluid replacement—Water must be available to athletes as needed. The following guidelines can be followed:
  o Before exercise: Drink 17 to 20 oz of water or a sports drink 2 to 3 hours before exercise. Drink another 7 to 10 oz of water or a sports drink 10 to 20 minutes before exercise.
  o During exercise: Drink early. Even minimal dehydration compromises performance. In general, drink at least 7 to 10 oz of water or a sports drink every 10 to 20 minutes. To maintain hydration, remember to drink beyond your thirst. Optimally, drink fluids based on amount of sweat and urine loss.
  o After exercise: Within 2 hours, drink enough fluid to replace any weight lost from exercise. Drink approximately 20 to 24 oz of a sports drink per pound of weight loss.

- Avoid diuretics—Substances that act as stimulants may increase your risk of heat illness. In addition, diuretics cause increases in fluid loss and can contribute to poor hydration states. Caffeine and ephedra are stimulants commonly found in over-the-counter nutritional supplements.

(continued)

Strategies for Preventing Heat Illness (continued)

- Utilize weight charts—Recording pre- and postpractice body weights will assist in determining the amount of fluid lost during a single practice session. In addition, it will allow the athletic trainer the opportunity to monitor hypohydration states for athletes who are not replacing lost fluids. Athletes who lose 5% or more of their body weight over a period of several days should be evaluated medically and their activity restricted until they are rehydrated.

- Identify athletes at risk—Previous history, poor acclimatization, poor fitness, increased body fat, athletes who are febrile (have a fever), poorly hydrated athletes, and those with a history of pushing themselves to capacity are at an increased risk and should be monitored appropriately.

- Educate—Participants, coaches, and support personnel on the signs and symptoms of heat-related illness. The responsibility for a safe environment is shared and not the sole domain of the athletic trainer.

Adapted from:

The NCAA Sports Medicine Handbook Guideline 2C Prevention of Heat Illness. Revised June 2002. 2006-2007 NCAA Sports Medicine Handbook; 2006:28-31 and Casa D, Armstrong LE, Hillman SK, et al. National Athletic Trainers' Association position statement: fluid replacement for athletes. *J Athl Train.* 2000;35(2):212-224.

EXERTIONAL HYPONATREMIA: TOO MUCH FLUID REPLACEMENT?

The need for a proper fluid replacement plan has been discussed as an essential prevention strategy throughout this chapter. However, there is a condition that can result if an exerciser develops an imbalance between fluid (too much) and sodium (too little). Exertional hyponatremia occurs when sodium levels drop below 130 mmol/L.[7] Athletic trainers may encounter exertional hyponatremia in events that last greater than 4 hours such as marathons and other endurance events. The underlying cause is usually a failure to replace sodium lost through excessive sweating.

The classic patient is a slow running marathoner in a warm environment who is on the course for a long period of time and uses only water as a fluid replacement. Women seem to be at higher risk than men. This condition is common in ultra-endurance athletes (9% to 29%). Participants who have increased body weights are also at risk. The resulting osmotic imbalance causes intracellular swelling that produces several complications, including the following[7,8]:

- ✓ Altered mental status
- ✓ Headache
- ✓ Vomiting
- ✓ Lethargy
- ✓ Swelling in the extremities
- ✓ Pulmonary edema
- ✓ Cerebral edema
- ✓ Seizures

It is essential to differentiate between hyponatremia and heat stroke. Unlike heat exhaustion or heat stroke, hyperthermia is often mild in hyponatremia cases (eg, rectal temperature less than 40°C). While recognition of hyponatremia can be difficult, suspicion should be high under the circumstances described previously. Exertional hyponatremia can be fatal if it is unrecognized or treated improperly.

If hyponatremia is suspected, the emergency plan should be activated with the patient immediately transported to an emergency facility. Determination of serum sodium levels is critical to determine the treatment course to correct the fluid imbalance. A patient suspected of hyponatremia should be transported to a medical facility. If blood sodium levels cannot be determined onsite, rehydration should be avoided until a complete medical evaluation takes place. The delivery of sodium, certain diuretics, or IV solutions may be necessary. All will be monitored in the emergency department to ensure no complications develop.

ACCLIMATIZATION

In addition to the availability of fluids and proper hydration, acclimatization appears to have the greatest impact on preventing heat-related illnesses. Individuals must acclimatize themselves to the heat. Heat acclimatization refers to the physiologic adaptations that improve heat tolerance. Several physiologic adaptations take place as acclimatization improves and include the following:

- ✓ Improved peripheral blood flow
- ✓ Earlier onset of sweating
- ✓ Greater volume of sweat

Table 12-3
Physiologic Effects of Heat Acclimatization

Improved cutaneous blood flow ——————————→ Better peripheral heat dissipation

Lower threshold for start of sweating ——————→ Earlier onset of evaporative cooling

Increased sweat output ——————————————→ Maximize evaporative cooling

Lower salt concentration of sweat ——————————→ Decreased electrolyte loss

---

All of these adaptations will assist with improved heat dissipation. The acclimatized individual must be properly hydrated to keep these systems functioning at an optimal level. Table 12-3 outlines some of the physiologic responses to heat acclimatization, while Table 12-4 provides the heat stress index and gives recommendations for activity in the heat.

COLD INJURIES

At cold temperatures, the body essentially has 2 compartments that are critical to maintaining proper body temperature. In the cold, you can think of the body as 2 distinct areas: the core and the shell. The body core, which includes the internal organs, must be kept between the extremes of 75°F to 105°F; it usually is kept a constant 99°F. The shell can be thought of as the skin, muscles, and extremities. Temperatures in these areas fluctuate widely. Adjustments in blood flow and muscle activity (ie, shivering) are designed to protect the core temperature. The shell is vulnerable to cold injuries that damage the skin and underlying tissues (ie, frostnip, frostbite), while the body core can be compromised by hypothermia. Understanding these conditions is essential for any health care provider who cares for physically active individuals who are exposed to the elements.

HYPOTHERMIA

Hypothermia is defined as a significant drop in body temperature. It can occur with rapid cooling, exhaustion, and fatigue. Hypothermia can be classified in 3 categories: mild, moderate, and severe and defined as a core temperature below 35°C (95°F). A drop in temperature is sensed by the hypothalamus, causing the physiologic responses of vasoconstriction in the skin to decrease heat loss and the activation of skeletal muscles to cause shivering. Shivering helps generate heat to elevate body temperature.

ⓘ Hypothermia

Category	Body Temperature
Mild	32.2°C to 35°C (90°F to 95°F)
Moderate	26.6°C to 32.2°C (79.9°F to 90°F)
Severe	26.6°C (<79.9°F)

Classification predicts mortality. Up to 50% of severe cases result in death.

Cold temperatures alone are not the only factor that can contribute to hypothermia. Wind and dampness play a significant role. Natural wind or a head wind caused by running can cause a wind chill factor that changes the perceived "coldness" to the skin. The Wind Chill Index illustrates the cooling effects of wind velocity on bare skin for different air temperatures. For example, an air temperature of 25°F (4°C) with a 10-mile per hour wind has the same effect as calm air at 9°F (-13°C). Because of wind and dampness, hypothermia can occur in temperatures well above freezing.

Heat produced by the body is lost through radiation with the majority being lost through the head and neck. Your grandma knew what she was saying when she told you to wear your hat and scarf. A significant amount of heat is also lost through evaporation in the skin and respiratory tract. In cold temperatures as muscle fatigue takes place, the amount of heat lost will exceed the heat held in the body and the beginning of hypothermia sets in. If patients cannot be removed from the environment and be properly rewarmed, the consequences may be catastrophic. Hypothermia can progressively lead to decreases in neuromuscular function, cardiac irregularities, coma, or even death.

Table 12-4

The Heat Stress Index

Athletic trainers can use a sling psychrometer to determine dry-bulb and wet-bulb temperatures at the site of participation to determine the relative humidity. The Heat Stress Index evaluates the relative degree of heat stress. The resultant temperature on the chart is the heat sensation felt for a given humidity and temperature. Recommendations can be made based on the findings. The 1996 Olympic Marathon race in Atlanta was moved to an early morning start time to avoid heat-related stress. This decision was reached following close monitoring of the weather conditions over a 24-hour period. The graph below shows the heat stress when you compare the relative humidity to air temperature.

	Air Temperature (°F)									
	70°	75°	80°	85°	90°	95°	100°	105°	110°	115°
Heat Sensation										
0%	64°	69°	73°	78°	83°	87°	91°	95°	99°	107°
10%	65°	70°	75°	80°	85°	90°	95°	100°	105°	111°
20%	66°	72°	77°	82°	87°	93°	99°	105°	112°	120°
30%	67°	73°	78°	84°	90°	96°	104°	113°	123°	135°
40%	68°	74°	79°	86°	93°	101°	110°	123°	137°	151°
50%	69°	76°	81°	88°	96°	107°	120°	135°	150°	
60%	70°	76°	82°	90°	100°	114°	132°	149°		
70%	71°	77°	85°	93°	106°	124°	144°			
80%	72°	78°	86°	97°	113°	136°				
90%	73°	79°	88°	102°	122°					

Recommendations for Activity

Heat sensation below 90°F	No adjustments needed
Heat sensation 91°F to 104°F	Increase rest breaks and fluid intake and monitor for signs of heat illness
Heat sensations 105°F to 129°F	Adjust practice time or activity, decrease intensity unless acclimated, monitor for heat illness, and change wet clothing during breaks
Heat sensation 130°F and above	Consider suspending activity or changing time of day. Extreme caution must be taken because the risks for heat illness are high

Adapted from McArdle WD, Katch FI, Katch VL. *Essentials of Exercise Physiology.* 2nd ed. New York: Lippincott, Williams & Wilkins; 2000.

COLD-RELATED INJURIES: SKIN AND TISSUE

When skin is exposed to cold, a spectrum of tissue damage can take place from superficial skin issues to deep tissue damage due to frostbite. Recognizing the signs and symptoms and a willingness to take quick action are essential to avoiding serious injury.

Chilblains

Chilblains is a superficial cold injury that results from prolonged exposure to the cold, particularly wet conditions. A common scenario for chilblains is someone hunting or hiking in cold, wet socks for an extended period. There will be redness of the skin, swelling, a burning or tingling, and pain in the toes and fingers. People with circulatory insufficiencies are also more prone to this injury. It can be prevented by avoiding the exposure, and the initial treatment is to gently warm the tissue and make appropriate clothing adjustments.

Frostnip

Frostnip is a common condition that affects the face, fingers, and toes. It is characterized by numbness and cyanotic (blue) discoloration due to vasoconstriction. Patients experience numbness and burning superficially while deeper tissues remain soft and pliable. Simple rewarming by covering the exposed extremities and moving out of the cold temperatures is the most effective technique for treating frostnip. Rubbing of the tissues is not recommended. Hyperemia (increased blood flow and redness) will follow the rewarming period. Patients should be

Severe Hypothermia: You Are Not Dead Unless...

In cases of moderate to severe hypothermia, the course of action is to warm the patient to a normal body temperature. Proper action includes the following:

- Activate EMS immediately
- Prevent further heat loss
- Start IV fluids warmed to at least body temperature
- Perform CPR only if cardiac arrest is definite
- Monitor ABCs (prepare to activate life-saving protocols)

When core temperatures fall below 95°F, finding a pulse can be challenging so 2 things must be kept in mind:

- CPR should only be performed if cardiac arrest is definite. Take a pulse every minute and check several sites to determine if a pulse is truly absent. Extreme bradycardia (slowed heart rate) can produce a very faint pulse. Starting CPR when a pulse is present could initiate ventricular fibrillation.
- No patient is dead until he or she is warm and dead. Miraculous recoveries have been documented in hypothermia patients; death should never be assumed until all life-saving measures have been attempted on a warm patient.

Remember that all but the most mild of hypothermia cases should be transported to an emergency care facility.

Bibliography

Bowman WD. Safe exercise in the cold and cold injuries. *Team Physician's Handbook*. 3rd ed. Philadelphia, PA: Hanley & Belfus; 2002:144-151.

advised that some skin may flake and peel afterward. Prevention is key for those who have had pervious frostnip experiences.

Frostbite

Frostbite can be divided into 2 categories: superficial and deep. Frostbite occurs when the tissues are exposed to cold and freeze. The actual freezing of the tissue and formation of the ice crystals in the tissue can cause serious damage or lead to necrosis (tissue death). Superficial frostbite involves the skin and the superficial layers of subcutaneous tissue. When affected, the skin will appear hard, pale, cold, and waxy.[6] With rewarming, the tissues will feel numb and then have a burning or stinging sensation. Previous exposure to frostbite will increase sensitivity; additional precautions must be taken to avoid exposure in the future.

Deep frostbite is a medical emergency and requires immediate attention. Deep frostbite means that the tissues have been frozen at a deep level. The area will be cold, pale, and waxy not unlike superficial frostbite. The difference is the level of frozen tissue and the extent of the damage. Aggressive rewarming using hot drinks, heating pads, and hot water bottles 100°F to 110°F (37°C to 43°C) is appropriate.[6] The rewarming of frostbite is very painful. Tissues may become red and swollen. Loss of tissue due to tissue death or secondary infection is common with frostbite.

PREVENTION OF COLD-RELATED INJURIES

The prevention of cold-related injuries focuses on the importance of dressing properly to control the environment near the skin and maintaining proper energy and fluid intake to avoid fatigue.[9] The following are recommended prevention strategies for hypothermia:

✓ Dress in layers and make every effort to stay dry. Wear a base layer that will not stay wet. Base layers should "wick" or move the perspiration away from your skin (eg, polypropylene). Cotton is a poor base layer since it holds moisture. Remember to dress in base layers to wick moisture, middle layers for warmth, and outer layers to stop wind. Your head should be covered to prevent excess heat loss. Base layers that wick can also help keep hands and feet warmer; use a sock or glove liner. When the temperature is below freezing, consider one layer of protective clothing for every 5 mph of wind.[6]

✓ Maintain proper energy levels. Eat properly; negative energy balance can impair your ability to generate heat. It is also important to stay hydrated during exercise in the cold. Dehydration can decrease blood volume, thus making less available for warming the tissue.[2]

✓ Fatigue and exhaustion increase susceptibility to hypothermia. People exercising in the cold need adequate rest and should be cautious about overexertion.

✓ Warm up properly prior to activity. Cold tissue has been shown to have a significantly shorter time to failure than warm tissue.[10]

✓ Use a mask or scarf to warm cold air prior to breathing. While this cold air does not damage lung tissue, it does make the lungs irritable and can activate bronchospasm. Coughing and burning sensations are common when very cold air passes through the throat and nasal pathways.

✓ Train with a partner in the winter. A simple orthopedic injury could turn deadly if you are on a trail run in the winter. Do not put yourself in a position where you may be exposed to the cold if you have an injury. The best way to do this is to train with someone.

Immediate Treatment of Hypothermia

✓ Move to a warm environment

✓ Remove wet clothing

✓ Wrap exposed parts with dry, warm materials

✓ Do not rub skin

✓ Rewarming agents—Oral in mild cases, IV saline in severe cases

✓ Hypothermia patients often have rapid vascular changes due to changes in the peripheral vasodilation with rewarming

✓ Personnel working with the hypothermic patient must be prepared for changes in blood pressure and cardiovascular instability in extreme cases

LIGHTNING

The third environmental consideration we will discuss is lightning. Of all weather-related hazards, lightning is the most consistent that can affect athletic events. The National Severe Storms Laboratory (NSSL) estimates that 100 fatalities and 400 to 500 injuries requiring medical treatment occur from lightning strikes annually.[11] Lightning strikes occur most often in the summer between late morning and early evening. These are times of year and times of day when athletic and outdoor activities frequently take place.[12] Athletic facilities are often open spaces with tall backstops and metal poles that surround them, making them targets for lightning strikes. Direct strikes are only one mechanism of lightning injury. Injury can occur from indirect mechanisms such as touching an object that is struck, being next to an object that has been struck, from the ground itself, or injuries that can occur from being thrown by the force of a strike.[12]

The key to lightning safety is prevention and education. Institutions must develop a lightning-safety policy that can provide written guidelines for safety during lightning storms. Ninety-two percent of NCAA Division I athletic departments responding to a survey did not have a formal, written lightning-safety policy.[13] The NATA has established a Position Statement on Lightning Safety for Athletics and Recreation. Table 12-5 provides recommendations for lightning safety. This list is only a summary. For more details, refer to the NATA position statement and the NCAA guidelines.

SUMMARY

Each environmental topic discussed in this chapter is united by the common themes of planning and prevention. Proper planning will greatly reduce your chances of injury. Establishing policies, following prevention guidelines, and recognizing the signs and symptoms of environmental illnesses are the responsibility of the athletic trainer. The athletic trainer must remain vigilant in his or her efforts to monitor and appropriately adjust to changes in the weather.

REFERENCES

1. Sullivan AJ, Anderson SJ. *Care of the Young Athlete*. Oklahoma City, OK: American Academy of Orthopaedic Surgeons & American Academy of Pediatrics; 2000.
2. McArdle WD, Katch FI, Katch VL. *Essentials of Exercise Physiology*. 2nd ed. New York, NY: Lippincott, Williams & Wilkins; 2000.
3. Plowman SA, Smith DL. *Exercise Physiology for Health, Fitness, and Performance*. Boston, MA: Allyn and Bacon; 1997.
4. Hillman SK. Introduction to athletic training. In: Perrin DH, ed. *Athletic Training Education Series*. Champaign, IL: Human Kinetics; 2000.
5. Casa DJ, Hillman SK, Armstrong LE, et al. National Athletic Trainers' Association position statement: fluid replacement for athletes. *J Athl Train*. 2000;35:212-224.
6. Arnheim DD, Prentice WE. *Principles of Athletic Training*. 13th ed. New York: McGraw-Hill Higher Education; 2009.
7. Binkley HM, Beckett J, Casa DJ, Kleiner DM, Plummer PE. National Athletic Trainers' Association position statement: exertional heat illnesses. *J Athl Train*. 2002;37(3):329-343.
8. Mellion MB, Shelton GL. Safe exercise in the heat and heat injuries. *Team Physician's Handbook*. 3rd ed. Philadelphia, PA: Hanley & Belfus; 2002:133-143.
9. NCAA Committee on Competitive Safeguards and Medical Aspects of Sports. NCAA. Cold Stress. 2005-2006 NCAA Sports Medicine Handbook: NCAA; 2005-2006:25-27.
10. Noonan TJ, Best T, Seaber AV, Garrett WE. Thermal effects on skeletal muscle tensile behavior. *Am J Sports Med*. 1993;21:517-521.
11. NCAA Committee on Competitive Safeguards and Medical Aspects of Sports. Lightning safety. In: *2006-2007 NCAA Sports Medicine Handbook*. Indianapolis, IN: NCAA; 2006:12-14.

Table 12-5
Lightning Safety Recommendations

A comprehensive lightning safety policy should include the following:

- A designated chain of command that establishes who should make the call to remove individuals from the athletic activity.
- Designate a weather watcher. This person will actively look for signs of threatening weather and notify the chain of command if conditions warrant.
- A method for monitoring local weather forecasts and warnings.
- Where the closest "safe structures or locations" are located near the athletic fields or playing areas.
  - Any building NORMALLY occupied or frequently used by people. Buildings with plumbing and/or electrical wiring that can act to electronically ground the structure. Avoid using showers for safe shelter and do not use the shower or plumbing facilities during a thunderstorm.
  - If a building is unavailable, any vehicle with a hard metal roof can serve as protection. The roof can dissipate the lightning strike. DO NOT TOUCH THE SIDES OF THE VEHICLE.
- Educate participants on how to minimize their body's surface area to help avoid a ground strike.
  - If a safe structure cannot be found, try to find a thick grove of small trees surrounded by taller trees or a dry ditch. Assume a crouched position with only the balls of your feet touching the ground, wrap you arms around your knees, and lower your head. MINIMIZE YOUR BODY'S SURFACE AREA, AND MINIMIZE CONTACT WITH THE GROUND! DO NOT LIE FLAT!
  - Avoid tall objects, metal objects, standing water, and individual trees. Never take shelter under a single tall tree.
- Be aware of how close the lightning is occurring. Use appropriate lightning detection technology or strike-to-bang method. Strike to bang means you should begin counting when you see the lightning flash and stop counting when the associated thunder is heard. Divide this number (in seconds) by 5 to determine the distance (in miles) to see the lightning strike.
- Establish criteria for suspension and resumption of activities.

Adapted from NCAA Committee on Competitive Safeguards and Medical Aspects of Sports. NCAA. Lightning Safety. 2006-2007 NCAA Sports Medicine Handbook; 2006:12-14. and Walsh KM, Benett B, Cooper MA, Holle RK, Kithil R, Lopez RE. National Athletic Trainers' Association position statement: lightning safety for athletics and recreation. *J Athl Train.* 2000;35:471-477.

---

12. Walsh KM, Benett B, Cooper MA, Holle RK, Kithil R, Lopez RE. National Athletic Trainers Association position statement: lightning safety for athletics and recreation. *J Athl Train.* 2000;35:471-477.
13. Walsh KM, Hanley M, Graner SJ, Beam D, Bazluki J. A survey of lightning policy in selected Division I colleges. *J Athl Train.* 1999;32:206-210.

WEB RESOURCES

National Athletic Trainers' Association
www.nata.org
Copies of position statements regarding fluid replacement, exercise in the heat, and lightning safety can be found at the NATA Web site.

National Collegiate Athletics Association
www.ncaa.org/wps/ncaa?ContentID=1446
Links to NCAA Health and Safety page provides copies of position papers, NCAA-sponsored research, and links to the *Sports Medicine Handbook.*

National Lightning Safety Institute
www.lightningsafety.com
The National Lightning Safety Institute (NLSI) is an independent, nonprofit consulting, education, and research organization that advocates a proactive risk management approach to lightning safety. Links to current information regarding safety issues, products, and other weather-related topics are provided.

National Weather Service
www.nws.noaa.gov
Weather information for all areas of the country updated and maintained by the National Weather Service (NWS). Site includes information about planning for weather-related emergencies, lightning safety, heat-related issues, cold, and many other topics.

Career Spotlight: Professional Bull Riders Association Athletic Trainer

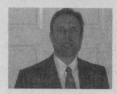

Tony Marek, MS, LAT

Manual Therapy Associates, Reno, Nevada

Professional Bull Riders Association-Athletic Trainer

My Position

I currently work as a certified athletic trainer with the Professional Bull Riders Association providing rehabilitative services, emergency care, and treatment of injuries. Injuries can include everything from extremity fractures to severe facial and cranial wounds. In this job setting, athletic trainers provide medical services at weekly events by traveling to 32 cities across the United States with a mobile sports medicine unit. We are a total mobile unit and each week we are required to set up an athletic training room and provide the same services that you would find in any collegiate or professional setting. Rehabilitation occurs on a weekly basis with athletes receiving rehabilitation protocols and reassessing the following week. Injuries are entered and tracked on a computer so that at year's end the sports medicine team can analyze injuries for frequency and severity and recommended safety changes.

Unique or Desired Qualifications

Working with professional bull riding requires the ability to think on your feet; specifically how to handle injuries and medical emergencies in extreme conditions. All members of the sports medicine team (ATCs and MDs) must be comfortable with a range of skills, from placing cowboys on a spine board to working in the mobile care facility. Working in this setting requires dedication to the profession and to the athletes we serve. I would venture to say that all of us who travel with the medical team could make more money, if that were the object, staying at home and working with our respective businesses. However, we view ourselves as a specialized team. All the athletic trainers hold a master's degree and have extensive experience, and the orthopedic physician we work with has additional training in trauma and plastics.

Favorite Aspect of My Job

There are many favorites to this job. Working with young, competitive, honorable athletes is perhaps the most enjoyable part of the job. Traveling with my colleagues and enjoying new cities makes this job a great adventure. In addition, working with young cowboys who are at the peak of their competitive level and trying to stay that way until at least age 30 (a 35-year-old bull rider is very, very "old"). The camaraderie with which these young men compete and yet pull for their fellow bull riders to achieve greatness is truly remarkable to be around. They have an appreciation for our services that is genuine and very rewarding; these athletes never fail to say "thank you."

Advice

My advice for athletic training students who would like to someday work with the sport of professional bull riding: study hard, listen to your mentors, don't be afraid to work events/sports outside your comfort level, and above all remember that the athletes you work with must trust you completely.

CHAPTER 13

FIRST AID AND
INITIAL INJURY CARE

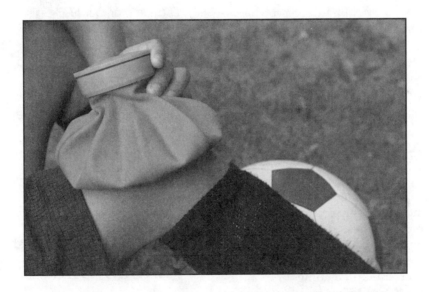

The next generation of athletic trainers must be better prepared to integrate into the health care system.

Sara D. Brown, MS, ATC
Clinical Associate Professor and Director,
Athletic Training Education
Boston University

Be prepared. The Boy Scouts of America have selected a great motto. It is hard to say just how many athletic trainers have scout training (boys or girls), but the ability to respond to a variety of first-aid situations is a foundational skill for the athletic trainer. Providing first aid and initial care is the first step in assisting your patient in his or her recovery. Proper basic first aid can be learned early in the athletic training student's educational program and can serve as a foundation for the development of advanced skills in the area of evaluation and the treatment and management of injuries. An athletic training educational program will require new students to be trained in basic first-aid skills and to possess up-to-date training in CPR. In Chapter 11, we discussed the importance of being able to recognize an emergency, perform an initial evaluation, and activate an emergency action plan. In this chapter, we explore some basic first aid and initial care steps commonly employed by athletic trainers. This chapter is an overview and cannot take the place of a basic first aid and CPR course.

Upon completion of this chapter, the student will be able to:

✓ Differentiate the factors to be addressed when caring for open and closed wounds

✓ Describe sterile technique and explain its importance in caring for wounds

✓ State the basic considerations for dressing and bandaging wounds

✓ Recognize the signs and symptoms of inflammation

✓ Classify and describe the mechanical forces associated with injury

✓ List the signs, symptoms, and first aid for shock

✓ Describe the principles of splinting and immobilization for musculoskeletal injuries

✓ Identify the risks of tetanus

✓ Compare the physiologic effects of cold and heat in the treatment of injuries

✓ Explain the proper steps for fitting crutches to aid in ambulation

✓ Describe CPR requirements for the certified athletic trainer

GENERAL FIRST AID: AN OVERVIEW

Earlier in the text we defined 2 types of emergencies that require first aid: a sudden illness and an injury. A sudden illness is a physical condition that requires immediate medical attention (eg, severe allergic reaction, heart attack, stroke). Injuries are defined as damage to tissues that occur from outside forces. Emergencies are either life threatening or nonlife-threatening. A life-threatening emergency impairs the ability to circulate oxygenated blood to all parts of the body. A nonlife-threatening emergency does not prevent the circulation of oxygenated blood but still requires medical attention.[1] For instance, a fracture to the ankle is not life threatening but requires medical attention.

Basic first aid is the care provided to someone who has sustained an injury or has developed a sudden illness until more advanced care can be obtained. Athletic training students just beginning in an athletic training education program should be trained in first aid. As students advance and receive more training, they can take on the role of a first responder. First responders are people who due to the nature of their jobs may find themselves caring for emergencies often. They are on the scene and have the supplies and equipment available to provide first-aid care on a regular basis. They are a transition between the basic first aid a trained citizen may provide and the advanced care emergency medical technicians (EMTs) are trained to provide.[1] Many athletic trainers who work in environments where acute care is common

pursue additional EMT training although it is not required for certification by the BOC.

In an athletic injury environment, first aid is sometimes thought of as initial care. Initial care is the care that is provided to an injured person immediately after the injury occurs. Initial care is an important first step in the overall treatment and rehabilitation of an injury. Reducing pain, controlling swelling, and protecting the tissues are initial care goals.

ⓘ Always Be Prepared: Emergency Cardiac Care

In Chapter 11, we referred to our need to be up-to-date on our ECC certification. It is a must when dealing with potentially life-threatening injuries. In this chapter, our discussion of initial care and first aid will focus on wounds and response to soft tissue injury. We must always be prepared to recognize an injury situation that may seem routine but can escalate to a full-blown emergency. Understanding wounds and recognizing signs and symptoms of shock are key elements.

Always expect the unexpected—you will never be surprised that way.

CLASSIFICATION OF OPEN VERSUS CLOSED WOUNDS

Athletic trainers are often called upon to provide care to skin injuries for athletic populations.[2] As the largest organ in the body, the skin is exposed to many injuries. The skin is made up of 2 layers: the epidermis and the dermis. When trauma to the skin causes a disruption or break in the continuity of the tissue, it is called a wound. A closed wound is one in which the skin is intact and the damage lies below the surface of the skin. A contusion is an example of a closed wound and most do not require medical attention. They should be treated with PRICE. However, not all contusions are minor injuries. A contusion that produces persistent pain, inability to move the limb, or swelling that affects circulation or sensation should be referred immediately.

There are a variety of open wounds that include damage to the outer layer of the skin. The forces that cause the injury or the resulting arrangement of the tissue once it has been injured determine how an open wound is classified. The descriptions provided next discuss some common open wounds, how they occur, and potential complications.

ABRASIONS

To abrade something means to scrape it against a rough surface. An abrasion is a common wound that results when the skin is scraped. Mats, rugs, court surfaces, asphalt, artificial turf, and equipment are common rough surfaces that can cause abrasions. The abrasion can be problematic due to the top layer of skin being scraped, exposing capillary beds. These beds are susceptible to dirt, debris, and bacterial agents that may cause a subsequent infection. An abrasion tends to ooze rather than bleed like other wounds. The patient's thinking that "It is just a scrape" may minimize abrasions. In reality, this type of wound can be easily infected and lead to a more serious problem. A common abrasion is the turf burn. Turf burns are caused by artificial playing surfaces. Like all wounds, the abrasion should be cleaned of debris, treated, and covered following universal precautions.

BLISTERS

Blisters are caused by repetitive friction. Rubbing of the skin causes the formation of fluid between layers of the skin. The athletic trainer must make a decision whether to drain the fluid from the blister or leave it to its own course. This decision is based on the comfort of the athlete and the location of the blister. Most often the blister will be drained using sterile technique followed by cleaning and covering of the area.

Proper fitting shoes, socks that help wick (remove) moisture, and the use of lubricants on hot spots are all good strategies to prevent blisters. The formation of calluses over areas of friction is common in active populations. This is particularly true for court sport athletes like basketball, racquetball, and tennis players. These calluses can become quite large and begin to form a blister between the callus and the soft epidermis below it. These blisters can be painful and difficult to treat. Calluses should be treated by shaving with a callus shaver, foot file, or pumice stone.

LACERATIONS

A laceration is a wound that results in irregular edges to the skin once it has been damaged. Lacerations occur when the tissues are torn by a sharp object or when direct pressure to the tissue caused it to break. Equipment edges or items in the field of play may cause a laceration. A common mechanism is the elbow to the eyebrow while rebounding the basketball. The pressure of the blow causes a jagged, lacerated wound. Lacerations, like any open wound, must be cleaned of debris, treated, and covered following universal precautions. Lacerations tend to bleed immediately and may cause damage to underlying tissue as well. The initial treatment and closing

of a wound will help determine if a scar will be visible. Direct pressure to stop bleeding, proper cleaning, and closure are appropriate initial treatments. Butterfly strips, Steri-Strips (3M Corp, St. Paul, MN), and wound closure strips are common dressings for lacerations. Since these wounds frequently occur in the facial region, it is important to be sensitive to the patient's appearance and refer him or her to a physician to determine the need for sutures.

INCISIONS

Incisions are wounds that result in very smooth edges. They occur when a very sharp and smooth object causes damage to the skin and possibly anatomical structures nearby. The most common incisions for which an athletic trainer cares are those that occur in patients who have had surgery. However, sharp edges of equipment, glass, and metal may cause wounds that have smooth edges. Incisions tend to bleed and must be referred to a physician for evaluation.

CARING FOR OPEN WOUNDS

DRESSINGS AND BANDAGES

As always, universal precautions should be adhered to when dealing with all open wounds (see Chapter 10). In caring for open wounds, it is important that they be covered to help control bleeding and to prevent infection. This is accomplished by using dressings and bandages. Dressings are pads placed directly on a wound to absorb blood and other fluids and to protect from infection. Most dressings allow for some air circulation to promote healing (eg, sterile gauze, nonstick dressings). If a wound needs to be protected from the air, an air-tight dressing called an occlusive dressing can be used. Bandages are any material that is used to wrap or cover a body part. Bandages hold dressings in place, apply pressure to control bleeding, protect the wound from dirt and debris, and provide support to an injured limb (eg, sling). Figure 13-1 shows examples of common dressings and bandages.

STERILE TECHNIQUE—
WOUND CARE

Sterile technique insures that the dressings are sterile and the area that covers the wound is not touched. This is done by holding only the corners of the gauze while cleaning a wound, never touching an ointment or antiseptic tube to the surface of the

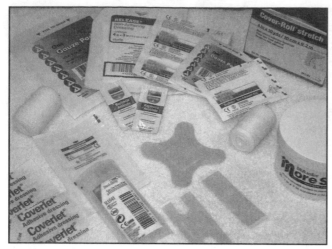

Figure 13-1. An assortment of dressings and bandages are available for proper wound care.

dressing, always opening dressings by the corner of the package to minimize exposure, and always using universal precautions.

MINOR WOUNDS

A minor wound can be treated using the following steps while adhering to sterile techniques[1]:

✓ Use disposable gloves or an appropriate barrier between your hand and the wound.

✓ Apply direct pressure to the wound using sterile gauze (the patient can often apply direct pressure while you are donning gloves).

✓ Irrigate the wound with a sterile water solution for several minutes (if not available, clean running tap water is acceptable). All wounds should be considered contaminated and thus cleaned appropriately. Irrigation can be performed using a large syringe (500 mL) and a sterile saline solution. This solution may be diluted with 3% hydrogen peroxide.

✓ Clean the area around the wound with mild antibacterial soap and water.

✓ Cover the wound with a sterile dressing (eg, nonstick absorbent pad) and a bandage (eg, roll gauze). Note: If the wound has been cleaned and does not need to be seen by a physician, an antiseptic/antibacterial ointment can be applied to the dressing. Clean moist dressings are associated with faster healing and less discomfort for patients than dry dressings. If available, a moist dressing such as a hydrocolloid or polyurethane semipermeable film should be used to cover the wound.

✓ Dressings should be inspected and changed often.

ⓘ Do I Need Stitches?

The decision to refer a patient for sutures can be a difficult call for the athletic trainer. Some simple guidelines can help. The patient likely needs sutures if:

● The edges of the wound do not align well

● The wound is over 1 inch in length

The following injuries ALWAYS should be referred and often require suturing:

● Bleeding that is difficult to control

● Any cut or wound that exposes tissue below the skin

● Embedded objects

● Human and animal bites

● Large punctures

● Wounds on the face that may leave a scar if left unattended

When in doubt, trust your gut. If you think the wound needs stitches, it likely does and you should refer the patient to a physician.

Tetanus—Better Safe Than Sorry

The micro-organism *Clostridium tetani* can cause tetanus when it infects open wounds. The organism can multiply in an environment that is low in oxygen, which makes puncture wounds and deep wounds at particular risk for infection. Over 1 million people in the world contract tetanus annually and up to 1 in 3 may die from the disease.[1] The organism produces a powerful toxin that can affect the CNS. Tetanus is sometimes called "lockjaw" due to the spasm that can occur in the muscles around the jaw. Once in the nervous system, the effects are irreversible. Developed nations with extensive immunization programs have all but eliminated the disease. Only 130 cases of tetanus were reported in the United States between the years 1998 and 2000 with a fatality rate of 18%.[3] The majority of cases are found in adults. It is recommended that adults receive a tetanus booster once every 10 years if they are between the ages of 19 to 49.[4] *C. tetani* is found in soils rich in organic matter and the feces of cows and horses. Thorough cleaning of all wounds is an essential first line of defense for prevention of tetanus as well as other potential contaminants. Athletic trainers must be aware of the immunization status of patients in their care. It is common practice for young adults to receive a tetanus booster if they sustain a wound. Consult with a physician if there is any question.

MAJOR WOUNDS

A major wound is one that has severe bleeding, an embedded object, or deep destruction of tissue. Steps for caring for such wounds include the following[1]:

✓ Activate the emergency plan by calling 911.

✓ Put on disposable gloves. If there is potential for blood to gush or splatter, use protective eyewear.

✓ Control bleeding:

  o Cover the wound with a dressing and press firmly on the wound with a gloved hand.

  o Apply a pressure bandage over the dressing to maintain pressure on the wound and hold the dressing in place.

  o Apply additional dressings if blood soaks through them but do not remove the bandages.

  o Pressure can be applied at brachial and femoral pressure points if needed.

✓ Monitor airway and breathing for the patient while awaiting EMS to arrive. Observe closely for breathing (slowing or growing rapid), changes in skin color, and alertness or restlessness.

✓ Position the patient to minimize shock.

✓ Keep the patient from getting chilled or overheated.

✓ Reassure the patient and continue to monitor his or her vital signs.

✓ Remove blood-soaked gloves and clothing with care and dispose of properly. Wash your hands thoroughly immediately after providing care.

SHOCK

Shock occurs when the circulatory system can no longer circulate oxygenated blood to all parts of the body. This is caused by a shift in fluid volume due to the dilation of blood vessels and the disruption of osmotic balance. During shock, the plasma moves from the vessels into surrounding tissues, causing circulation to slow. When oxygenated blood is not readily available, vital systems (eg, nervous, cardiac) are compromised. If left untreated, shock can be fatal. Shock can be associated with severe injury.

TYPES OF SHOCK

There are 7 types of shock: anaphylactic, cardiogenic, hypovolemic, neurogenic, psychogenic, respiratory, and septic.[5]

Anaphylactic	A life-threatening allergic reaction to a substance. Anaphylaxis may cause the airway to swell and affect the patient's ability to breathe. This type of shock is most associated with insect stings, food, and drugs.
Cardiogenic	Cardiogenic shock results from failure of the heart to effectively circulate oxygenated blood to all parts of the body. This can occur with heart attack.
Hypovolemic	Severe bleeding and loss of blood or plasma is the cause of hypovolemic shock. This can occur with bleeding wounds, burns, or with severe fluid loss due to vomiting and diarrhea.
Neurogenic	Disruption of the autonomic nervous system resulting in blood vessels expanding and causing a rapid drop in blood pressure. Fluid loss, trauma to the nervous system, and emotional distress are common causes of neurogenic shock. Syncope (fainting) is an example of neurogenic shock.
Psychogenic	Similar to neurogenic shock in that emotional circumstances cause a rapid drop in blood pressure due to temporary dilation of vessels reducing the normal amount of blood available to the brain.
Respiratory	Respiratory shock occurs when the lungs cannot supply enough oxygen to the blood. Severe trauma to the lungs (eg, pneumothorax) or injury to the mechanisms that control respiration can cause this type of shock.
Septic	Dilation of blood vessels caused by severe infection (usually bacterial).

SIGNS AND SYMPTOMS OF SHOCK

While the cause of shock may not be readily evident, it is essential that the athletic trainer recognize the signs and symptoms of shock, which include the following:

✓ Pale or ashen, bluish, cool, or moist skin

✓ Rapid breathing

✓ Rapid and weak pulse

✓ Excessive thirst

✓ Nausea or vomiting

✓ Restlessness and irritability

✓ Altered consciousness

NOTE: Shock is life threatening and requires immediate action. If any of the signs of shock are present, appropriate care should be initiated and an emergency action plan activated (see Chapter 11).

Emergency Action Steps: Check, Call, Care

If your initial care is emergency care, always follow these steps:

- CHECK the scene and the victim
- CALL 9-1-1- or your local emergency number (or have someone call)
- CARE for the victim

TREATMENT OF SHOCK

The treatment of shock will depend upon the cause. If there is any question, ALWAYS ACTIVATE THE EMERGENCY PLAN. In the event of shock:

✓ Monitor the patient's airway and breathing.

✓ Keep the patient from getting chilled or overheated.

✓ Elevate the patient's legs to keep blood circulating to the vital organs

  ○ If fracture is suspected, keep the patient's legs level until a splint has been applied.

  ○ If a cervical spine injury is suspected, the patient should be immobilized in the position in which he or she is found.

✓ Do not give the victim anything to eat or drink until the patient is seen by a physician.

Since psychological factors can influence shock, the following should be considered:

✓ Patients should be reassured and kept calm. Bleeding injuries and deformities should be shielded (or patients encouraged to look away).

✓ Onlookers should be kept at an appropriate distance as not to alarm the patient.

SOFT TISSUE INJURIES

In 2007, ankle sprain injuries alone represented an estimated 80,402 clinic, hospital, and emergency room visits for teenagers participating in sport and recreational activity.[6] Classification of these injuries and common mechanisms are discussed in detail in Chapter 5 and addressed throughout the text. Given the common occurrence of such injuries, athletic trainers with an understanding of the nature of soft tissue injury and the natural inflammatory processes that accompany these injuries can select the proper initial care interventions. In addition, recognizing the stages of the inflammatory process is the foundation for both immediate and long-term therapeutic interventions.

THE BASICS OF INFLAMMATION

While a complete understanding of the chemical reactions and hormone-mediated events in the healing process is beyond the scope of this text, it is essential to know some of the key components to guide proper first aid and initial care of injuries. Injured tissue responds with a predictable chain of physiologic events. The inflammatory process is a complex sequence of mechanical and chemical events that cause tissues to respond in a specific way. Alleviating some of the discomforts of the inflammatory process is the primary goal for most early treatment interventions following injury. It is imperative that the athletic trainer know the physiologic sequence of events associated with inflammation as he or she makes proper treatment choices for his or her patients. The healing process is divided into 3 distinct phases: inflammation, repair, and remodeling. Key physiologic changes and specific events are associated with each phase.

Acute Inflammatory Phase of Healing

Tissue injury causes a physical disruption of cellular structures, leading to a host of chemically mediated activities at the cellular level. During the inflammation phase, many of these chemically mediated processes overlap and occur simultaneously. These include the following[7,8]:

✓ Release of histamines, bradykinin, and serotonin in the area of injury. The net effect is an increase in capillary permeability around the injured site. In addition, pain receptors are sensitized and cause pain.

✓ Prostaglandins (PGE) are formed, allowing for continued permeability and the attraction of white blood cells to the area.

✓ Leukocytes (neutrophils and macrophages) help clean up damaged tissues through phagocytosis.

✓ Increased capillary permeability coupled with chemically mediated vasodilation causes fluids to lead into tissues and swelling to develop.

✓ As swelling increases, movement is inhibited and tension on the pain receptors causes discomfort.

The Cardinal Signs of Inflammation

The inflammatory process is a natural and needed response to injury. However, how an athletic trainer treats or manages an injury is dependent upon what stage of the inflammatory process is present. The recognition of temperature, color, and pain as indicators of injury can be traced back to the Roman and Greek origins of medicine. Almost 2000 years ago, the Roman physician Celsus recognized the warmth, redness, swelling, and pain associated with what now is known as "inflammation."

Allied health and medical professionals rely upon recognition of the signs of inflammation to determine appropriate referral and treatment strategies. The cardinal signs of inflammation often indicate an acute injury or the presence of infection. The indicators of inflammation are pain, heat, swelling, redness, and loss of function.

Indicator	Cause
Pain	Increased chemical activity and direct tissue damage
Heat	Increased metabolic activity
Swelling	Chemical and vascular changes allow fluid to leak into cellular spaces
Redness	Increased blood flow and increased metabolic activity
Loss of function	Inability to perform desired activities due to tissue damage, swelling, and pain

"Cardinal" Sign?

In astrology, a cardinal sign is a sign of the zodiac that initiates a change of season when the sun makes a passage into that sign. The word *cardinal* originates from the Latin word for hinge (that on which something turns or hinges). The cardinal signs mark the turning point of a temperate season. In the physiological use of the word, we can only guess that the "turning point of a temperate season" physiologically refers to the temperature, warmth, and redness associated with injury or infection.

Hmm, it kind of makes sense.

✓ Clotting factors eventually wall off the injured area and prevent blood loss in the area of injury.

✓ Unless aggravated by additional injury, the inflammatory phase lasts up to 5 days.

 ## When in Doubt, Fight Swelling

When all the physiologic outcomes of inflammation following injury are taken into account, the athletic trainer will find that one outcome must be vigorously fought on behalf of the patient. That outcome is swelling. Whether found in the tissues as edema or confined in a joint as an effusion, the net effects are always poor. Edema is formed by increased capillary permeability combined with plasma proteins in the region of injury, causing fluids to move into the tissue spaces. Effusion has a similar cause combined with intra-articular bleeding or increased synovial fluid production in response to joint irritation. No matter the cause, the adverse effects are many:

● Increased pain due to tissue or joint tension
● Inhibition of muscle activity
● Decrease in joint ROM
● Decrease in functional ability
● Compromise to healing tissues

The bottom line is that when tissues are swollen, the healing process cannot move forward and may become stagnant. The use of interventions to control swelling is of the utmost importance. Do not forget to protect, rest, ice, compress, and elevate.

When in doubt, always fight swelling!

Common interventions in this phase include ice to decrease chemical activities and reduce pain, compression to combat swelling, and protection to minimize secondary damage to injured tissues.

Repair Phase of Healing

As an injury moves from one phase of healing to the next, there is some overlap between phases. During the inflammatory phase, large white blood cells called macrophages help rid the injured area of debris and help neutralize the chemicals causing changes to tissue and sensitivity to pain. Once this is accomplished, the repair phase of healing can take place. Connective tissues repair through the formation of scar tissue (this is true for all connective tissues with the exception of bone). During the repair phase, the development of new tissue through the production of collagen and elastin and new capillary formation (angiogenesis) is seen. This new tissue is fragile and easily disrupted, making reinjury a concern during this phase. Key elements to the repair phase of healing include the following:

✓ Cells that can assist with the formation of new tissue (fibroblasts) are seen in greater numbers 3 to 5 days following injury.

✓ An increase in fibroblasts corresponds with a decrease in macrophages.

✓ Begin to see capillary buds forming in the endothelial cells.

✓ Start to see the formation of granulation tissue (ie, reddish granular tissue that "fills the gap" of the injury).

✓ Fibroblast cells produce an extracellular matrix of collagen and elastin.

✓ Collagen and elastin cells are distributed in a haphazard arrangement.

✓ Unless reinjury occurs, the repair phase can last up to 21 days.

Common therapeutic interventions during the repair phase include insuring that active inflammation is controlled as therapeutic choices may progress to the use of heat modalities. The cautious use of controlled and protected motion and functional movements are often during this phase as protecting fragile tissue is of importance.

Remodeling Phase of Healing

New and fragile collagen and elastin form a matrix of scar tissue. The formation of scar tissue is known as fibroplasia. This fragile tissue will begin to change and become stronger and more organized. At a cellular level, the term *remodeling* is most accurate in describing this phase of healing. During this phase, collagen fibers transition as some types of collagen are broken down and while new stronger tissue takes its place. Identifiers of the remodeling phase of healing include the following:

✓ Realignment and remodeling of tissue

✓ Increased organization and strength of the new tissue

✓ Scar contraction takes place as new tissue is laid down and organized

Several therapeutic interventions are designed to help this tissue align and become organized based on the stresses placed upon it. Functional movements, ROM exercises, and gradual weight bearing are just some examples of the influence of therapeutic exercise on this process.

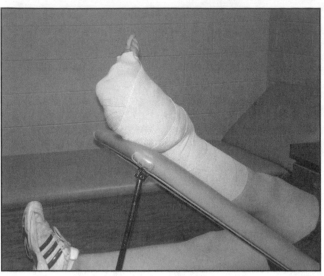

Figure 13-2. ICE. Ice, compression, and elevation are key elements in the treatment of acute injury.

IMMEDIATE CARE AND MANAGEMENT OF ATHLETIC INJURIES

The prospective athletic training student should have a basic understanding of the principles of immediate care of athletic injuries. The initial care following injury is designed to help combat swelling. Swelling is the common denominator for most acute injuries. Bleeding, synovial fluid, and the by-products of inflammation can all cause swelling. Swelling is detrimental to the healing process in a number of ways. Swelling can cause limitations in motion, inhibit the healing of tissues, and the increased pressure stimulates pain receptors. The PRICE concept is essential in the fight against swelling (Figure 13-2).

PRICE

(P) Protection

Appropriate splints, braces, slings, or immobilization devices should be used to protect the body part from further injury. Crutches may be used for ambulation to avoid the stress of weight bearing.

What Every Athlete Should Know About Over-The-Counter Pain Medications

As more people participate in sports and exercise, the number of people who sustain injuries associated with these activities also increases. People who injure themselves often use over-the-counter nonsteroidal anti-inflammatory drugs (OTC-NSAID) like Bufferin (Bristol-Myers Squibb, New York, NY) or Advil (Wyeth Consumer Healthcare, Richmond, VA) as part of their initial care following injury. Because these medications are available without being prescribed by a health care provider, many people do not know the appropriate use of these medications.

How OTC-NSAIDs work

When a person sustains an injury such as a sprained ankle or muscle strain, his or her body's inflammatory process begins immediately. Inflammation is the body's way of limiting the amount of tissue damage and protecting the body against further injury. The signs and symptoms of inflammation include swelling, redness, localized warmth, and pain. At the cellular level, there is an abundance of physiologic responses occurring, including vasodilatation of tissues and increased swelling. The enzymes that trigger these physiologic effects are called Cox-1 and Cox-2. NSAIDs such as Advil and ibuprofen have an anti-inflammatory effect by inhibiting these enzymes. NSAID also can reduce pain and fever.

OTC pain relievers that are not NSAID, such as acetaminophen (Tylenol, Johnson & Johnson, New Brunswick, NJ), are also commonly used to treat acute injuries. Tylenol has an analgesic effect (pain relief) and reduces fever but does not have anti-inflammatory functions.

When to Use OTC-NSAID

OTC-NSAID can be used to treat both acute and chronic injuries. There are 2 main reasons to use OTC-NSAID in the treatment of athletic injuries: to decrease excessive inflammation that can prolong the rate of healing and to decrease pain associated with the inflammation that allows for earlier rehabilitation. OTC-NSAID have been used to treat and decrease pain, inflammation, tenderness, and stiffness, which may lead to an earlier return to activity. Recent studies have shown that OTC-NSAID may promote short-term muscle healing and function, but no long-term benefits have been demonstrated. The OTC-NSAID alone will not accelerate the restoration of function and return to activity; rather, it may allow for a more comfortable and effective rehabilitation program.

Over-the-Counter Nonsteroidal Anti-Inflammatory Drugs

Active Drug	Common Trade Name
Acetylsalicylic acid	Aspirin, Ascriptin (Novartis AG, Basel, Switzerland), Bufferin, Excedrin (Novartis AG)
Ibuprofen	Motrin (Ortho-McNeill Pharmaceuticals, Titusville, NJ), Advil, Nuprin (Bristol-Myers Squibb))
Ketoprofen	Orudis KT (Wyeth Consumer Healthcare), Actron (Bayer HealthCare, Leverkusen, Germany)
Magnesium salicylate	Doan's Analgesic (Novartis AG)
Naproxen sodium	Aleve (Bayer HealthCare)

Contraindications and Possible Side Effects

Numerous studies have shown that OTC-NSAID decrease inflammation that may ultimately decrease pain. Is this truly beneficial? Does the use of anti-inflammatory medications actually have a negative effect on the inflammatory process and delay healing and return to sports? These questions are debatable. There is some evidence that has shown that while OTC-NSAID may speed recovery after acute soft tissue injuries, long-term healing may be compromised. This still remains a controversial issue.

There are numerous side effects that should be considered when taking OTC-NSAID. OTC-NSAID can increase bleeding in certain situations. For example, many athletes take an Advil or ibuprofen prior to activity. If an athlete would sustain an injury during activity and had taken an OTC-NSAID before that activity, he or she may be at risk for further injury. OTC-NSAID inhibits platelet aggregation, increasing the risk of bleeding. If an athlete strains a muscle, he or she can be at risk for increased bleeding within the injured tissues. If an athlete sustains a head injury, he or she may be at risk for a subdural hematoma (bleeding in the brain), which is a medical emergency. (continued)

What Every Athlete Should Know About Over-The-Counter Pain Medications (continued)

OTC-NSAIDs, like other common medications, are not free from side effects. The most common side effects associated with OTC-NSAID include stomach problems such as nausea, ulcers, and gastrointestinal bleeding. These side effects are mostly seen in long-term OTC-NSAID use. One way to help decrease the risk of these problems is to eat food when ingesting the OTC-NSAID.

Recommendations

These recommendations are not meant to replace the guidance of a physician or other medical professional. Consult a physician or other medical professional prior to taking any medication.

First, to be beneficial, OTC-NSAIDs should be taken on a consistent basis. Regular consumption of these medications is necessary for the active ingredients to take effect and suppress pain, fever, and inflammation. Taking medications in doses that are too low or not consuming them often enough will allow the dosage to dissipate quickly and not achieve maximum potential. Conversely, consuming medications in large doses or too often causes toxic levels of medication to build within the body, increasing the possibility for internal damage to the body.

By taking the medication according to the directions on the container, pain relief, fever reduction, and anti-inflammatory effects occur with low risk of reaching toxic levels. It is recommended that OTC-NSAIDs not be consumed for more than 14 days so that the progress of the healing may be checked under "normal" conditions.

Second, OTC-NSAIDs should be used in conjunction with an appropriate rehabilitation program. These medications should only be used as an aid to correcting an underlying problem. For example, a cross-country runner who repeatedly sustains "shin splints" and only takes these medications to help with the pain and/or inflammation will continue to have recurrent problems until the biomechanical dysfunction or training errors are corrected. Fallen arches, weak musculature, inappropriate or inadequate shoes, sudden increases in miles run, and changes in running surfaces are all possible underlying problems that may contribute to the instigation of the "shin splints" but are not solved by simply consuming any of these medications.

Third, the possibility of adverse effects associated with these medications should be weighed against the possible benefits. As mentioned earlier, OTC-NSAIDs, especially aspirin, can prevent clotting of blood. There can be a danger of fresh injuries that are treated immediately with OTC-NSAIDs to have blood pooling greater than injuries not initially treated with OTC-NSAIDs.

Similarly, there is evidence that use of OTC-NSAIDs during early rehabilitation has short-term beneficial effects but, as studies have begun to show, there are often either no long-term benefits or the long-term healing is hindered with the use of early OTC-NSAIDs.

Finally, OTC pain medications should NOT be utilized without the guidance of a physician under the following conditions:

- You have had previous stomach problems (dyspepsia, gastrointestinal bleeding, ulcers)
- You are taking anticoagulant medications
- You have had previous kidney dysfunction
- You have suffered previous liver damage
- You have sustained a recent head injury
- You are taking any other medications
- You have sustained a new injury
- You are aspirin sensitive
- You are dehydrated

Any questions or concerns about the use or the effects of these medications should be directed to a physician, pharmacist, athletic trainer, physical therapist, or other qualified medical personnel.

Bibliography

McKinley J, Nissenbaum D. UW Health Sports Link Sports Updates Information Series. Over-The-Counter Pain Medications. Patient Education Handout. 2007.

Table 13-1

Physiologic Effects of Heat and Cold

Physiologic Effects	Heat	Cold
Pain	Decrease	Decrease
Spasm	Decrease	Decrease
Edema	Increase	Decrease
Metabolic activity	Increase	Decrease
Capillary blood flow	Increase	Decrease
Collagen extensibility	Increase	Decrease

(R) Rest

Rest applies to the injured body part. Athletic trainers will employ the concept of active rest. Active rest allows for rest of the injured part while continuing to work other body parts and maintain cardiovascular fitness.

(I) Ice

The use of ice for acute injuries is widely supported. It is commonly used to provide pain relief, decrease the metabolic activity at the injured site, and promote local vasoconstriction. Studies suggest that ice has a greater impact on pain relief than swelling.

(C) Compression

Compression can have a tremendous impact on decreasing swelling. The purpose of compression is to reduce the space available for swelling by applying pressure to the injured area. This can be accomplished with elastic wraps, foam pads, and specific therapeutic devices. Elastic wraps must be applied with even pressure. Patients should use caution when sleeping to loosen wraps that can become constrictive.

(E) Elevation

Gravity will cause edema to pool in our extremities. To combat swelling following an injury, the extremity should be elevated to assist with lymphatic drainage and venous blood flow. Gentle muscle contraction can also assist with venous return. The extremity should be elevated well above the level of the heart.

Note: Ice, compression, and elevation are best used in combination to maximize the benefit. Any patient with a history of circulatory insufficiency, decreased sensation at the injured site, open wounds, or a history of allergic reactions to cold should not use cold treatment.

As part of a comprehensive athletic training education program, athletic training students will take courses in the use of therapeutic modalities. A modality is a method of therapy, or an apparatus used for therapy, that is designed to elicit a desired physiologic response. Students will learn the common physiologic responses, clinical conditions to which specific modalities can be applied, as well as the actual clinical skills needed to apply them. The physiology is the key. The athletic trainer must know the underlying physiology associated with injury and the desired physiologic responses of the modality. The application of ice, compression, and elevation is performed with knowledge of the desired physiologic responses. Table 13-1 compares the physiologic effects of ice and heat. The decision when to apply heat to an injury is often a conundrum for the average person. However, the athletic trainer is aware of the physiology of injury and the physiologic effects of hot and cold. Therefore, the decision must be made based on the status of the injury and the desired outcome. Apply heat too soon and the increase in blood flow could lead to greater amounts of swelling. However, once the swelling has subsided, heat may be beneficial to improving the ROM and bringing nutrients to the injured site. A variety of thermal, electrical, and mechanical modalities can be used in the care of athletic injuries. Students pursuing a degree in athletic training will be required to take coursework and demonstrate proficiency in the use of such modalities.

INJURIES TO BONES AND JOINTS

Intervening with appropriate first aid for bone and joint injuries is a common practice for athletic trainers. In 2007, it was estimated that over 10,000 lower leg fractures were treated at hospitals and emergency rooms for teenagers participating in sport and recreation, and over 34,000 knee sprain or strain injuries were estimated for this same time period.[6] While acute bone trauma is not as common as ligamentous injuries, the need to properly recognize bone trauma and provide appropriate prehospital care for bone injuries is an essential first-aid skill. Familiarity with splinting materials and techniques will allow for quick decision making when confronted with potential fracture.

THE BASICS OF SPLINTING

The use of splints is likely one of the oldest injury interventions on record. Tree limbs and branches have been used for centuries to temporarily support injuries to bone. While modern materials have allowed us to eliminate such primitive techniques, the

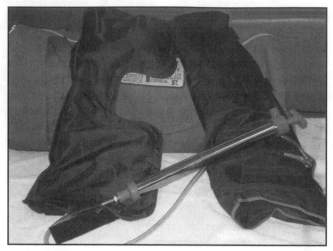

Figure 13-3. Vacuum splints should be kept at either courtside or on the sideline for easy access in the event of an injury.

principle remains the same: provide rigid support above and below an injured bone.[9] A variety of splints are available to athletic trainers. Rigid, padded, flexible, and vacuum splints are common pieces of emergency equipment that should be readily available for the athletic trainers who may encounter acute bone trauma (Figure 13-3). Padded and rigid splints made of foam or cardboard are commonly used for upper and lower extremity fractures. Additionally, there are types of rigid splints, such as ladder splints and SAM splints (SAM Medical Products, Houston, TX), that can be bent to better conform to the shape of the affected extremity.

Vacuum splints are essentially large air bladders filled with semirigid material that becomes rigid when the air is "vacuumed" out after the splint is wrapped around the affected extremity. Vacuum splints are effective, relatively easy to use, and quick to apply. Traction splints for the femur and pneumatic garments to stabilize the pelvis are commonly used by most EMS and paramedical emergency response professionals. Athletic trainers facing such injuries may be better served to call for EMS support and transport when fractures to the femur and pelvis are suspected.

The basic principles of splinting are as follows[1,9]:
- ✓ Splint only if you have to move the injured person and can do so without causing further injury and pain.
- ✓ Splint the injury in the position you find it. Do not move, straighten, or bend the injured part in a prehospital setting.
- ✓ Splint the injured area and the joints or bones both above and below the site of injury.

- ✓ Always check for proper circulation (pulse, sensation, warmth, and capillary refill) before and after applying the splint.
- ✓ If possible, remove any clothing that may impede the splint's working properly.
- ✓ If there are open wounds or exposed bone, bandage appropriately.

Some specific splinting guidelines include the following[9]:
- ✓ Fractures of the humerus and radius/ulna
  - ○ After assessing motor function and alignment, splint the arm under or along the fractured area.
  - ○ For a fractured humerus, the splint should rest at the upper arm and span the length between the shoulder and elbow.
  - ○ For a fracture to the radius and/or ulna, the splint should rest under or along the forearm and span the length between the elbow and wrist.
  - ○ Secure above and below the fracture.
  - ○ Use triangular bandages to make a sling (supporting the shoulder and arm) and swathe (holding the arm against the chest) to immobilize the limb.
  - ○ Reassess motor function after applying the splint.
  - ○ A roll of gauze should be placed in the hand of the affected arm to limit movement of the fingers and wrist.
- ✓ Tibia/fibula fractures
  - ○ Lower leg fractures are immobilized without traction splints.
  - ○ After assessing motor function and alignment, place a long splint under or along the side of the affected leg.
  - ○ Immobilize above and below the fracture and secure the foot in the position of function.
- ✓ Vacuum splints (see Figure 13-3)
  - ○ When using vacuum splints, place the injured extremity inside the splint.
  - ○ The pump is used to draw air out of the splint, which compresses it, making it rigid.
  - ○ The splint will conform to the patient and reduces pressure on the area.
  - ○ When using vacuum splints, make sure to keep the patient's fingers and/or toes exposed to assess motor function.
  - ○ Vacuum splints must be checked periodically during transport to ensure there are no leaks. Leaks in the splint diminish its rigidity and effectiveness.

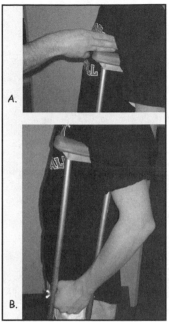

Figure 13-4. (A) Proper spacing between the axilla and crutch pad and (B) an appropriate angle at the elbow are important considerations in proper crutch fitting.

crutches provide support to swing the unaffected extremity through. Caution should be used to avoid placing pressure on the axilla and to instead use the hand grips to control crutch placement and movement. Light toe touching or partial weight bearing follows a similar process as the injured leg and crutches are put forward together to allow for partial weight bearing. Four-point walking is a technique often used for gait training. It involves starting with the feet together and moving one crutch forward followed by the one step forward with the opposite foot. This process is repeated with the opposite crutch and foot.

Crutch Fitting

Visit the Web site for video of proper crutch fitting and examples of the assisted ambulation gaits described above.

CRUTCH FITTING

In several instances, athletes may need to use crutches to assist with ambulation. The athletic trainer must be able to provide a proper fit and instruct the patient on crutch use. Crutches are commonly used for nonweight bearing, partial weight bearing, and gait training for patients with lower extremity injuries. It is imperative that crutches are fit properly to allow for safe and effective use. The following guidelines should be followed to insure proper fit (Figure 13-4):

✓ The athlete should wear shoes similar to those he or she will use with the crutches.

✓ The shoulders should be relaxed and level with the head held in an upright position.

✓ Crutch tips should be placed approximately 6 inches lateral and 2 inches anterior from the anteriolateral aspect of the shoe.

✓ Crutch length should be adjusted to allow 2 to 3 finger-breadths between the crutch and the axillary fold.

✓ Hand grips should be adjusted to allow 20 to 30 degrees of elbow flexion.

✓ The wrist should be held straight when adjusting the hand grip.

It is not enough to properly fit the patient with crutches; the athletic trainer must provide appropriate instruction for ambulation. Walking gaits with crutches will vary depending upon the goal of the crutch use. A swing gait for nonweight bearing is used when the injured extremity is held off the ground and the

Patients may be more comfortable or may progress to using only one crutch or a cane. When using one crutch or a cane, use the following guidelines:

✓ The top of the cane should fit to the level of the greater trochanter of the femur or to the ventral wrist fold with the arm resting at the side.

✓ The elbow should be in slight flexion during cane ambulation.

✓ The crutch/cane should be used on the side opposite the affected extremity. This allows for the weight to be distributed away from the injured body part (Figure 13-5).

Navigating stairs is a sometimes daunting task for patients using crutches. However, it can be made easier by remembering the simple phrase: "Good Guys Go Up and Bad Guys Go Down." This means that when going up stairs, you should place the unaffected extremity on the up step and then follow with the affected extremity and the support of the crutches. When going down the stairs, you place the affected extremity and the crutches down together and lower your unaffected extremity to the next step. Patients should be instructed to proceed slowly and use the handrail for additional assistance.

SUMMARY

The ability to provide initial care and proper first aid is a foundational athletic training skill that can be learned early in the athletic training curriculum. In addition to CPR and advanced rescue techniques, athletic training students should be competent in wound

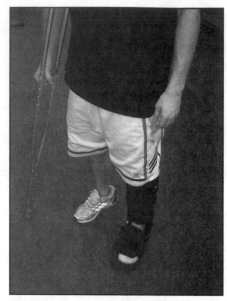

Figure 13-5. Patients who use one crutch often do so incorrectly. The single crutch should be placed on the opposite side of the injured extremity. This allows weight to be taken off the extremity during assisted ambulation.

recognition and care, treatment of acute inflammation (PRICE), recognizing and treating shock, proper splinting techniques, and fitting crutches to aid ambulation. All first-aid and initial care techniques are guided by the emergency action plans. Initial care is dictated by the ability to recognize and understand the underlying physiology of the inflammation and healing process. Understanding this process is the cornerstone to further study in treatment and rehabilitation of injuries and conditions.

REFERENCES

1. The American National Red Cross. *First Aid—Responding to Emergencies*. 4th ed. Stamford, CT: Staywell; 2006.
2. Foster DT, Rowedder LJ, Reese SK. Management of sports-induced skin wounds. *Journal of Athletic Training*. 1995;30:135-139.
3. Centers for Disease Control and Prevention. CDC summary: tetanus (lockjaw, *Clostridium tetani* infection). Available at www.cdc.gov/ncidod/diseases/submenus/sub_tetanus.htm Accessed July 25, 2008.
4. Luke A, d'Hemeourt P. Prevention of infections diseases in athletes. *Clin Sports Med*. 2007;26:321-344.
5. Prentice WE. *Arnhiem's Principles of Athletic Training*. 13th ed. New York: McGraw-Hill Higher Education; 2009.
6. Consumer Product Safety Commission National Electronic Injury Surveillance System. Available at www.cpsc.gov/LIBRARY/neiss.html. Accessed July 25, 2008.
7. Houglum, P. *Therapeutic Exercise for Musculoskeletal Injuries*. 2nd ed. Champaign, IL: Human Kinetics; 2005.
8. Starkey C. *Therapeutic Modalities*. 3rd ed. Philadelphia, PA: FA Davis Co; 2004.
9. Perkins TJ. Fracture management: effective prehospital splinting techniques. *Emerg Med Serv*. 2007;36(4):35-37, 39.

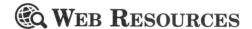 WEB RESOURCES

American Red Cross
www.redcross.org
A comprehensive Web site that covers the range of educational and disaster response programming carried out by the American Red Cross. Local chapter searches by zip code are available.

Centers for Disease Control and Prevention
www.cdc.gov
A comprehensive Web site that provides information on healthy living, environmental issues, diseases and conditions, traveler's health, workplace safety, and more.

Career Spotlight: Research Coordinator

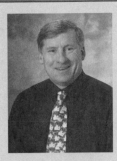

Tim McGuine, PhD, ATC

Research Coordinator

University of Wisconsin Health–Sports Medicine Center

Madison, Wisconsin

My Position

I am employed to coordinate the sports medicine research program for the University of Wisconsin–Health Sports Medicine Center. The research program has 2 distinct aspects. These include the clinical component and the sports medicine outreach (athletic training) component. The clinical research component includes research that is conducted in the sports medicine outpatient clinic. Research in the clinic includes studying methods to diagnose and treat specific injuries. The sports medicine outreach component involves field research conducted in middle and high schools as well as sports and recreational facilities. Typical research focuses on observational and analytic epidemiology as well as injury prevention trials.

My role is to work with a wide variety of staff from the UW Medical School, UW-Madison Campus, and UW Health Sports Medicine Center to facilitate sports medicine research. Specific duties include planning prospective research studies, assisting with grant writing and IRB submissions, coordinating data collection activities, and assisting with data analysis. I also administer a sports medicine research grant fund that distributes research funds to our staff.

Unique or Desired Qualifications

An athletic trainer who aspires to this role should possess a wide variety of work experiences. Knowing first hand what it is like to work with high school athletes and coaches as well as treating patients every day in an outreach clinic provides me with a unique viewpoint on what type of research needs to be done and how best to carry it out. In addition, the person should have a thorough understanding of a wide variety of research methodologies. Finally, this role requires an ability to work with individuals (medical professionals, academicians, and health care administrators) from various departments who may not fully appreciate the importance of conducting effective sports medicine research. This is a challenge that needs to be met and overcome on a daily basis.

Favorite Aspect of My Job

Quality sports medicine research (especially a study conducted in real-life athletic settings) is extremely difficult to carry out. Therefore, it is very rewarding to see the research process as it unfolds through typical steps that include beginning with an idea, progressing to a full-fledged research proposal, undergoing IRB scrutiny and approval, obtaining research funding, collecting and analyzing the data, and publishing the results in a peer-reviewed medical journal.

Advice

I would advise athletic training students who want to work in this type of position to embrace the notion that sports medicine is a dynamic field that requires a commitment to lifelong learning. I would also encourage these students to embrace the idea that preventing and treating injuries that occur in young athletes will improve the quality of life for these young athletes and help reduce health care expenditures in the United States.

CHAPTER 14

COMPONENTS
OF REHABILITATION

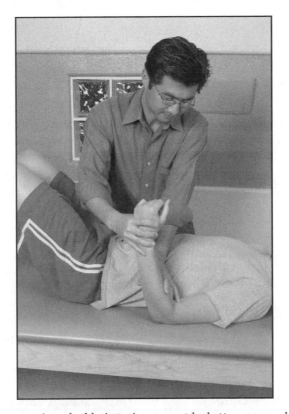

The next generation of athletic trainers must be better prepared to be versatile in the patient population that they treat. Be trained and comfortable with treating physically active people across the lifespan and demonstrate that we are the experts of that type of care for physically active people of all ages.

Marjorie Albohm, MS, ATC/L
President–National Athletic Trainers' Association

The skills possessed by an athletic trainer are utilized in many ways and some skills are utilized in many phases of the athletic trainer's daily duties. For example, the very same evaluation skills required for initial assessment and diagnosis of injuries are essential skills needed for the treatment and rehabilitation process. Prior to the initiation of a treatment program, the athletic trainer must determine the injury status (acute or chronic), affected structures, and the presence of any contraindications in order to determine the most appropriate treatment, rehabilitation, and reconditioning program for the patient. Rehabilitation of athletic injuries requires clinicians to possess skills that allow them to control pain, restore ROM to injured joints, restore muscle strength and endurance, and regain neuromuscular control and proper

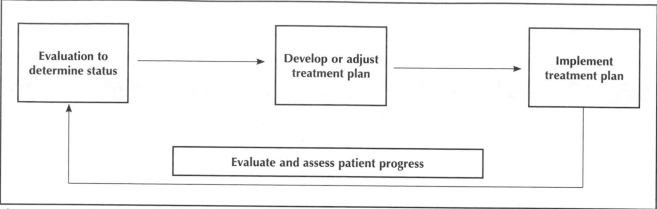

Figure 14-1. Feedback loop.

balance. In addition, the athletic trainer must have the ability to apply these skills in a progressive and functional fashion to assist the patient in returning to his or her desired level of activity as soon as is safely possible. Much like the use of therapeutic modalities, rehabilitation requires a keen awareness of the physiology of healing and the effect injury has on the function of joints and related structures. While an extensive discussion of rehabilitation and therapeutic exercise is beyond the scope of this text, an overview is warranted.

Upon the completion of this chapter, the student will be able to:

- ✓ Describe the feedback loop process in rehabilitation
- ✓ Discuss the components of a rehabilitation program
- ✓ Identify the types of resistance exercise
- ✓ Describe common tools and techniques utilized to achieve treatment goals in a rehabilitation program
- ✓ Explain the difference between closed and open kinetic chain exercises
- ✓ Discuss the importance of objective data in making return-to-activity decisions
- ✓ Explain the key components of a balance training program
- ✓ Describe the historical role the arthroscope has played with advancing sports medicine and its impact on rehabilitation

REHABILITATION: THE FEEDBACK LOOP PROCESS

Initiating a rehabilitation program involves planning. While health care professionals may use many of the same techniques and therapeutic exercises for treating similar conditions, each patient represents an individual case that must be treated appropriately. This includes the understanding that we need to consider the needs of the person before the injury. The old adage, "Treat the person, not the injury" is true. You are treating someone with an ACL injury, not treating an ACL injury. This is not a subtle difference. Early in their professional development, students can often find themselves relying on "cookbook" methods of rehabilitation. These should be avoided. While protocols and common treatments may serve as a guide, students will need to develop their evaluation skills to help set the stage for what the patient needs. Evaluation is the cornerstone of the feedback loop process. An example of a rehabilitation feedback loop is provided in Figure 14-1.

The feedback loop allows for adjustment and changes to the rehabilitation program. Knowing how to adjust, when to accelerate the program, and when to pull back is what differentiates the rehabilitation professional from someone "following a cookbook." The need for constant feedback and adjustment as the patient progresses to his or her goals is the essence of the feedback loop.

ESTABLISHING PATIENT GOALS

Rehabilitation programs can be divided into specific components. Each component can be considered a short-term goal such as regain strength, re-establish balance, etc. Long-term goals are "big picture" goals. These include return to preinjury health status, return to daily activity, return to training, return to practice, and return to competition. However, long-term goals may seem far away for the athlete just out of surgery who has swelling, pain, and limited motion in his

Table 14-1

Types of Resistance Exercise

Isometric	Resistance exercises held in a static position. Isometrics are often used in the early stages of a rehabilitation program to retard atrophy. Strength gains are limited to the angle of the performed exercise.
Isotonic	Exercises that provide resistance through a ROM while the muscles change length (shorten and lengthen). Manual resistance, bands and tubing, free weights, and weight machines all are commonly used for isotonic exercise. These exercises are the cornerstone of PRE and therapeutic exercise.
Isokinetic	Isokinetic exercises rely on controlling a fixed speed of contraction while varying resistance through the range of motion. Isokinetic devices often are used to assess strength at the later stages of a rehabilitation program. These devices are often connected to computer programs that allow for assessment of torque, power, and work.

or her ankle. To make the program manageable, it is necessary to divide it into specific objectives that are sequential steps. When each objective is met, the athlete can progress further in the rehabilitation program. This allows the athletic trainer to build progressions in such a way as to guide the patient toward recovery. It is essential that specific criteria be met before advancing in the program. Criteria for advancement may be as simple as eliminating swelling, having an active ROM measurement equal to the opposite limb, testing at 75% strength as compared to the opposite side, performing a functional running test without pain within a predetermined time—the possibilities are endless. Athletes are goal oriented and rehabilitation programs should be developed with this approach in mind.[1]

 Therapeutic Exercise

Most of us exercise for fitness. We do strength training, cardiovascular, maybe some yoga. We exercise for our physical and mental health—for our overall conditioning. When we exercise for the purpose of restoring the body to its normal function after an injury, it is called *therapeutic exercise*. Therapeutic exercise is the cornerstone of injury treatment and rehabilitation.

RANGE OF MOTION

The discussion of PRICE stresses the battle line that must be drawn against swelling. Swelling is a common cause of limitations in ROM. Other items that can affect ROM include pain, muscle weakness, or an intra-articular obstruction. There are a number of specific therapeutic exercises and rehabilitation skills that are used to assist with regaining ROM. Passive exercise, hands-on joint mobilization, soft tissue mobilization, and active motion exercise (stationary bike, pool exercises, etc) are just a few of the tools used to improve motion. At the heart of this rehabilitation component is the need for the athletic trainer to know exactly what is causing the limitation in ROM.

STRENGTH, ENDURANCE, AND POWER

When the term *therapeutic exercise* is used, most people tend to think about regaining strength. Strength is a measure of the muscle's ability to exert a maximal force against a resistance. *Therapeutic exercise* is an umbrella-type term that refers to any exercises used in a rehabilitation program. Several types of strength exercises can be used in a rehabilitation program. Isometric, isotonic, and isokinetic resistance can all play a role (Table 14-1). Strength exercises fall under the category of progressive resistance exercises (PRE). PRE rely on gradual increases in muscle demand in order to achieve a desired outcome. This is the SAID principle (specific adaptations to imposed demands). This principle states that tissues will respond to the demands placed upon them. To get stronger, muscles must adapt to increased loads. Following injury, this "load" may be just the force of gravity as the patient moves through a ROM. As the patient gets stronger, the athletic trainer may apply manual resistance (use his or her hands), the patient may then progress to weight equipment or some other strength device. The key is progression. PRE exercises allow patients to work through a full ROM and utilize both concentric (muscle shortening) and eccentric (muscle lengthening) contractions.

ℹ️ Did You Know?

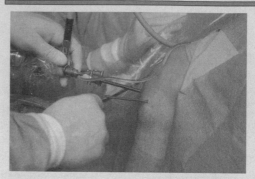

Arthroscopy

Pepper Burruss, PT, ATC, the long-time head athletic trainer for the Green Bay Packers of the NFL, frequently speaks to college students about the athletic training profession and specifically about being an athletic trainer in the NFL. One of his best talks is *Sports Medicine in the NFL A-Z*, a discussion of how sports medicine has changed during his time in the league. Right up front with the letter "A" is arthroscopy. Arthroscopic surgery may be the biggest innovation in orthopedic sports medicine in the past 30 years.

Arthroscopy is a minimally invasive surgical procedure. It has become so familiar that it is simply referred to as "getting scoped." The small (4 to 5 mm in diameter) tube-like instrument can be inserted into the patient's joint and, when fitted with fiber optic equipment, allows the surgeon to see the joint on a video monitor. Small arthroscopic tools can be inserted to allow for surgical procedures that are minimally invasive, cause less pain and less tissue damage, and yield shorter recovery periods. While arthroscopic procedures are best known in the knee and shoulder, they also can be performed on the wrist, elbow, hip, and ankle. Rehabilitation has been faster and less painful since the use of arthroscopy. The "scope" may have made an impact on sports medicine as a surgical tool in the past 30 years, but would you believe that the first arthroscopy was done over 90 years ago?

In 1918, Professor Kenji Takagi of Tokyo University performed the first arthroscopy of the human knee with a cytoscope on a cadaver. He was motivated by a desire to better understand the inside of the knee joint not for orthopedic reasons but to help tuberculosis patients. At the time, tuberculosis was causing many Japanese to suffer from "stiff knee." By 1936, he had developed a way to obtain color pictures and movie (pre-video) of the interior of the knee joint.

Dr. Eugene Bircher was the first to use the arthroscopy on live patients 1 year after Takagi's procedure. In 1922, he reported published results on his "arthroendoscopy" using a laparoscopic device. The next 2 decades saw many pioneers experimenting with this new technology. Skeptics were plentiful given many complications with poor technology and equipment. The onset of World War II brought development to a halt. It was not until the 1950s when Dr. Masaki Watanabe (a former student of Takagi) began to make several contributions to the field of arthroscopy.

Watanabe developed the first true arthroscope and performed the first recorded surgical procedure to remove tumor cells from the suprapatellar pouch. He also performed a partial meniscectomy (removal of the meniscus). In 1957, he published the first edition of the *Atlas of Arthroscopy*.

Further developments came at the University of Toronto in the 1970s. Drs. Jackson and Abe had studied Watanabe's techniques and started the *Journal of Bone and Joint Surgery*, which is now a widely respected journal in orthopedics. During the late 1980s, a move beyond just using the arthroscope for diagnostic purposes and the development of surgical techniques expanded widely thanks to improvements in technology. Articles in the literature during this time frame of developing procedures read as a who's who of modern orthopedic sports medicine. Many new surgical instruments and techniques were developed during this time period. Instruments that allowed for grasping tissue, smoothing surfaces, cutting and shaving, and aligning structures during ligament reconstruction all advanced as the use of the arthroscope increased.

Yes, in the A-Z talk, "A" definitely stands for arthroscope. Today, there are over 1.5 million arthroscopic procedures performed annually, and the technique has forever changed orthopedic surgery in sports medicine. Not bad for something someone tried nearly 100 years ago.

In addition to regaining strength, it is important to address the components of endurance as well as power. Muscular endurance refers to the muscle's ability to perform over a period of time without fatigue. Resistance exercises that are performed using lower resistance and increased time or repetition help build endurance. Power refers to the amount of work performed over a period of time. Athletes who are powerful tend to be explosive and can generate large amounts of force in a short period of time. A comprehensive rehabilitation program should address all 3 components (strength, endurance, and power) to best prepare the patient for functional activities and to return to a preinjury status.

Closed and Open Kinetic Chain Exercises

The parts of the body can be viewed as a series of segments joined together like links in a chain. The links connect and move at the various articulations. This is easily visualized when you stop and think of the parts that make up your upper and lower extremity. The concept of an open or closed kinetic chain exercise is defined by what is happening at the distal segment of the chain. For example, in a squat or leg press-style exercise, the foot is the distal segment and is fixed on the ground or press plate to form a closed kinetic chain. If you sat in a chair and performed a knee extension exercise, the distal segment would move freely through space and form an open kinetic chain.

The choice of using closed versus open kinetic chain exercises in rehabilitation has received attention in recent years. Exercising with a closed kinetic chain exercise requires the use of multiple joints. For example, the squat exercise impacts the ankle, knee, hip, and trunk in the kinetic chain. The ability to create co-contractions of supporting muscle groups and to decrease shear forces at a joint are thought to be a benefit of the closed kinetic chain exercise. Closed kinetic chain exercises are not exclusive to the lower extremity. It is common to use therapeutic closed chain exercises in the upper extremity to assist with joint stability by stimulating co-contractions (eg, a push-up position). Open chain exercises such as throwing and kicking can generate high velocities at a joint but lower overall forces. When segments work in an open chain, they are nonweight bearing.

It is essential for athletic trainers in rehabilitative settings to select therapeutic exercises that best approximate the actual demands of the patient's activities. This will likely include both open and closed kinetic chain exercises. However, the selection of which exercises, when to apply them, and at what quantity is dependent upon many therapeutic decisions. The skilled athletic trainer will have to take into account many factors, including the goals of the program, stages of tissue healing, and the functional demands when selecting a therapeutic exercise.

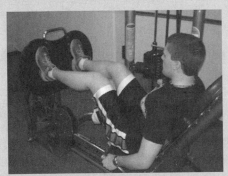

Closed Kinetic Chain Leg Press Exercise

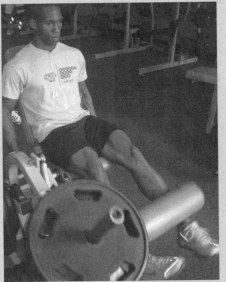

Open Kinetic Chain Leg Extension Exercise

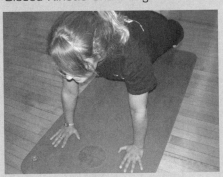

Closed Kinetic Chain Upper Extremity Exercise

NEUROMUSCULAR CONTROL AND BALANCE

Our CNS is constantly taking in information from peripheral mechanoreceptors located in our joints, tendons, ligaments, and muscles. These receptors send information to the CNS that then responds by initiating specific motor responses. Signals sent from the peripheral receptors to the CNS travel what are called afferent pathways. The motor response from the CNS to the muscles travels an efferent pathway. This relationship between the nervous system and the muscular responses that allow for coordinated

Core Stability

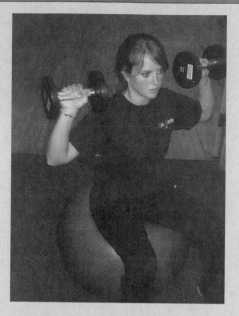

The *core* is a common term used to describe the "trunk" of the body. The trunk includes all of the body except the head, neck, and extremities. Trunk muscles help provide stability for dynamic movement of our core and also provide a stable platform for movement at the extremities. Good core stability allows the trunk and spinal segments to move while under some dynamic protection (dynamic stability) and allows for good postural positioning (static stability).

Improvements in core stability have been associated with improved sports performance and are widely used in rehabilitation and injury prevention programs. Beyond just core strength, core endurance seems to be associated with injury protection as well, specifically in the protective nature associated with lumbar spine injury. Bridging programs, unstable surfaces, Swiss balls, and foam rolls are commonly used to promote core stability. In addition, it is not uncommon to manipulate traditional strength exercises to specifically address core stability (eg, dumb bell exercises while seated on a Swiss ball, squat style movements on a balance board surface).

As always, the athletic trainer designing and implementing a therapeutic rehabilitation program will need a clear understanding of the stages of tissue healing, desired program outcomes, and the functional demands the patient will face when designing and prescribing therapeutic exercise. Addressing the core stability is one key component of such a program. Theories and practices in therapeutic exercise are constantly changing. This is an area for CE long after the certification process.

movement is called *neuromuscular control*.[1] Proprioception is the ability to determine the position of a joint or limb in space. If patients are injured or immobilized for extended periods of time, they will have proprioceptive deficits and demonstrate a decline in neuromuscular control.[1] If not addressed, these neuromuscular deficiencies can lead to reinjury. Specific exercises that stimulate the mechanoreceptors and cause desired neuromuscular responses are an essential component to the rehabilitation program. The use of balance boards for both upper and lower extremity exercises are the most common; however, a wide range of creative exercises are used to help enhance afferent stimulation and efferent response. For simplicity, these exercises are often called "proprioceptive exercises;" however, they encompass much more than that and are aimed at the entire neuromuscular picture.

Balance is a complex process that involves the integration of muscular forces, neurological sensory information from mechanoreceptors, and biomechanical information.[2] Balance is the ability to maintain our center of gravity (COG) over a base of support. The range we can move our COG and maintain balance is called our limits of stability (LOS).[2] When we move our COG outside of our LOS, we must initiate a balance strategy to avoid falling. These strategies include adjusting joint position at the hip, knee, and ankle or stepping to prevent a fall.[2]

The control of balance involves the organization of sensory information gathered from afferent receptors, vision, and vestibular (inner ear) input. The ability to maintain balance in a variety of positions and changes to our base of support (one leg or two legs) is a common need in athletic endeavors. In addition, changes to the surfaces that provide support can also affect balance. Athletic events often occur in environments where the surfaces are inconsistent or uneven, thus the need to emphasize neuromuscular control and specifically balance in the entire rehabilitation program. Exercises that require adjustments to sensory input, changes in surface, and incorporate moving the COG to various positions can help train different components of postural control system.

FUNCTIONAL PROGRESSION AND FUNCTIONAL TESTING

Function is currently one of the more bandied-about terms in rehabilitation. *Return to function, functional exercise, functional rehabilitation,* and *functional training* are all common terms that may hold different meaning to whoever is using them. However, at the center of this discussion is a desire to utilize rehabilitation techniques and outcome measures that are

Balance Training Program

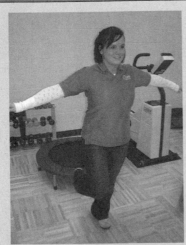

Ankle sprains are the most common musculoskeletal injuries that occur in athletes. Sports that require sudden stops and cutting movements such as basketball and soccer cause the highest percentage of these injuries.

A recent study[1] conducted by UW Health Sports Medicine researchers found that a balance training program implemented in the preseason and maintained throughout the season reduced the risk of ankle sprains in male and female high school soccer and basketball players by 40%.

The Balance Training Program to Reduce Risk of Ankle Injuries

Phase	Surface	Eyes	Exercise (each performed for 3 to 5 repetitions)
I Week 1	Floor	Open	Single leg stance
		Open	Single leg stance, while swinging the raised leg
		Open	Single leg squat (knee flexed 30 to 45 degrees)
		Open	Single leg stance while performing functional activities (dribbling, catching, kicking)
II Week 2	Floor	Closed	Single leg stance
		Closed	Single leg stance, while swinging the raised leg
		Closed	Single leg squat (knee flexed 30 to 45 degrees)
III Week 3	Wobble board	Open	Single leg stance
		Open	Single leg stance, while swinging the raised leg
		Open	Single leg squat (knee flexed 30 to 45 degrees)
		Open	Double leg stance while rotating the board
IV Week 4	Wobble board	Closed	Single leg stance
		Open	Single leg stance, while swinging the raised leg
		Open	Single leg squat (knee flexed 30 to 45 degrees)
		Open	Single leg stance while rotating the board clockwise and counterclockwise
V Week 5+	Wobble board	Closed	Single leg stance
		Open	Single leg squat (knee flexed 30 to 45 degrees)
		Open	Single leg stance while rotating the board clockwise and counterclockwise
		Open	Single leg stance while performing functional activities (dribbling, catching, kicking)

Note: Phases I to IV are performed 5 days per week. Phase V is performed 3 days per week for the rest of the season. Each exercise is performed 30 seconds per leg. Athletes should alternate legs to allow a rest period of 30 seconds between repetitions.

Reference

1. McGuine TA, Keene JS. The effect of a balance training program on the risk of ankle sprains in high school athletes. *Am J Sports Med.* 2006;34(7):1103-1111.

Treatment Options for a Torn ACL

The athletic trainer with responsibilities for rehabilitation of postoperative patients will need to be familiar with the repair techniques utilized by orthopedic surgeons to correct injuries like a tear to the ACL. A big part of understanding the rehabilitation needs will begin with understanding the surgical repair.

Surgery is not always indicated for, nor desired by everyone who tears his or her ACL. In some cases, it is possible to do well by following a rehabilitation program and avoiding activities that require cutting and/or pivoting movements.

If surgery is chosen, it is recommended that the patient undergo a preoperative therapeutic exercise program to regain normal knee ROM, decrease pain and swelling, and strengthen the musculature around the knee. This may last 3 to 6 weeks but will allow the postoperative course to progress faster.

Surgical reconstruction involves replacing the torn ACL with a graft. The 2 most common grafts used are the patellar tendon graft and the hamstring tendon graft.

The patellar tendon graft is usually taken from the knee that has the torn ACL. In this procedure, the central third of the patellar tendon is removed along with a bone plug at each end of the tendon. One bone plug is taken from the patella and the other is harvested from the tibia. Tunnels are drilled in the femur and the tibia near the normal attachment sites for the ACL.

The patellar tendon graft is then threaded through the tunnels so that it is placed where the original ACL was located. The bone plugs of the graft are then anchored with screws into the femur and tibia. Because of its strength, the patellar tendon graft is often recommended for patients who will be returning to high-demand sports such as football or basketball.

The disadvantage of the patellar tendon graft is that patients occasionally have problems with anterior knee pain or patellar tendonitis because of the location from which the tendon graft was taken. The hamstring graft is a preferred graft choice for patients who will be required to kneel frequently after surgery (eg, a carpenter).

Removing the central third of the patellar tendon often causes more immediate postoperative stiffness than using a hamstring graft. This may require more initial work with ROM exercises.

The hamstring tendon graft is also usually taken from the knee that has the torn ACL. A strip of tendon is taken from 2 muscles, the semitendinosus and gracilis. These 2 muscles are located on the back of the knee on the inner (medial) side. The 2 tendons are then put together to make one graft. This graft does not have attached bone, although bone may be added to it. Tunnels are drilled in the femur and the tibia near the normal attachment sites for the ACL. The hamstring graft is then threaded through the tunnels so that it is placed in the location of the original ACL. The graft is anchored in the tibia and femur with either screws or buttons. The advantage of the hamstring graft procedure is that there is usually less postoperative pain and tendonitis. The hamstring graft procedure is often recommended for patients who will be returning to an active lifestyle, but participation in high-demand sports such as soccer or basketball is less frequent.

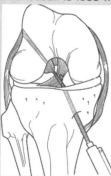

One bone plug is harvested from the patella and the other is harvested from the tibia.

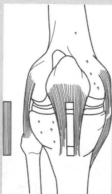

Tunnels are drilled in the femur and the tibia near the normal attachment sites for the ACL.

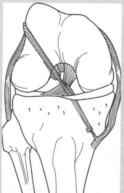

The patellar tendon graft is then threaded through the tunnels so that it is placed where the original ACL was located. The bone plugs of the graft are then anchored with screws into the femur and tibia.

Adapted with permission of UW Health, Madison, WI. from Rehabilitation Guide. Anterior Cruciate Ligament Reconstruction.

representative of the actual demands that an active individual will face. A rehabilitation program for a physically active patient should incorporate sports-specific functional training and activities. To this direction, the functional progression is an effective component of a rehabilitation program. A functional progression is a succession of activities that simulate actual motor and sport skills, enabling the athlete to acquire or reacquire the skills needed to perform athletic endeavors safely and effectively.[3] A functional progression for a basketball player with an ankle injury might include riding a bike, walking in a pool, walking on dry land, jogging straight ahead, starting and stopping on the court, starting and stopping while dribbling the ball, getting in a defensive position and moving side to side, jumping to mimic shooting and rebounding, actual shooting and rebounding, progression to full speed drills, progression to actual parts of the practice, to full participation. Sports-specific components make up parts of the progression. This method is only one part of a comprehensive rehabilitation approach and should enhance not replace the items listed above.

A second consideration under the general heading of function is functional testing. Functional testing and measures of rehabilitation outcomes are used to determine if a patient can progress in his or her rehabilitation program or to determine his or her readiness to return to competition. Functional testing should operate under the guiding principle of specificity of training, meaning that the measure or test should be reflective of the methods used for physical training as well as demands that will be placed on the patient in his or her chosen endeavor.

CARDIOVASCULAR FITNESS

No rehabilitation program is complete without attention to cardiovascular fitness. Athletes who are unable to practice and compete due to injury will lose cardiovascular fitness rapidly due to inactivity. It is essential that alternative methods of aerobic exercise be introduced into the rehabilitation protocol as soon as possible. Stationary bikes, upper body ergometers, and pool exercises are all viable options to address this need. Early initiation of fitness activities may also help to motivate the athlete and assist with compliance to the treatment protocol. However, the athletic trainer must be creative and find ways to eliminate the monotony associated with some of these activities.

RETURN TO ACTIVITY

The final component to consider in the rehabilitation program is the decision to return the patient to activity. The decision to release a patient from your care must be done in consultation with the physician

 Wii Therapy: Fad or the Future?

Virtual activities as a rehabilitation tool? The Nintendo Wii (Nintendo Company Ltd, Redmond, WA) was originally a popular holiday item that stores could not keep in stock. The video game requires movement from the players using a hand-held device. They can control virtual tennis racquets and try to bowl a strike on the flat-screen alley or many other sport choices. The fact that it requires some movement beyond just a quick thumb has some rehabilitation specialists reaching for the video game as a therapeutic tool.

Multiple stories have appeared in the popular press discussing the value of the Wii for hand-eye coordination and its use in assisting patients who have had strokes or suffer from Parkinson's disease. Not surprisingly, it has been helpful with increasing rehabilitation compliance and creating a positive sense of accomplishment for patients who struggle with what they cannot do.

The Wii therapy can be useful in fine and gross motor skills, strength, stability, coordination, and weight bearing. It may also be helpful with problem solving, memory, and decision making. Some speculate that in the near future virtual games in concert with biomechanical movement analysis will be common place in the sports conditioning and rehabilitation environments. Until that day, Wii therapy is improving the public perception of video games thanks to creative therapists and athletic trainers who are looking to find new ways to challenge patients.

No word yet on whether you can convince your insurance company to buy you one!

guiding the rehabilitation program. The physician will want to see information from functional progressions and functional tests. The athletic trainer must oversee criteria for return to activity. These criteria will contain specific physical parameters such as full pain-free ROM, strength comparable to the opposite extremity as measured in an objective fashion, and the result of a functional physical test. Developing valid and reliable functional tests that can be used for upper and lower extremity injuries is currently an active area of research in sports medicine.

TOOLS AND TECHNIQUES USED IN REHABILITATION

To achieve the desired outcomes in a rehabilitation program, the athletic trainer will use a variety of techniques to address the physical limitations or functional short comings presented by the patient. In the course of any injury or postoperative treatment, a rehabilitation specialist may rely on any number of exercises to restore and enhance motion, strength, neuromuscular function, and activity-specific movement. While any good athletic training education program will provide students with a foundation of skills to use in the rehabilitation domain, continuing professional education will be essential to stay abreast of the latest trends in rehabilitation. The informed practitioner wants as many "tools" as possible in his or her "therapeutic tool box." Over reliance on any one therapeutic approach may create a narrow focus and not address the whole scope of a patient's problem.

The techniques outlined below are representative of a variety of therapeutic tools available to the practicing athletic trainer. It is beyond the scope of this text to provide instruction in these techniques. However, learning the basic purpose and common uses is a good first step in establishing a strong foundation for future study in this area.

- ✓ Aquatic exercise—The use of water as a therapeutic tool goes back to the earliest of times. The unique environment of water allows for the manipulation of buoyancy and hydrostatic pressure to aid in ROM, strength, power, and functional movement patterns.[4] Water exercise can be initiated early in the rehabilitation process since the buoyancy can alleviate some of the stress normally found with dry land exercises. An assortment of flotation devices is available to assist with water rehabilitation.

- ✓ Gait analysis—Observation of a patient's gait pattern is a common practice. In rehabilitative settings, it can be useful to record walking (or running) gait in order to identify underlying causes of injuries and conditions.

- ✓ Joint mobilization—Mobilization of the joint involves hands-on techniques used to improve joint mobility or to decrease joint pain by restoring accessory motions. When joints move, the joint surfaces move across one another based on the shape of the moving bone. Gliding and rolling movements take place at the joint surfaces. If these movements are limited, overall joint function will not be achieved. Mobilization techniques are used to reduce pain, improve motion, and loosen capsular structures. Some joint mobilization techniques are quite simple while others will require some CE. The movements are applied with low force in a rhythmic fashion called *oscillations* while isolating the joint and stabilizing surrounding structures.

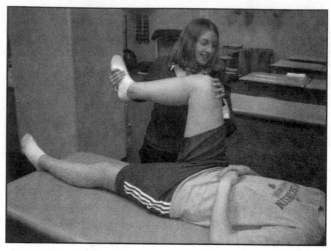

Figure 14-2. Muscle energy techniques can be used to address functional leg length discrepancies from a rotated innominate bone.

- ✓ Muscle energy—Muscle energy techniques are used to treat joint malalignments. Muscle energy techniques rely on specific and controlled voluntary contraction of a muscle against a counter-force provided by the practitioner followed by a passive stretch.[5] Malalignment may be caused by muscle spasm, a weak muscle overpowered by a stronger muscle, or restrictions in mobility. Muscle energy techniques are frequently used for the sacroiliac region to treat rotations (anterior or posterior) of the innominate (Figure 14-2).

- ✓ Neural mobilization—Neural mobilization is a manual therapy technique that stretches neural and connective tissue structures to affect neural symptoms, restore tissue balance, and improve function. Neural mobilization should be used with extreme care due to potential irritation of nerve tissues and should only be performed by a trained practitioner.

- ✓ Plyometrics—Plyometrics are performed by lengthening a muscle followed by a sudden shortening to increase power. Plyometrics can be performed using medicine balls in the upper extremity and they are commonly used in the lower extremity using boxes for landing and explosive jumping exercises. Plyometrics are also called stretch-shortening exercises (Figure 14-3).

- ✓ Proprioceptive neuromuscular facilitation (PNF)—PNF techniques are hands-on therapeutic movement patterns that use tactile, auditory, and proprioceptive stimulation to achieve desired muscle responses. Methodical contractions, relaxations, holds, and repetitive patterns can be used to improve strength and flexibility (Figure 14-4).

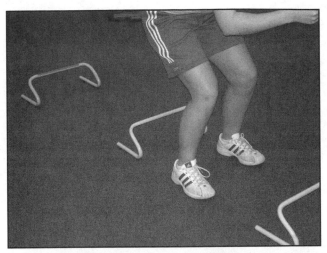

Figure 14-3. Plyometrics are commonly used to train explosive movements. In a rehabilitation setting, they can help patients slowly regain form as they attenuate forces.

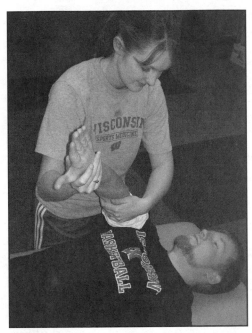

Figure 14-4. PNF is a common manual therapy strength technique.

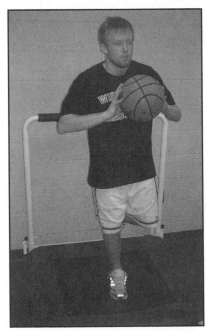

Figure 14-5. Functional sport activities can be included in the rehabilitation program to recreate specific movement patterns.

✓ Soft tissue mobilization—A variety of tissue mobilization techniques qualify as soft tissue mobilization. Massage is the most recognized form of soft tissue mobilization. Massage techniques can relax muscles, improve blood and lymph flow to reduce edema, alleviate pain, and improve motion. Myofascial release is similar to massage in that is seeks to relieve restrictions in tissue mobility through manual contact with the goal of improving movement and decreasing pain.

✓ Sport or activity specificity—As patients improve and progress through a rehabilitation program, exercises should increasingly become more sport or activity specific. Specificity will allow for better functional return to activity and alleviate boredom in the rehabilitative process (Figure 14-5).

SUMMARY

The development of foundational knowledge and skills in the treatment, rehabilitation, and reconditioning domain is an essential component of an athletic training education program. Students completing such a program should be well prepared to practice as entry-level professionals. However, CE is a key element of learning and refining skills that can enhance the athletic trainer's ability to address patient needs. A commitment to the acquisition of new skills and improving existing skills should be a career-long dedication. Athletic trainers in treatment and rehabilitation settings must utilize the feedback loop process to make adjustments to treatment plans based on new information. Program adjustments will require the creative implementation of therapeutic exercise and development of functional activity-specific programming. Evaluative skills are the cornerstone to determining initial patient needs and for assessing patient improvements. Proper development of realistic goals coupled with objective criteria for return to activity will provide benchmarks for patient progress.

REFERENCES

1. Prentice WE. *Arnheims's Principles of Athletic Training.* 13th ed. New York, NY: McGraw-Hill Higher Education; 2009.
2. Guskiewicz K. Regaining balance and postural equilibrium. In: Prentice WE, ed. *Rehabilitation Techniques in Sports Medicine.* New York, NY: WCB/McGraw-Hill; 1999:107-131.
3. McGee M. Functional progressions and functional testing in rehabilitation. In: Prentice WE, ed. *Rehabilitation Techniques in Sports Medicine.* New York, NY: WCB/McGraw-Hill; 1999:266-283.
4. Thein JM, Thein-Brody LA. Aquatic-based rehabilitation and training for the shoulder. *Journal of Athletic Training.* 2000;35(3):382-389.
5. Houglum P. *Therapeutic Exercise for Musculoskeletal Injuries.* 2nd ed. Champaign, IL: Human Kinetics; 2005.

Sample Rehabilitation Protocol

The MCL is located on the inside or medial aspect of the knee. It is commonly injured in contact sports from a blow to the outside of the knee.

The LCL is located on the outside or lateral aspect of the knee. It is not as frequently sprained as the MCL but can be injured when a force is applied to the inside of the knee. Isolated sprains may occur to either ligament, but other knee joint structures can be injured at the same time as the MCL or LCL.

Note: This protocol should serve only as a guide and is presented to illustrate common exercises and treatment options for a common knee injury. In treating a real patient, the athletic trainer could make multiple changes to this protocol based on the evaluative findings.

Treatment and Rehabilitation of MCL or LCL Sprains

Days 1 to 3

- Rest: Decrease or eliminate activity
- Ice: Apply ice for 15 to 20 minutes several times each day
- Compression: Use an elastic bandage to control swelling. Start at mid-calf and wrap upward to the thigh
- Elevation: Elevate the injured limb higher than heart level to assist the removal of swelling
- Crutches with partial weight bearing are indicated if the athlete cannot walk without pain or a limp
- A knee immobilizer is indicated for comfort
- Quad sets: 4 sets of 25, 2 to 3 times per day
- Straight leg raises: 4 sets of 25, 2 to 3 times per day

Days 4 to 7

- Cold whirlpool and ROM (biking motion while in the water) may be used at days 5 and 6 if swelling has decreased for 2 consecutive days
- Continue compression and elevation for swelling
- Continue quad sets and straight leg raises

Day 8 (if 90 degrees of knee flexion is present)

- Continue warm whirlpool and ROM
- Begin exercise bike or swimming (kicks) 15 to 20 minutes
- Exercises:
  - Continue quad sets and straight leg raises
  - Leg curl, 4 sets of 15
  - Leg press, 3 sets of 10 to 15
- Ice and compression after exercise

Day 14 (If full ROM is present)

- Continue:
  - Whirlpool
  - Exercise bike/pool
  - Strengthening exercises, increase weight and lower to 8 to 10 reps for leg curls and leg press
- Begin prescribed running program
- Ice after activity

The athlete must have the following to return to participation:

- Full ROM
- No pain
- No swelling
- Completed the entire prescribed running program

Adapted with permission of UW Health, Madison, WI. UW Health Sports Link Sports Updates Information Series. Treatment and Rehabilitation of MCL or LCL Sprains. Patient Education Handout 2007.

Career Spotlight: Physician Extender–Athletic Trainer

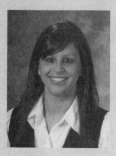

Shari A. Khaja, MS, LAT

Senior Athletic Trainer

UW Health Sports Medicine, Madison WI

My Position

I provide athletic training services for the University of Wisconsin Hospital and Clinics under the direction of a designated sports medicine physician. This includes direct patient contact primarily for the evaluation and treatment of medical and musculoskeletal pathology consistent with the scope and practice of athletic training clinical competencies as defined by the NATA-BOC and the State of Wisconsin Athletic Training Affiliated Credentialing Board. As a clinical physician extender, I evaluate and treat patients from pediatric to geriatric populations. My position involves coordinating new and existing physician extender clinical staff orientation and education. I serve as clinical education coordinator for issues relating to HIPAA (Health Insurance Portability and Accountability Act) and JCAHO (Joint Commission on Accreditation of Health care Organizations) compliance. I also assume responsibility for developing and directing the athletic training internship program.

A wide variety of internal and external contact relationships are involved in performance of the duties of this position, and a high degree of independence in creating and enhancing these relationships is expected. Internal contacts include other members of the athletic training and sports rehabilitation staff, physicians, nursing personnel, fitness center staff, exercise physiology staff, preventive cardiology staff, radiology staff, public relations personnel, legal counsel, and a variety of clerical staff. External contacts include physicians, athletic trainers, and physical therapists from other institutions, academic athletic training programs, patient and/or athlete family members, coaches, athletic directors, equipment vendors, case managers and insurance representatives. I also play a lead role in the development of clinical support staff, athletic training internship students, and volunteer workers.

Unique or Desired Qualifications

Minimum qualifications for this position include the following:

- Athletic training licensure or eligibility for athletic training licensure in the state of Wisconsin
- Athletic training certification by the BOC
- UW Athletic Training Education Program Approved Clinical Instructor (ACI)

Unique qualifications would include previous experience in an orthopedic clinic setting, strong written and verbal communication skills, knowledge of computer-related skills, as well as excellent understanding of audiovisual and technological programming for maintaining Web site interactions. It is also of benefit to pursue further educational experience in an administrative or business-related field.

Favorite Aspect of My Job

The favorite aspect of my job is working with so many different individuals in a wide variety of settings, including business, education, administration, and health care. Although it can be somewhat challenging at times to find balance, my position also allows me to seek out unique opportunities for athletic trainers to evolve the profession in different settings and avenues.

Advice

It is not always about the grades, the accolades, or natural talent. If you have what it takes and the desire to achieve, success will ensue.

CHAPTER 15

TAPING AND BRACING

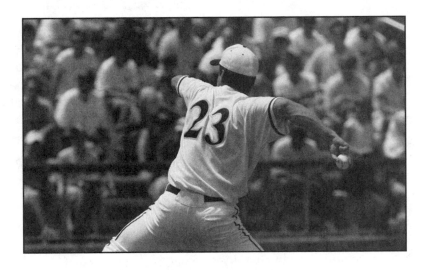

Expect the unexpected. If you can be prepared and expect the unexpected, you will have thought through the "what ifs" and be ready for anything that comes down the line.

Kevin Guskiewicz, PhD, ATC
Associate Professor Department of Exercise and Sport Science
Director, Sports Medicine Research Laboratory
University of North Carolina–Chapel Hill

The application of adhesive tape is often the image that comes to mind when people think of athletic training. It is too bad really. Not that there is anything wrong with the judicious application of athletic tape; this chapter is dedicated to the topic. The reality is that taping only makes up a small portion of the athletic trainer's professional duties, yet it is the one visual image people often have of the profession. Certified athletic trainers spend much more professional time on things like injury assessment, initial care and management, and rehabilitation. In addition, the efficacy of some taping techniques under specific conditions has been questioned in the literature.[1-3] While some techniques have shown to be useful, a large number remain untested and rely solely on clinical observation (anecdotal) evidence for their use.

Despite some of these uncertainties, there are enough well-supported uses of taping, bandaging, and bracing that they should be considered foundational skills for the athletic training student. Learning these techniques and developing proficiency can serve as a foundation upon which other skills can be built. It is usually through the application of preventative taping techniques that students are provided with their first opportunity to interact with patients and use their skills in "real world" clinical settings. Developing confidence in this area will aid the athletic training student as he or she progresses to more advanced athletic training skills.

Upon completion of this chapter, the student will be able to:

✓ Describe the types of adhesive tapes used in athletic training settings

✓ Differentiate between taping and bandaging

✓ Describe the uses, materials required, general application technique, and precautions for a variety of taping techniques

✓ Explain the pros and cons of taping and bracing of the ankle

✓ Explain the proper use of compressive wraps in the management of injury

TAPING

Adhesive taping in an athletic training setting has many uses:

✓ Securing dressings and compressive wraps

✓ Providing preventative support for joints during activities

✓ Supplying support following injury

✓ Securing protective padding

The most common taping technique that seeks to provide preventative support for a joint is the ankle taping. The goal of any preventative technique is to limit the motion of the body part by applying the taping technique. While the biomechanical ability to fully support a joint with tape has been questioned, studies have demonstrated that proprioceptive feedback of injured ankles is enhanced with taping.[4] Taping should not be confused with bandaging. Bandages are strips of cloth or other material that are used to dress wounds and hold dressings in place. The most common type of bandage used in athletic settings is the elastic bandage, which is used for compression and support.

EVIDENCE-GUIDED PRACTICE: BANDAGING, TAPING, AND BRACING

Taping skills are readily identified within the practice domain of the athletic trainer. However, very few taping skills have been subjected to the rigors of clinical trials research to evaluate their efficacy. Most have been developed and their efficacy described by anecdotal evidence—most often based on athletic trainer observations and patient feedback. A recent review of clinical trials examining functional treatment strategies for acute lateral ankle ligament injuries in adults is useful when looking at the tape versus brace issue.[5]

 ## Tearing the Tape

When you observe someone who has taped for many years, he or she has the ability to "make it look easy." Truth be told, he or she had just as much trouble when he or she started out. Like with any other skill, your ability to tear the tape will improve with practice. One of the most difficult tasks for the beginner is tearing tape. Nonelastic white cotton tape can be torn quite easily; some elastic tapes can be torn by hand while others will require taping scissors. Visit the companion Web site and watch the video on tearing tape. Keep these guidelines in mind:

● Place your fingers close together

● Try to handle only the edge of the tape

● Place tension on the tape by pulling it apart

● Snap your fingers in the opposite direction

● Wrinkled or folded tape will not tear – try another spot along the edge

Be patient and practice. Once you can tear a whole roll without problems, you will be ready to start taping.

This clinical trial only looked at data from randomized clinical trails that included functional treatment strategies such as bracing, taping, and using elastic bandages. Of the numerous studies examined, only 9 met the criteria for inclusion (fully randomized and compared different treatment options). These 9 represent 892 participants and examined outcomes such as return to sport, return to work, pain, swelling, objective instability, subjective instability, ROM, and satisfaction. Some of the findings include the following[5]:

✓ Tape versus elastic bandages—In the early stages of injury, the use of tape is not supported. The use of an elastic bandage will lead to fewer complications to the skin. No significant difference was noted in any other outcomes.

✓ Tape versus semi-rigid ankle support—No significant differences were found on any of the outcomes between taping and use of a semi-rigid ankle support.

✓ Tape versus lace-up ankle braces—No significant differences were found on any of the outcomes between taping and use of a lace-up ankle brace other than finding less swelling at short-term follow-up when using a lace-up ankle brace.

Keep in mind the above Cochrane Review only looked at randomized clinical trails that included bandaging, bracing, or taping as part of the functional treatment. They only examined studies that looked at treatment, not what happens after the injury. Many

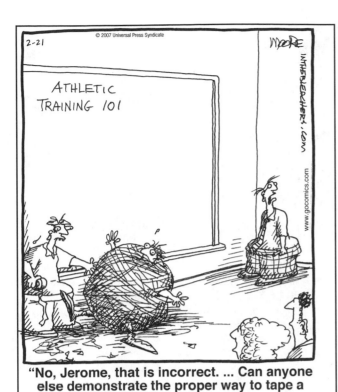

2-21   © 2007 Universal Press Syndicate

ATHLETIC
TRAINING 101

"No, Jerome, that is incorrect. ... Can anyone else demonstrate the proper way to tape a basketball player's ankle?"

studies have looked at taping versus bracing under a range of conditions to better assess the protective quality. A recent review paper identified some pertinent findings[6]:

- ✓ The use of either tape or braces reduces the incidence of ankle sprains.
- ✓ The use of tape or braces may result in less severe ankle sprains. However, braces seem to be more effective in preventing ankle sprains than tape.
- ✓ It is not clear which athletes are to benefit more from the use of preventive measures: those with or those without previous ankle sprains.
- ✓ The efficacy of shoes in preventing ankle sprains is unclear. It is likely that newness of the footwear plays a more important role than shoe height in preventing ankle sprains.
- ✓ Proprioceptive training reduces the incidence of ankle sprains in athletes with recurrent ankle sprains to the same level as subjects without any history of ankle sprains.

It is noteworthy that the overwhelming majority of the taping-versus-bracing discussion focuses on the ankle. It is clear that more research is needed to examine the efficacy of many other taping techniques. In the mean time, we can safely say the following:

- ✓ The cost benefit and ease of use may make ankle braces a better alternative to taping.
- ✓ Taping efficacy is dependent upon the skill of the practitioner and the desired time needed for protection. Taping can provide protection to the ankle similar to a brace but not for as long a period of time. As time passes after application, the efficacy of the taping becomes limited.
- ✓ Athlete concerns about decreased performance from taping or bracing do not appear to be valid.

Strong anecdotal evidence for the use of specific taping techniques will continue to require that the skilled athletic trainer is proficient in their application. In addition, as literature becomes available to support or refute the use of specific techniques, athletic trainers will need to be willing to adjust accordingly in the interest of evidence-guided practice.

SUPPLIES USED FOR TAPING

A wide variety of athletic tapes are available for use by athletic trainers. Nonelastic white cotton cloth athletic tape is the most common tape used to provide support and secure bandages. This tape is available in 0.5-, 1-, 1.5-, and 2-inch widths of various quality grades. Made of cotton linen, several factors influence the quality and price of the tape. These include the number of fibers per inch, quality of the adhesive, and how easily it comes off the role (winding tension). Nonelastic tape is used for everything from taping hockey sticks to taping ankles; however, you would not want the same quality for those jobs. Cost, personal preference, and ease of use will influence most purchases. Personal experience places winding tension and quality of the adhesive as prime considerations in selecting tape. Adhesive that sticks to the layers of tape below or leaves large amounts of adhesive on the skin (adhesive transfer) can be problematic. Application of nonelastic tape requires instruction followed by practice since it does not easily conform to the body. Knowing the "angles" to get the tape to go where you want it to go is a learned skill. This tape is also constrictive; if it is applied improperly (ie, around a muscle belly), it can cut off circulation and damage surrounding tissue.

Elastic tape easily conforms to body parts, making it a good choice for a range of tasks. Elastic tapes come in varying strengths and are often used in combination with nonelastic tapes to provide additional support (see variations described next). Elastic tapes are available in 1-, 2-, 3-, and 4-inch widths. Some have an adhesive backing much like nonelastic tape, while others adhere only to themselves. The latter are commonly used to hold dressings and bandages in place. Other lighter-weight elastic tapes that may not be useful in supporting a joint are valuable in securing protective pads and equipment. Like all taping supplies, personal preference, desired use, and cost will influence purchasing.

Other essential taping supplies include underwrap, heel and lace pads, spray adherents, and protective ointment or lubricant. Underwrap is an ultra thin, foam-like product that can provide protection over superficial bony areas and prominent tendons. While taping to the skin can provide the greatest amount of support, repeated applications may cause skin irritation. Use of underwrap that is anchored to the skin can cut down on this problem. Heel and lace pads are small squares of foam or gauze with a thin layer of protective ointment or lubricant to protect the skin from blisters. A spray adherent can aid in improving the adhesion of the tape. Caution should be used to insure athletes do not have a skin allergy to the adherent. Proper cleaning and removal of all adherent and tape adhesive will help prevent skin irritations.

Additional supplies needed for safe and effective taping include a razor for hair removal, tape scissors for cutting tape, and tape cutters for tape removal.

How to Use This Chapter

To make the most of the material presented in this chapter, students should do the following:

- Review the various taping and bandaging techniques outlined
- Visit the Athletic Training Foundations Web site to watch step-by-step video of each technique
- Combine video viewing with instruction from a proficient athletic trainer
- Be patient and keep practicing.

PRECAUTIONS AND SAFETY CONSIDERATIONS

The following precautions should be considered when applying tape to a patient:
  ✓ Make sure there are no underlying skin irritations or skin conditions that would prevent safe use of a spray adherent or adhesive tape.

General Taping Guidelines

Some considerations for applying elastic and nonelastic adhesive tape:

- Always be sensitive to patient position—proper position of the ankle, contraction of a muscle belly, slight knee flexion, etc. These factors can influence the efficacy of the technique and contribute to proper application and patient comfort.
- Use anchors to secure above and below the joint you are stabilizing. Subsequent strips of tape are applied from, and attached to, the anchors.
- Always overlap tape by half to maximize strength and avoid gaps in the tape.
- Do not tape continuously with nonelastic tape because this can constrict the extremity and disrupt circulation.
- Avoid wrinkles and gaps in the tape by smoothing the tape as you go.
- Insure that the skin is clean, dry, and healthy prior to taping.
- Tape to the skin for maximum support.

  ✓ Caution should be taken to insure proper tension and avoid cutting off circulation to the extremity. The mid-foot is a common area for applying the tape "too tight."
  ✓ Smooth application free of wrinkles will help prevent blisters and cuts.
  ✓ Avoid using nonelastic tape around a muscle. Use elastic tape or only circle the nonelastic tape half the circumference.
  ✓ When using underwrap, be sure to secure the tape to the skin using a large enough area to avoid skin irritations.
  ✓ Taping of an acute injury for the purpose of returning to play is largely contraindicated. The presence of bleeding and swelling heighten the opportunities for diminished circulation if the application is too tight.

TAPING TECHNIQUES

The taping techniques outlined next are representative of those commonly used by athletic trainers. This list corresponds with the videos available on the text's companion Web site. While there are countless variations and other techniques to learn as you progress in athletic training, this group will provide an excellent starting point for any athletic training student. Each technique is presented with the purpose, supplies needed, application guidelines, variations, and precautions. A photo of the completed taping techniques is also provided. All taping techniques require the skin to be clean, dry, preferably shaved, and free of any irritations.

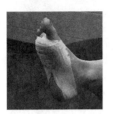

LONGITUDINAL ARCH

Purpose

Longitudinal arch taping is used to support the longitudinal arch of the foot under a variety of conditions. The taping can be used to support the arch as part of a treatment program or return-to-activity plan for a sprain injury. Taping the longitudinal arch is commonplace as an adjunct to plantar fascitis treatment and is also frequently used to assist with treatment of common lower leg injuries such as medial tibial stress syndrome, posterior tibialis tendonitis, and the catch all "shin splints."

Supplies

✓ Spray adherent
✓ 1-inch adhesive tape

Application

✓ Apply an anchor strip around the metatarsal heads at the "ball" of the foot.

✓ A series of overlapping "X" patterns using 1-inch adhesive tape are then applied as follows:

○ Stating at the first metatarsal head, looping the calcaneus, and ending back at the same starting point.

○ A second "X" pattern is applied from the first metatarsal head, again looping the calcaneus, and finishing at the 5th metatarsal head (making a full "X" pattern).

○ The third strip begins at the 5th metatarsal head and ends at the 5th metatarsal head.

○ This pattern allows for an overlapping pattern that covers the arch. The size of the patient and the desired level of support dictate the number of strips.

✓ Applying a horseshoe strip from the lateral to medial anchor helps complete the taping.

✓ Closure strips are then applied from the lateral to medial across the bottom of the foot starting and ending at the horseshoe strip. The closure strips should extend from one tape width distal to the calcaneus up to the ball of the foot.

Precautions

The longitudinal arch taping is applied directly to the skin. The bottom of the foot is often sweaty so care should be taken to be sure the foot is clean, dry, and free of any skin irritation. Take care to allow spray adherent to dry and become tacky prior to application.

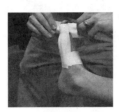

TURF TOE

Purpose

Turf toe is an injury to the first metatarsophalangeal (MP) joint. It is named due to the common occurrence on hard artificial surfaces. The injury involves pain, swelling, and irritation to the 1st MP joint secondary to excessive hyperextension of the great toe. The purpose of the turf-toe taping is to support the 1st MP joint and prevent excessive hyperextension.

Supplies

✓ Spray adherent
✓ 1-inch nonelastic adhesive tape
✓ 1.5-inch nonelastic adhesive tape
Variations to the turf toe:
✓ 1-inch elastic adhesive tape

Application

✓ Spray adherent should be applied to a clean and dry foot that is free of skin irritation.

✓ One or 2 anchor strips are placed around the mid-foot using 1.5-inch nonelastic adhesive tape.

✓ An anchor strip is placed around the great toe; this anchor should cover the IP joint and base of the great toe.

✓ Hold the toe in a neutral position while overlapping 1-inch adhesive tape strips are applied from the distal to the proximal anchor working in a lateral to medial direction. NOTE: Some turf toe tapings will use strips that overlap from the plantar aspect of the foot up to the dorsal surface in an effort to provide greater support.

✓ The number of strips applied will be dependent upon the size of the patient and the desired level of support.

✓ Apply closing strips around the great toe and the middle of the foot to finish.

✓ Variation: 1-inch elastic tape is often used to support the 1st MP joint using a crossing pattern that runs from the mid-foot anchor around the MP joint and back to the anchor. Despite many variations, the goal is the same—secure the 1st MP from excessive motion.

Precautions

Care should be taken not to place the distal anchor above the IP joint of the great toe. If this should happen, excessive flexion of the toe may occur and provide discomfort for the patient.

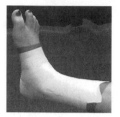

PREVENTATIVE ANKLE TAPING

Purpose

The purpose of the preventative ankle taping is to provide support from the common inversion ankle sprain injury. The efficacy of this taping will be dependent upon several factors, including how the tape job is anchored, the time between application and the activity, and the previous injury history of the patient. The use of preventative taping has been explored in the literature mostly as it is compared to ankle bracing (see above). Despite some of the advantages that bracing may provide, taping of the ankle is still commonplace due to athlete preference and the common use of variations to this procedure following injury.

Note: There are countless variations of the preventative ankle taping. The one outlined below and presented on the companion Web site is a variation of the basket weave taping technique. Students will see many variations among the professionals they encounter.

Supplies

✓ Spray adherent

✓ Pre-tape wrap

✓ Heel and lace pads with ointment/skin lubricant

✓ 1.5- or 2-inch nonelastic adhesive tape

Variations to the preventative ankle taping may utilize:

✓ 2- or 3-inch elastic adhesive tape

✓ 3-inch moleskin

Application

The position of the patient during the ankle taping is extremely important. The ankle should be held in a neutral 90-degree angle throughout. The contentious athletic trainer will need to remind the patient to hold this position.

✓ Underwrap—Following the application of spray adherent and the placement of heel and lace pads, underwrap should be applied beginning at the foot and continuously applied to an area just above the ankle.

✓ Anchor strips—Apply 3 to 5 anchor strips on the lower leg by beginning a few inches above the underwrap (no higher than the base of the gastrocnemius). Work toward the ankle, overlapping each strip by half. Remember, the lower leg is not a cylinder. You will need to angle the tape slightly so it does not wrinkle or gap in the back.

✓ Heel locks—Lateral and medial heel locks are applied to the ankle. Students should practice applying heel locks one at a time. Once they are proficient at this, they can be applied continuously.

✓ Stirrups and horseshoes—Stirrups and horseshoes are applied in an alternating fashion (this pattern is called a basket weave). Anchor the stirrup from the medial anchor to the lateral anchor. The stirrup should hit the posterior third of the medial and lateral malleoli. Two or 3 stirrups will be applied (depending on the size of the athlete). Students can give a slight tug just before laying down the tape on the lateral anchors. To prevent an inversion sprain, stirrups should be applied medial to lateral. Each stirrup should overlap the previous one by half (anteriorly). When completed, the entire malleolus should be covered on each side. Horseshoe strips are applied in an alternating pattern with each stirrup. They are applied from the anchor at the base of the foot around the heel and back to the anchor on the midfoot (medial to lateral).

✓ Closures—Closure strips can be applied to any open areas of the foot or lower leg (except the bottom of the heel, which will remain exposed).

✓ Variations—Common variations to the ankle taping involve using different materials to enhance the support of the tape job. Moleskin for stirrups and strong elastic adhesive tape for heel locks are common substitutions.

Precautions

Applying the mid foot anchor too tightly is the most common problem with ankle taping. In addition, sloppy or wrinkled tape application can lead to hot spots or blisters for the patient. Great care should be taken to make sure an adequate area of skin is exposed if you wish to anchor the taping to the skin surface (2 to 3 tape widths). Anchoring the tape job to too small an area of skin may cause damage to the exposed skin as the adhesive tape pulls due to motion at the ankle joint. Lastly, students are encouraged to practice sufficiently and have their skills evaluated by a qualified athletic trainer before taping athletes in actual practice or competition environments.

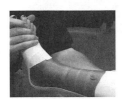

ACHILLES TENDON TAPING

Purpose

The Achilles tendon taping helps limit dorsiflexion of the ankle. By limiting dorsiflexion, pressure can be alleviated from a strained or inflamed Achilles tendon. Chronic Achilles tendon irritations can be particularly difficult to manage. While taping support is helpful, it is not a replacement for appropriate rest and therapeutic treatment.

Supplies

- ✓ Spray adherent
- ✓ Pre-tape wrap
- ✓ Heel and lace pads with ointment/skin lubricant
- ✓ 1.5- or 2-inch nonelastic adhesive tape
- ✓ 2- or 3-inch elastic adhesive tape (depending upon the size of the athlete)

Application

The Achilles tendon taping begins very similar to the preventative ankle taping:
- ✓ Spray adherent is applied to a clean and shaved ankle. Heel and lace pads and underwrap are applied as described previously.
- ✓ Anchors to the base of the gastrocnemius and forefoot should be applied using 1.5- or 2-inch nonelastic tape.
- ✓ Once the anchors are in place, the patient should then drop his or her ankle into plantar flexion (yep, that thing we never want to do while taping the ankle!).
- ✓ A 2- or 3-inch piece of strong elastic tape is then measured from anchor to anchor.
- ✓ Apply the elastic tape at the proximal and distal anchor and secure it with nonelastic tape. Allow the patient to return to the 90-degree position.
- ✓ Place closure strips using 1.5- or 2-inch flexible elastic tape.
- ✓ Variations—If supporting the ankle, in addition to taking pressure off the Achilles tendon heel locks, use elastic tape. It is also a common practice to use a heel lift to take additional pressure off the Achilles tendon.

Precautions

If using a heel lift with the Achilles tendon taping, be sure to place the lift in both shoes to avoid creating a leg-length discrepancy.

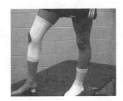

KNEE MCL TAPING

Purpose

Taping of the knee is not a common practice for the athletic trainer. As a rule, the use of knee braces coupled with the ineffectiveness of most tape jobs to this joint have made taping the knee almost obsolete. There are 2 exceptions to this rule: taping of the patella to affect patellar tracking (see p. 278) and taping of the MCL.

The MCL protects the knee from valgus forces (ie, when someone lands on the outside of the knee) and also assists in preventing anterior movement of your tibia on the femur.

Supplies

- ✓ Spray adherent
- ✓ Underwrap
- ✓ Heel and lace pads with ointment/skin lubricant
- ✓ 1.5- or 2-inch nonelastic adhesive tape
- ✓ 3-inch elastic adhesive tape
- ✓ 2- or 3-inch flexible elastic tape

Application

- ✓ Position the patient with the knee flexed (approximately 15 degrees) and the hip slightly flexed (a heel lift can help position the athlete).
- ✓ Apply spray adherent to dry, clean, shaven, and healthy skin. Note: This tape job must be anchored to the skin to be effective.
- ✓ Use 2 lubricated heel and lace pads behind the knee to help prevent irritation in this area.
- ✓ Apply underwrap to cover the upper third of the gastrocnemius, knee, and lower third of the thigh.
- ✓ Use a strong 3-inch elastic tape to create anchors at the mid calf and mid thigh. Apply 2 anchors overlapped by half for each.
- ✓ Using 2-inch adhesive tape, apply an "X" pattern over the MCL. Be careful to stay one fingerbreadth away from the patella. Apply 2 or 3 "X" patterns (depending on the size of your athlete).
- ✓ Apply an additional "X" pattern using 3-inch elastic tape. Once completed, secure the 3-inch elastic tape with 2-inch nonelastic tape.

Patella Taping

Mechanical alterations in the smooth tracking of the patella in the femoral groove can be a source of great discomfort for many active individuals. This maltracking and associated discomfort is known as patellofemoral stress syndrome (see Chapter 6). Some patellar maltracking can be corrected using a specific taping technique. Improvements in patellar position may allow for pain reduction during participation or may provide an improved environment to allow for improved comfort during rehabilitation. This technique is known as the McConnell taping. This taping examines the side-to-side movement of the patella, tilt or height of the lateral border of the patella, and both the rotation and anteroposterior alignment of the patella.

While the technique is fairly simple, the evaluative skills used to identify patellar orientation take practice. The example provided below demonstrates one common application to improve lateral glide. The procedure requires 2 types of specialty tape produced by Biersdorf (Hamburg, Germany). These are called Leukotape and Fixomull. The Fixomull serves as a base to which the Leukotape will be placed.

Example: McConnell Taping for Lateral Patellar Glide

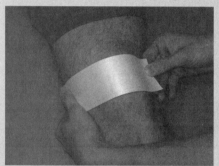

Base to which Leukotape will be applied.

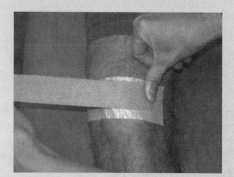

The tape is placed one thumb width from the lateral patellar border pushing the patella medially in the frontal plane of movement.

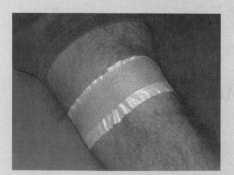

The tape is then secured to the medial aspect of the joint.

✓ Cover the entire tape job with a flexible elastic tape, and secure the ends with white tape.

Precautions

During the MCL taping, precaution should be taken to keep the patella open and insure that the tape job does not interfere with movement of the patella in the femoral groove. There are many braces available on the market designed to support the MCL. Many athletic trainers and patients will be more comfortable with such a product rather than an extensive taping procedure. However, individual patient comfort and desired activity may make this tape job useful for a short period of time as part of a return-to-activity plan.

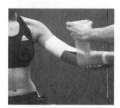

ELBOW

Purpose

The elbow taping is designed to prevent hyperextension of the elbow. Forced hyperextension can result in soft tissue injury to the anterior anatomical structures of the elbow joint. Severe hyperextension can result in bony injury to the ulna or humerus. More severe forced hyperextension may cause an anterior dislocation—a rare event. The hyperextension taping often is used to protect the patient as he or she returns to activity. This taping must be anchored to the skin to be effective.

Supplies

✓ Spray adherent
✓ Underwrap
✓ Heel and lace pads with ointment/skin lubricant
✓ 1.5-inch nonelastic adhesive tape
✓ 3-inch elastic adhesive tape
✓ 2- or 3-inch flexible elastic tape

Preparation and Application

The patient must be positioned with the elbow in slight flexion. The patient should also make a fist to flex the bicep and allow for adequate anchoring without constriction. The taping surface should be shaved free of hair at the upper and lower arm to allow proper anchoring of the tape. Have the athlete make a fist to contract the biceps muscle and prevent constriction. After spray adherent is applied to clean, dry, and healthy skin, the following steps should be followed:

✓ Apply anchor strips around the biceps and forearm using either elastic or 1.5-inch adhesive tape. If using adhesive tape, remember to make

half circular strips to complete the anchor and avoid constricting the muscle. Elastic tape can be safely applied around the entire arm.

✓ Make a "bridge" or "check rein" out of 1.5-inch overlapped tape. The number of strips will depend upon the size of your patient. It is also permissible to make an "X" pattern using a strong elastic tape.

✓ Attach the check rein strips using 1.5-inch tape at each anchor strip. Hint: Using a couple of heel and lace pads over the antecubital fossa (anterior elbow) can prevent irritation to the skin under this friction point.

✓ Secure the upper and lower portions of the tape job with strong elastic tape.

✓ Use a flexible elastic tape or a compression bandage to cover the tape job and secure with adhesive tape.

Precautions

The amount of motion limited by this taping procedure must be checked repeatedly to insure proper support. Elbow tapings can easily come loose due to the repeated contraction of the biceps.

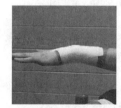

WRIST

Purpose

The wrist taping is used to provide general support to the gliding articulations of the wrist. The wrist taping can also be used to limit either flexion or extension based on the use of check-reign style strips that cross the wrist joint and attach to an anchor that is secured around the hand.

Supplies

✓ 1-inch nonelastic adhesive tape
✓ 1.5-inch nonelastic adhesive tape
✓ 1-inch elastic adhesive tape
✓ 1.5- or 2-inch flexible elastic tape

Preparation and Application

There are several variations of taping for the wrist. Each tape job involves the placement of circular strips in support of the wrist joint. Skin should be clean, dry, and healthy. Adherent is not often used for taping of the wrist. The patient's hand should be placed in a neutral position with the fingers spread. Taping of the wrist is easy and a good confidence builder for students. The accompanying video on the Web site shows several variation of the wrist taping.

Precautions

Given the number of extensor and flexor tendons that cross the wrist, applying the tape too tightly can have consequences for athletes who need fine movements with the hand. To avoid this, it is essential for the patient to keep the fingers spread while the tape is being applied.

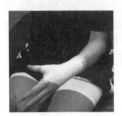

THUMB

Purpose

Sprains to the thumb frequently involve hyperextension of the MCP joint and may involve a valgus force that injures the ulnar collateral ligament (UCL). A complete rupture of the UCL will require anatomical restitution through a surgical repair. The taping of the thumb will vary depending on the severity of the injury and the activity of the patient. The greater the fine motor movements needed, the more difficult to tape the thumb securely.

Supplies

Taping the thumb is usually done in combination with taping the wrist. Common supplies include the following:
- ✓ 1-inch nonelastic adhesive tape
- ✓ 1.5-inch nonelastic adhesive tape
- ✓ 1-inch elastic adhesive tape

Preparation and Application

The key pattern to the thumb taping is the figure-of-8 that circles the wrist and the MCP joint. For many injuries, this simple taping combined with taping of the wrist is sufficient to support the wrist. If additional support is desired, the taping can be "closed" by attaching individual 1-inch taping strips to anchors on either side of the MCP and base of the thumb. Both variations of this common taping technique are provided online.

Precautions

The "web" of skin that sits between the thumb and 2nd digit can become very tender if the strips of adhesive tape are too tight or if the edges cut into this delicate skin. This can be avoided by having the patient spread his or her fingers wide during the tape procedure and to fold the edges of the tape that crosses this area. A small amount of lubricant can also be helpful; however, too much lubricant will interfere with the adhesive and may impact the effectiveness of the procedure.

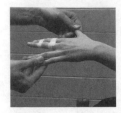

FINGERS

Purpose

Fingers are most often taped to provide support to the adjacent finger following a sprain to the PIP joint. This taping style is known as a "buddy taping." This taping can use the adjacent finger as a splint while still allowing flexion and extension. Athletes who must wear removable gloves for their sport activity will need to have the finger taped around the specific joint. This can be accomplished using a strong elastic tape that wraps around the finger and is held in place by nonelastic tape.

Supplies

Most finger taping applications can be completed with 1-inch adhesive tape. Smaller patients may require this tape to be split into smaller widths. If compression of the finger is the goal, 2- or 3-inch elastic adhesive tape can be applied to provide compressive support.

Preparation and Application

To buddy tape, simply secure the fingers by applying the tape just proximal to the PIP joints and between the PIP and DIP joints. This will allow for flexion and extension of the joint while still providing support. If compression is the goal, the desired width of strong elastic tape can be wrapped around the entire finger and secured with nonelastic tape.

Precautions

It is important to never leave the 2nd and 5th digit unsecured when using the buddy taping technique. Secure either the 4th and 5th fingers or the 2nd and 3rd—never buddy tape the 3rd to the 4th because it places the free fingers at risk of injury. Chapter 7 outlines a variety of serious finger injuries that require physician evaluation and special splinting or, in some cases, surgical repair. If in doubt to the seriousness of a finger injury, always refer the athlete for consultation.

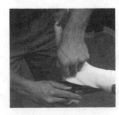

PROPER TAPE
REMOVAL

Careful removal of all tape and adhesive residue following use is essential for skin health. After a practice or competition, athletes should remove their tape using surgical scissors with a safety edge or a commercial tape cutter. Care should be taken to use the scissors or tape cutter in such a way as to avoid boney prominences. A small drop of lubricant will help glide the tape cutter. Care

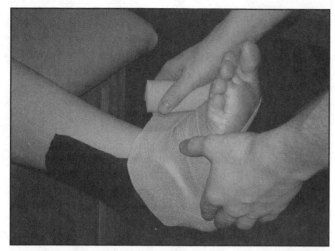

Figure 15-1. The use of a compressive wrap is a common practice to combat edema and effusion following injury. Note the distal to proximal pattern and the exposed toes to allow for circulation to be monitored.

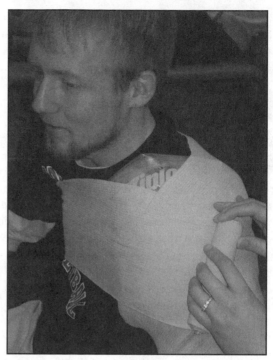

Figure 15-2. The shoulder spica is a versatile pattern that can be used to secure ice packs or hold protective pads in place over the AC joint.

should be taken when removing the tape from the skin; tape-remover products may be helpful. Some athletes find that wetting the tape in the shower is also helpful. Upon removal of the tape, athletes should carefully wash the area as to remove all adhesive residue. Athletic trainers who are taping athletes on a regular basis can inspect for evidence of skin irritation before applying tape. Persistent skin irritation may require trying alternative tapes, different adhesives, or in some cases referral to the physician for a consultation on specific rashes.

ELASTIC BANDAGES AND COMPRESSION WRAPS

The use of elastic bandages and compression wraps is common in many sports medicine settings. Elastic bandages are used to apply an even amount of compression to help reduce swelling and to provide support to muscle tissues. They are used postinjury as supporting devices that are not strong enough to offer any significant level of protection to anatomical structures. However, when properly applied, they are invaluable in assisting the recovery process post injury. Elastic bandages come in a variety of widths and lengths that allow the athletic trainer to make an appropriate selection based on the desired body part being treated.

When applying an elastic wrap for compression, specific guidelines should be followed:
- ✓ Apply the wrap from distal to proximal to best combat gravity and assist with the reduction of edema.

- ✓ Overlap the elastic bandage by one half and apply in a circular fashion.
- ✓ Apply the elastic wrap with modest tension to avoid constricting circulation.
- ✓ Check the circulation in the extremities often to insure the wrap has not been applied too tightly.
- ✓ Do not allow the patient to sleep in a tight elastic wrap since the compression may be too tight in this relaxed state.
- ✓ A compression pad, such as a horseshoe of foam or felt at the ankle, may be used to assist with compression (Figure 15-1).

THE SPICA PATTERN

The spica pattern is a commonly used figure-of-8 pattern used with a variety of elastic bandages. When applying the spica pattern, one loop of the figure-of-8 is smaller than the other based on the involved body part. For example, a shoulder spica can be used to secure an ice bag or hold a protective pad in place. A shoulder spica wraps an elastic bandage around the humerus and around the trunk of the body with an "X" pattern where the wrap crosses over the AC joint (Figure 15-2). A very common application is the hip spica. The hip spica requires an extra long elastic wrap (usually 4-inch width) being wrapped around the thigh and the waist to provide support to muscle injuries at the groin and hip flexor. Two common hip spica applications are provided next.

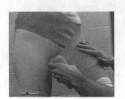

GROIN SUPPORT

Purpose

The hip spica for groin support is used to allow patients with newly injured groin or adductor strains to ambulate with greater comfort and to apply compression to newly injured soft tissue. This wrap is also applied to provide additional support during return to activity.

Supplies

✓ Extra long elastic wrap (4- or 6-inch width)
✓ 1.5-inch nonadhesive tape to secure the wrap

Application

The key to proper application of the groin support is the starting position of the patient. The patient should stand on a table with his or her weight on the uninjured extremity. The injured limb should be internally rotated. The wrap should be applied as follows:

✓ Start at the upper third of the thigh and pass the rolled elastic wrap toward the midline of the body and around the back of the thigh.

✓ After one complete wrap around the thigh, bring the wrap up and around the lower abdomen to the opposite iliac crest, and back down and around the thigh. This will create a crossing pattern over the thigh.

✓ Continue this pattern until the wrap is completely applied. Leave enough wrap so that it may be secured using half circles of 1.5-inch non elastic tape. ALWAYS secure the wrap around the thigh. Attempting to secure the wrap around the waist is not effective.

Hint: For the groin support, the patient has an internally rotated limb, the pattern will have a "down and around" feeling in supporting the groin. This is the opposite of the hip flexor "up and around" pattern seen below,

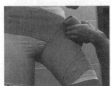

HIP FLEXOR SUPPORT

Purpose

The hip spica for hip flexor support is used to allow patients with newly injured hip flexor strains to ambulate with greater comfort and to apply compression to newly injured soft tissue.

This wrap is also applied to provide additional support during return to activity.

Supplies

✓ Extra long elastic wrap (4- or 6-inch width)
✓ 1.5-inch nonadhesive tape to secure the wrap

Application

The key to proper application of the hip flexor support is the starting position of the patient. The patient should stand on a table with his or her weight on the uninjured extremity. The injured limb should be forward in a slight hip flexed position. The wrap should be applied as follows:

✓ Start at the upper third of the thigh and pass the rolled elastic wrap to the outside of the thigh, around the back of the thigh, and up toward the iliac crest. This up-and-back pattern is the opposite of the pattern described for the groin.

✓ After one complete wrap around the thigh, bring the wrap up and around the lower back toward the opposite iliac crest, and back down and around the thigh. This will create a crossing pattern over the thigh.

✓ Continue this pattern until the wrap is completely applied. Leave enough wrap so that it may be secured using half circles of 1.5-inch non elastic tape. ALWAYS secure the wrap around the thigh. Attempting to secure the wrap around the waist is not effective.

Hint: The hip spica procedure is also useful when applying compression to a new hamstring injury. The added support around the waist helps keep the wrap in place. The only modification is greater coverage of the hamstring musculature. The distal to proximal guidelines still apply.

BRACES AND SUPPORTS

A variety of commercial braces and supports are available for use in the sports medicine setting. To discuss them all is outside the scope of this introductory text. However, ankle braces and knee braces seem to garner the most attention. The role of preventative ankle braces has been discussed earlier in this chapter. The use of a lace-up or rigid ankle support can be an effective tool in prevention of injury and is also useful for providing support during the return-to-activity phase of a rehabilitation program. When properly applied, ankle braces can, over time, be a lower cost alternative to preventative taping. Figure 15-3 provides examples of common ankle braces and knee supports.

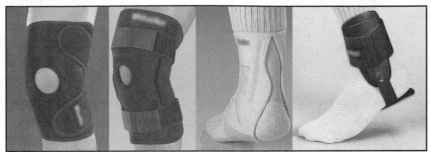

Figure 15-3. Examples of preventative ankle braces and knee supports.

Knee braces can take on many varieties. The postoperative hinged knee brace is commonly used to assist with ambulation following a surgical procedure. Many knee braces are available to help patients prevent knee injury and to protect specific structures during sport activity and rehabilitation. These braces are known as functional knee braces. There is not full agreement in the literature regarding the need for these braces, even after surgical reconstructions.[7,8] Many braces designed with lateral supports are available. These braces aim to protect the MCL and LCL and are frequently worn in American-style football. As mentioned, the efficacy of these braces is not universally accepted. In addition, there are countless Neoprene (DuPont Performance Elastomers, Wilmington, DE) sleeves and supports designed to provide warmth, compression, and modest support to the knee joint. Some neoprene sleeves are specifically designed to support the patella. Open holes and lateral buttresses are built into the sleeve to help control tracking.

SUMMARY

The techniques presented in this chapter and on the companion Web site are designed to give students an overview of common methods and to establish a foundation for supervised development of skills. The use of taping and bracing in sports medicine needs further study to fully evaluate the efficacy of specific techniques and to allow for greater reliance on evidence-based practice. Great care must be taken in the selection of the taping materials and the application of the techniques in the interest of patient comfort and safety. Students should strive to master these foundational skills because they can be a source of great confidence and allow for initial patient interactions in an athletic training environment.

REFERENCES

1. Verbrugge JD. The effects of semirigid Air-Stirrup bracing vs. adhesive ankle taping on motor performance. *J Orthop Sports Phys Ther.* 1996;23(5):320-325.

2. Jerosch J, Thorwesten L, Bork H, Bischof M. Is prophylactic bracing of the ankle cost effective? *Orthopedics.* 1996;19(5):405-414.

3. MacKean LC, Bell G, Burnham RS. Prophylactic ankle bracing vs. taping: effects on functional performance in female basketball players. *J Orthop Sports Phys Ther.* 1995;22(2):77-81.

4. You SH, Granata KP, Bunker LK. Effects of circumferential ankle pressure on ankle proprioception, stiffness, and postural stability: a preliminary investigation. *J Orthop Sports Ther.* 2004;34(8):449-460.

5. Kerkhoffs GM, Struijs PA, Marti RK, Assendelft WJ, Blankevoort L, van Dijk CN. Different functional treatment strategies for acute lateral ankle ligament injuries in adults (review). The Cochrane Collaboration. *The Cochrane Library.* 2007;4.

6. Verhagen EA, van Mechelen W, de Vente W. The effect of preventive measures on the incidence of ankle sprains (Review). *Clin J Sports Med.* 2000;10(4):291-296.

7. Baker BE. The effect of bracing on the collateral ligaments of the knee. *Clin Sports Med.* 1990;9(4):843-851.

8. McDevitt ER, Taylor DC, Miller MD, et al. Functional bracing after anterior cruciate ligament reconstruction: a prospective, randomized, multicenter study. *Am J Sports Med.* 2004;32(8):1887-1892.

PREPARING FOR SUCCESS

CHAPTER 16

LOOKING AHEAD

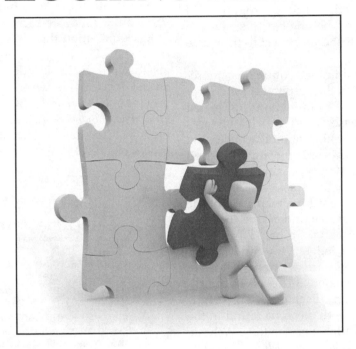

Maintain a vision for your profession that expects the best, have a positive vision and strive for that.

Sandra J. Shultz, PhD, ATC, CSCS
Associate Professor
University of North Carolina–Greensboro

When planning for a career, it is often helpful to take a look at what milestones you will need to reach as you pursue your goals. In athletic training, there may be several: gaining acceptance into a CAATE-accredited program, advancing through the various stages of clinical development, graduating with your degree, successfully completing the BOC exam, selecting and pursuing graduate or professional education, and finding an athletic training position. Looking ahead to these goals can serve as a compass for the beginning student. Keeping these goals in focus can help you stay the proper course in your chosen academic field. This chapter is designed to help you think about some of those things that are around the bend.

Upon completion of this chapter, the student will be able to:

- ✓ Appraise the issues facing future athletic trainers
- ✓ Explain various formats for developing a résumé
- ✓ Describe the proper format for a cover letter
- ✓ Identify steps to prepare for the BOC examination
- ✓ Discuss the various graduate education options available to athletic training students

PREPARING FOR CERTIFICATION

While is may seem that the actual BOC certification exam is too far off in the future to discuss in an introductory book, it does warrant discussion given that certification is a required step for entry into the profession. A complete history of the certification process is presented in Chapter 2. Students completing a CAATE-accredited athletic training program will meet the requirements and be eligible to sit for the BOC examination on the test date closest to their date of graduation.

Preparing for the examination requires a comprehensive plan to capitalize on the preparation your program will provide. The BOC examination is designed to provide a thorough assessment of a candidate's knowledge and decision-making abilities concerning the practice of athletic training. The computer-based exam is made up of 2 question types: multiple choice and hybrid. The examination assesses whether a particular candidate has sufficient understanding of the principles, practices, and science underlying the practice in the domains of athletic training. Hybrid-style questions incorporate knowledge with clinical decision making. Test questions are written, validated, and reviewed by a panel of content experts in coordination with psychometricians. Each question is referenced to at least 2 textbooks that can be found in the BOC Exam References (available on the BOC Web site at www.bocatc.org). The BOC *Role Delineation Study* serves as the blue print for the BOC certification exam. This study identifies the domains for the practice of athletic training (see Chapter 1). The link between the *Role Delineation Study* and the BOC exam ensures that the exam validly reflects the skills and knowledge needed for entry-level athletic trainers.[1] No student should prepare for the certification examination without an assessment of strengths and weaknesses based on the most recent *Role Delineation Study*.

To assist with preparation for the examination, the BOC Web site offers clear instructions to candidates in the *Candidate Handbook*. The BOC Web site offers self-assessment examination for students who are preparing for the BOC certification exam. The self-assessment exams contain questions that were written by content experts who develop the actual BOC certification examination. The intent is to help identify strengths and weaknesses by specific domain. The self-assessment could also be used by athletic trainers who wish to assess CE needs.[1] These on-line exams also help students feel comfortable with the exam process. While the items are similar in style and reflect the same content, no self-assessment questions will ever appear on the actual BOC certification exam.

In preparation for the exam, a number of study guides are published by a variety of publishers. These guides can be helpful in gaining familiarity with the style of questions used in the test and reducing anxiety about the testing procedures. Study guides can assist in learning about the exam and planning a strategy for studying. However, a focused comprehensive study plan should be devised under the guidance of your program's director and CIs. Reading a study guide is not a substitute for actual studying! The student should keep in mind that information in some guides may be incorrect due to changes in the BOC examination that take place after their publication. The BOC does not endorse any study materials that are available outside of the BOC Web site. Students with questions regarding the certification process should visit the BOC's Web site and study the *Candidate Handbook* with care; these items will reflect the most accurate information on the certification process.

 Stay Up-to-Date on Certification Issues

There seems to be lots of myth and folklore about the BOC examination. How it is developed and scored, or even how you apply. Lots of this folklore grows from the fact that the exam is stressful to some candidates and when we are stressed, we do not always think in a logical manner. Misinformation is everywhere. Do not allow yourself to fall into this trap. If you need the most up-to-date information about the certification process, get it from the source: www.bocatc.org. Having your facts straight about the exam process will allow you to stay focused on the task at hand, studying and being successful.

GRADUATE EDUCATION

Students looking beyond their athletic training program may wish to consider an advanced degree. The decision to pursue a master's or doctoral degree should be made after considerable thought regarding your career goals. Graduate education is commonplace among athletic trainers, with approximately 70% holding an advanced degree.[2] Individuals with career aspirations that include teaching at the college or university level will need a minimum of a master's degree. Teaching at the university level may require doctoral training. Students looking ahead to graduate education should be aware of the guiding principles of graduate study and how they apply to athletic

The Next Generation

Looking ahead is the theme and title of this chapter. What are some of the things that athletic trainers do now that they will not do in the future? What are some items that we do not do now that we need to prepare for? Professions are not static; they are constantly changing and evolving. Portions of our current practice change and evolve as the profession progresses. With this in mind, a group of experienced athletic trainers were asked what the next generation of athletic trainers must be better prepared to do. As we look ahead to the future, you may find some direction in their answers.

"The next generation of athletic trainers must be better prepared to ..."

- Understand advanced technology, read and interpret diagnostic studies such as MRI and CT, and continue to maintain pace with surgical advancements with respect to rehabilitation.
- Deal with a diverse society as part of their clientele (by diverse I mean in the sense of cultural and ethnic diversity).
- Market themselves by being prepared to work in multiple settings.
- Continue to work as hard and respect the profession as much as their predecessors.
- Market themselves.
- Integrate into the health care system.
- Be prepared to document the outcomes of their clinical interventions.
- Be flexible with the variety of settings where they seek employment.
- Focus on the key elements that comprise the practice of athletic training
- Work in other health care environments where they can be appropriately remunerated for their services.
- Defend what it is they do. The way to do this is through educational reform and research.

training. The Council of Graduate Schools (www.cgsnet.org) describes graduate study in this way:

- ✓ Students must deal with subject matter at the leading edge of their disciplines, a territory characterized by different and often opposing points of view.
- ✓ They must learn to question what they read and write in a manner that is both rigorous and evenhanded.
- ✓ They must maintain high standards for the criteria of proof, and they must be not only willing, but also eager to test their ideas in a forum of their peers and colleagues.
- ✓ Graduate study, at its best, should allow students to hone their own skills and learn to engage in and contribute to the continuing discussion that defines the current consensus in their field.

Students exploring educational information on the NATA Web site will notice links to advanced graduate programs in athletic training. These are programs that have been reviewed and approved by the NATA. These programs are designed for students who have completed entry-level preparation in athletic training, are already certified or eligible for certification, and have a desire to expand the depth of their athletic training knowledge. The NATA Education Council's *Standards and Guidelines for Post-Certification Graduate Education in Athletic Training* states that the philosophy of postcertification graduate education is[3]:

> *The mission of a post-certification graduate athletic training education program is to expand the depth and breadth of the applied, experiential, and propositional knowledge and skills of entry-level certified athletic trainers, expand the athletic training body of knowledge, and to disseminate new knowledge in the discipline. Graduate education is characterized by advanced systematic study and experience—advanced in knowledge, understanding, scholarly competence, inquiry, and discovery*

Most of these programs require clinical assistantships that allow graduate students to seek additional clinical experience in a variety of settings (secondary schools, intercollegiate athletics, and clinical settings). Many programs require graduate students to complete a master's thesis or research-oriented project as part of the graduate program. Admission criteria will vary by individual program but most will examine cumulative grade point average, Graduate Records Examination (GRE) scores, a personal essay stating reasons for graduate study, a cover letter, résumé, and letters of recommendation.

A directory of postcertification programs can be found on the NATA Web site at www.nata.org.

It is still a widespread practice for universities to fund graduate-assistant positions that allow graduate students to get additional clinical experience while providing service to the intercollegiate athletic program. In exchange for this service, students are provided with a stipend and often full tuition remission. Students must then find an area of study to pursue a master's degree. While some degree programs are particularly useful, the downside of such an assistantship is that there is no guarantee of a meaningful connection between the clinical and academic program. Students must explore these graduate options with care. By contrast, the NATA-approved program can allow for greater depth of knowledge in the chosen discipline of athletic training.

Graduate Education in Athletic Training

Why Pursue Graduate Education in an NATA-Approved Graduate Program?

- To become an expert in athletic training, students need advanced education in athletic training.
- Critical thinking skills, coursework, clinical opportunities, and mentoring are more focused toward the athletic training profession.
- Knowledge that accredited programs meet established standards and undergo rigorous external review.
- Athletic training research experience develops the skills and mindset necessary to practice in the spirit of evidence-based medicine.

Issues to Consider for Graduate Training in Other Disciplines

- There is nothing "wrong" about pursuing education in another discipline provided it will meet your professional needs.
- Studying in a different area will broaden your knowledge but will not necessarily provide depth and context in the domains of athletic training.
- A research opportunity may be present but may provide irrelevant context and/or limited clinical skill development.

Adapted from Ingersoll CD, Geick JH. Why certified students should enroll in an accredited graduate program. June 2003 NATA Symposium Graduate Education Session. Available at http://www.nataec. org/AcademicPrograms/PostProfessionalEducat ion/tabid/97/Default.aspx. Accessed March 17, 2008.

In addition to the advanced master's programs, some universities offer doctoral-level training in the area of athletic training or sports medicine. This evolution is reflective of the increased academic stature afforded these programs. While it is not uncommon for doctoral students with athletic training backgrounds to study in related disciplines (eg, biomechanics, epidemiology), in the past is was necessary for athletic trainers to seek out degrees in related fields. Now doctoral students can enjoy areas of study and research much closer to their clinical interest in athletic training.

Students should explore all of the options available to them for graduate study to help determine which path aligns best with their goals. The prospective graduate student should seek advice from as many current professionals as possible to best determine what kind of graduate program he or she desires. Ask direct questions, speak to current graduate students of a program that interests you, use on-line resources, talk to alumni, review research that comes from a given program, and make a campus visit if at all possible. If you have done your homework, you will have a sense of what type of program is best for you.

Dual Credentials

It is not uncommon to find certified athletic trainers who hold dual credentials. One of the most common combinations is the athletic trainer/physical therapist (ATC/PT). While historically the relationship between these allied health groups has not always been positive, we are hopeful for improved relations as state regulation helps better define roles and boundaries for all allied health practitioners. While the ATC/PT combination is not uncommon, it is not a requirement of any kind. Each profession is well defined and can stand on its own.

In addition to considering graduate education, students may wish to consider other credentials, certifications, or areas of advanced qualification to better market themselves for the wide range of employment settings available to the athletic trainer. Common dual credentials or qualifications may include EMT, certified strength and conditioning specialist (CSCS), physician's assistant (PA), registered dietician (RD), massage therapist, orthopedic technician, and many other possibilities. These additional qualifications may require passing a certification exam (CSCS), a semester of work followed by an examination (EMT), or an entire second degree (PT, RD, PA). Something as straightforward as becoming a CPR/first-aid instructor may assist in your marketability for a given position.

Students should look carefully at their future goals and determine if they wish to pursue additional training. Keep in mind the athletic training education program is designed to help you become a certified athletic trainer and prepare you appropriately to work with physically active populations. Students should plan accordingly but not get too far ahead of themselves. Be prepared to focus on athletic training for the entire course of the educational program.

Do not get an athletic training certification (or any certification or degree) just to "have more letters after my name."

Gather advice, plan ahead, and determine the path that best fits your goals.

TECHNOLOGY AND ATHLETIC TRAINING

No discussion that looks toward the future would be complete without some mention of technology. Over the last few decades, athletic training has seen several technological advances in the form of better equipment, changes in modalities, and the ability to organize information. Ironically, recent years have seen a movement toward manual "hands-on" therapy, functional exercise, and less emphasis on machines. Despite this, technology is an integral part of the athletic training professional landscape. The use of technology as a means to increase the number of CE opportunities available to certified athletic trainers continues to grow.

The acquisition and dissemination of information are areas where technology has already had a tremendous impact on the athletic training educational and work environments. The proliferation of the Internet and widespread availability of electronic mail have already had an impact of how athletic trainers communicate. The ability to participate in on-line discussion groups, collaborate with colleagues, and share information instantly has become commonplace. The availability of educational materials in an on-line format is steadily growing. As Internet users become more knowledgeable and comfortable with technology, their expectations for on-line educational materials will increase. As expectations change, the Internet will continue to evolve from a place where documents were simply displayed to a media-rich interactive learning environment.[3] On-line learning allows for the selection of various media (text, graphics, video, audio, animation, etc) to best fit the learning goals. Active acquisition of information, competencies, and skills can be achieved through interaction that extends beyond passive reading of materials.[4]

Students in athletic training education programs will need to be comfortable using technology as part of their learning experience. On-line discussion groups, directed assignments, and Web-based projects can provide a link between the classroom and the clinical experience. The on-line environment also allows for student-centered learning. Students can access information from a variety of locations and at their own pace. Modules on specific topics that are important for the student but not frequently seen in a clinical setting lend themselves well to on-line environments.

The computer literate student must reach beyond the basic computer skills of email, Internet searching, word processing, and social networking to do much more. Students must have the ability to maximize their abilities to retrieve and evaluate research as evidence-based practices gain greater acceptance.

Students will need to maximize collaborative web-based environments in application-driven ways rather than specifically in social networking. Students with the ability to design their own Web-based materials, create effective presentations, use a wide range of software (spreadsheets, databases, and statistics), and manipulate various media forms (video, audio, and still images) will be very well equipped to use technology to maximize their educational experience and will improve their marketability.

 ## What Does Your Facebook Page Say About You?

Done a Google Search Lately?

Social networking sites have become quite popular in recent years. Facebook.com (Facebook, Palo Alto, CA) began as a place for college students to post pictures and share common interests and is now very popular. Recent news reports show that the site has become a tool for potential employers. This has experts discussing the legality of such use and young job-seekers nervous.

It is not uncommon that employers routinely conduct Web searches to find background information on job candidates. Companies have furthered this practice by using Facebook and other social networking sites.

Lance Choy, Director of the Career Development Center at Stanford, commented, "Employers might be able to confirm background information." He added, "Some students write about their interests, and employers might want to check on whether this supports their job application. Some employers might try and learn something about the student's personality and whether it would be appropriate for the job. However, there is information on Facebook that is not relevant to the job but may be used inappropriately by employers to assess a candidate."

The use of Facebook by businesses has raised ethical concerns. Students contend that snooping on a social networking site is like listening in on conversations among friends. The practice of tagging photos also can be problematic as what might be fun college humor during your junior year spring recess may not look so great to a prospective employer.

Certainly, social networking sites were not designed for employer use. However, students should monitor what they put on the public portion of the site. Monitor photos, keep track of tags, and be very careful about the personal disclosure in the public domain. Just because everyone can see it does not mean that everyone should. Be careful how you portray yourself—you do not know who might be looking.

Table 16-1

Action Words for Résumé Writing

achieved	constructed	explained	motivated	reported
acquired	contracted	forecasted	negotiated	researched
adapted	converted	formed	obtained	resolved
addressed	coordinated	founded	operated	reviewed
administered	created	generated	organized	selected
analyzed	cultivated	guided	originated	separated
anticipated	demonstrated	hired	oversaw	set up
assembled	designed	implemented	performed	simplified
assisted	developed	improved	planned	solved
audited	devised	informed	prevented	surveyed
budgeted	discovered	insured	produced	staffed
calculated	doubled	interpreted	programmed	supervised
centralized	drafted	interviewed	promoted	taught
changed	edited	launched	provided	tested
collaborated	eliminated	maintained	publicized	trained
composed	enforced	managed	published	used
condensed	established	marketed	recruited	
conducted	expanded	minimized	reorganized	

Adapted from National Association of Colleges and Employers. Your guide to résumé writing: action words. Available at http://jobweb.com/Résumé/help.aspx?id=280&terms=action+words+for+résumé+writing. Accessed March 11, 2009.

RÉSUMÉ WRITING

It can be argued that a section on résumé writing is premature for an introductory book that will be used by students trying to decide if athletic training is the career choice for them. I have to disagree. Too often a résumé is thought of as something you put together when you are at the end of your undergraduate program. I can understand that viewpoint because you will need to refine and develop a résumé as graduation approaches. However, your undergraduate career and the experiences you gather in your athletic training education program will become the content of that résumé. It is never too early to start developing your résumé and selecting experiences based on how they will help you develop as a prospective athletic trainer and how they can be used on your résumé. If an undergraduate student has an understanding of how to develop this important document, he or she will be well prepared to evaluate specific experiences and determine if they are relevant to demonstrating his or her strengths, values, interests, specific skills, and career priorities.

Prior to developing your résumé, some of the basics of résumé writing should be reviewed. Students must remember the following[5]:

✓ A résumé is often the first impression you make on a potential employer or graduate program director

✓ Résumés are screening devices and therefore they need to be visually appealing, clear, concise, and comprehensive.

✓ Use quality paper and equipment

✓ The primary purpose of the résumé is to get you an interview

✓ Résumé readers are often looking for key words such as *experience, success, responsibility*, or action verbs (Table 16-1)

There are several formats for developing a résumé. These include the chronological résumé, functional résumé, and the combination résumé. Chronological résumés are most often used if an individual has significant work experiences. This will not likely be the case with a recent college graduate. Functional résumés allow you to categorize achievements from different areas under one heading. In addition, the

AT Student
2000 N. University St. #1
Anytown, WI 53703
(608) 555-1234 atstudent@students.edu

OBJECTIVE: To further develop my athletic training skills by obtaining a position as a graduate assistant in a Division I intercollegiate setting while pursing a master's degree in a related field of study.

EDUCATION   University of Higher Education
Bachelor of Science, May 2009
Major: Kinesiology-Athletic Training
CAATE-Accredited Athletic Training Education Program
GPA: 3.91   GRE: 1980 (700 Q, 610 V, 670 A)

EXPERIENCE
8/07-Present   **University of Higher Education Athletic Training Student**
Intercollegiate clinical experience with football, softball, swimming and diving, men's and women's basketball, wrestling, crew and women's soccer participating in the evaluation, treatment and rehabilitation of injuries under the supervision of certified athletic trainers.
Level III senior athletic training student with women's soccer program; gained experience as a first responder as well as independent travel, packing, and informal instruction of introductory athletic training students.

Summer 2006   **University of Higher Education Summer Camps**
Provided triage and first aid at summer camps for boys' soccer, boys' basketball, girls' basketball, volley ball, and wrestling while in communication with camp counselors, coaches, and parents.

Summer 2005   **United Way Volunteer/Camp Counselor Anytown, USA**
Oversaw activities and games for participants with cognitive challenges. Coordinated first aid program and provided triage and first aid for participants and counselors.

AFFILIATIONS   National Athletic Trainers' Association—Student member 8/07 to present
Great Lakes Athletic Trainers' Association—Student member 8/07 to present

CERTIFICATIONS   **HONORS**
Red Cross CPR   2008 Alex Henweigh Scholarship
First Aid   2009 Mya Kneehurts Scholarship
NATA-BOC anticipated May 2009   Dean's List 7 semesters

References provided upon request

Figure 16-1. Sample functional résumé.

functional résumé allows you to highlight skills, experiences, and qualifications that are gained in areas not always related to employment. These may include internships, clinical experiences, and volunteer work. Functional résumés are appropriate for new college graduates who may lack significant experience in their field.[6] A sample functional résumé for an athletic training student is presented in Figure 16-1.

A combination résumé is sometimes called a targeted résumé. This résumé starts with a summary of skills and qualifications followed by a chronological work history. The combination résumé allows you to highlight specific skills and qualifications then backs them up with a work history. An example of a targeted résumé for an athletic training student is provided in Figure 16-2. This résumé is best if you have more experience; however, it can be adapted for the recent graduate if he or she wishes to quickly identify skills that are directed to a specific position. Students will need to explore different formats to determine which one best fits their personal situation. The student's own experience and the nature of the job or program to which he or she is sending the résumé will help determine the best fit.

AT Student
2000 N. University St. #1
Anytown, WI 53703
(608) 555-1234 atstudent@students.edu

Summary

- Proven skills in the area of injury evaluation and treatment
- Effective program planning skills
- Fluent in Spanish
- Manage time effectively

Education

University of Wisconsin-Madison
Major: Kinesiology – Exercise Science
Emphasis: Athletic Training (CAATE-Accredited Program)
Cumulative GPA: 3.87/4.0
Expected graduation date: May 2009

Experience

Athletic Training Student (August 2005 to Present)
University of Wisconsin-Madison
- Worked under the supervision of certified athletic trainers in the prevention, treatment, and rehabilitation of athletic injuries
- Mentored Level I and Level II student athletic trainers
- Gained athletic training experience with Division I football, track and field, and softball teams
- Provided athletic training coverage to high school athletes attending football and basketball summer camps

Step Aerobics Instructor (May 2004 to December 2004)
University of Wisconsin-Madison
- Lead and motivated participants in aerobic exercise classes
- Educated participants on proper exercise techniques

Hospital Volunteer (June 2007 to August 2007)
Door County Memorial Hospital, Sturgeon Bay, Wisconsin
- Gained knowledge of responsibilities of physical therapists and athletic trainers while observing them in an outpatient rehabilitation setting
- Utilized bilingual skills in patient interaction

Affiliations

National Athletic Trainers' Association—Student member 2007 to present
Wisconsin Athletic Trainers' Association—Student member 2007 to present

Certifications	**Honors**
Red Cross CPR	2007 Alex Henweigh Scholarship
First Aid	2007 Mya Kneehurts Scholarship
NATA-BOC anticipated May 2009	Dean's List 7 semesters

References provided upon request

Figure 16-2. Sample targeted résumé.

RÉSUMÉ HEADINGS AND CATEGORIES

Contact Information

Your name must be clearly identified in a larger font than the rest of the résumé's font. Use your complete name and avoid nicknames. List your address, phone number, and email address. If your address may change, you should also include a permanent address. If you list an email address, it must be an address that you check regularly. Also, select an email that is professional and appropriate. If you have a Web site that addresses your professional goals, then it is appropriate to include a URL. If your Web site consists of pictures of your dog and your last camping trip, do not bother listing it.

Objective/Summary

Your objective is a brief statement that describes the job, program, or type of organization for which you are looking. This is optional and may not be necessary if you include a cover letter. However, athletic training students with very specific goals (ie, graduate school) should include a clear objective. The objective is an essential component of the functional résumé. The summary is a summary of skills or abilities that show what you can do for an employer. Targeted résumés include a summary of skills that should distinguish you from other candidates.

Sample objectives:

✓ To secure an entry-level athletic training position in an interscholastic setting that utilizes my clinical, organizational, and communication abilities. Skilled in evaluating, managing, and rehabilitating athletic injuries and illnesses. Excellent interpersonal skills.

Sample summary:

✓ Proven skills in the area of injury evaluation and treatment

✓ Effective program planning skills

✓ Fluent in French and Spanish

✓ Manage time effectively

Education

In this section you should list schools, degrees, and dates with the most recent first. You should also list specific courses or programs that enhance your marketability. List your highest degrees first. Students who are nearing graduation and applying for positions can list a date they expect the degree to be conferred. Additional categories such as "Related Coursework" may be needed if it can be used to appropriately describe your talents.

Honors and Activities

List relevant awards and honors. Undergraduate students will need to determine if awards earned in high school are relevant. It is unlikely you will wish to list any awards you received prior to entering your undergraduate program.

Relevant Experience

This section is sometimes listed as Related Experience, Athletic Training Experience, or Work Experience. Experiences should be prioritized to best meet your stated objective. Most often the experiences will be chronological with the most recent presented first. Students should describe their experiences in a way that conveys to the reader what skills they can bring to the position. These descriptions should include action verbs such as *coordinated, implemented, organized, achieved,* etc (see Table 16-1).

Don't Lie!

There have been several high profile examples of late of a degree that was not quite finished, a less-than-truthful accounting of work history, or maybe an inflation of academic performance. From high profile coaching jobs to the head of the USOC, résumés are under the microscope. Does the average athletic training job have the same level of public scrutiny? It is doubtful. However, the damage that can be done to your reputation and the harm it can cause your career by being less than honest will follow you forever. It is simple—be honest. Integrity and honesty are what you do when you think no one is looking. Maintain the highest level of professionalism possible. Do not pad your résumé. Hard work and dedication will always stand out.

Other Possible Categories

Professional affiliations can be listed as a category. A student who has been a member of a state or national organization for an extended period of time shows dedication and consistent interest in the profession. Certifications such as CPR, first aid, and BOC should be listed. If you have applied to take the BOC examination and have a confirmed date, you can list your test date on the résumé or list that the certification is anticipated on a specific date. NEVER misrepresent your certification status; it is a violation of the NATA *Code of Ethics.*

Getting Help

The samples provided and the suggestions listed above can serve as a guide to get started. Students should seek advice concerning the résumé development from their athletic training education program's faculty and athletic trainers on their campus. Most campuses have career centers or Web resources that can assist with the process. Take the time to get help and edit with care. Edit. Edit. Edit. Nothing stands out like incorrect information or misspellings on your résumé.

Date

Specific Individual
Position, Address (School, Clinic, ...)
Street
City, State, and Zip Code

Dear _____:
First Paragraph. State who you are and the reason you are writing. Explain a little about your interest and indicate how you learned about the position (use "network" sources).

Second and Third (if needed) Paragraphs. Be specific about why you are interested in the position. Briefly summarize some of your strongest qualifications for the position. Consider the point of view of someone reading the letter. Illustrate both clinical and academic strengths. Show what you have to offer to the position, not just what the position can offer you.

Closing Paragraph. Refer to your résumé, which will be enclosed. Declare you interest in an interview and offer to provide further information upon request.

Sincerely,

Your name (type written) – include signature as well

Enclosure

Figure 16-3. Cover letter template.

WRITING A COVER LETTER

The cover letter is a formal letter to a prospective employer that essentially "covers" your résumé. It is the first item that an employer will see and provides you with an opportunity to present yourself in a way that best fits the position being offered. You can use the cover letter to do the following:

✓ Sell yourself and show you "fit" the position you desire

✓ Demonstrate your ability to organize your thoughts and get to the point

✓ Include your professional objective

✓ Call attention to your skills and abilities

✓ Show you meet specific requirements

✓ Explain specific circumstances in your résumé

A cover letter should be properly addressed, provide an introduction, a body that outlines your qualifications, an action paragraph, proper closing and handwritten signature. Figure 16-3 provides a common cover letter template. Figure 16-4 provides an example of a cover letter used for an application for a graduate assistant position in an athletic training environment. Table 16-2 gives a list of cover letter Dos and Don'ts.

SUMMARY

Although students should avoid getting too far ahead of themselves, looking ahead can help students map where they want to go. This chapter has addressed specific issues facing future athletic trainers as well as provided information on common issues that affect students toward the end of an educational program. Learning résumé skills, writing cover letters, understanding the certification process, and thinking about graduate education will help students keep an eye on the future while they make the most of the present.

October 7, 2008

Mr. Hal Hireme
Head Athletic Trainer
University of Anytown
Anytown, USA 11233

Dear Mr. Hireme:

I am submitting my résumé in response to the announcement for a graduate assistant that was provided to me by Dr. Ed Ucator, the program director at Mytown University. I will be graduating in May from Mytown University's CAATE-accredited athletic training program. I am interested in a graduate position that will allow me to continue my education in a related field while gaining further clinical experience as a graduate assistant.

My preparation at Mytown has provided me with the opportunity to combine rigorous class work with extensive clinical experiences in an NCAA Division I athletic environment. I have gathered clinical experiences with volleyball, football, swimming, track and field, and crew. The athletic training program has allowed me to develop the strong clinical and interpersonal skills needed to be an asset to your sports medicine team. In addition to my clinical skills, I have served as a tutor and lab assistant for our introductory athletic training class. My cumulative GPA is 3.5/4.0 and I have achieved GRE scores of 590 (verbal), 620 (quantitative), and 660 (analytical).

I would enjoy the opportunity to be a part of your sports medicine team and would welcome the opportunity to prove myself in an interview. My résumé with a list of references and contact information is enclosed. A copy of my transcript, GRE scores, and the requested letters of recommendation have been forwarded to you. My availability for an interview is at your convenience.

Sincerely,

AT Student

Enclosure

Figure 16-4. Sample cover letter.

Table 16-2

Dos and Don'ts for Cover Letters

- Write to an individual, never to just an address or title. It is okay to use networking sources to introduce yourself in the opening paragraph. However, do not be a "name dropper." Only use the resource if it is appropriate (see Figure 16-4).

- Write in such a way that the reader will know you have done your homework and you have a genuine grasp of the available position. Be professional. Do not gush.

- Write each cover letter separately, even if you use a common framework. Personalize the letter with sentences that reflect your sincere interest in the specific position.

- Use natural language in simple, clear sentences. Do not try to impress the reader with unusual vocabulary or complicated sentence structure.

- Express your capabilities with confidence, but avoid exaggerating your level of experience. A week of basketball summer camp does not equal extensive experience with that sport.

- Finish with a strong closing that indicates the action you desire, such as a request for an interview or your intention to call. This action must be specific for the position you are seeking.

- Check and recheck (and then check again!) your letter for correctness with regard to spelling, punctuation, and sentence structure. Be sure to have someone who is a good writer review your letter with you.   (continued)

Table 16-2 (continued)

Dos and Don'ts for Cover Letters

- Make sure your final letter is completely professional in appearance. Use standard business letter format, standard type, on good stationery. That baby blue paper might look good in the store but will not be very professional. Use a high-quality laser printer.

- The letter should reflect you—your personality, confidence, and desire to be an athletic training professional. Use words that reflect action and confidence. The reader should sense why you are a good "fit."

 ## Advice and Wisdom for the Athletic Training Student

Building a foundation for a successful career in athletic training requires students to grow and develop through many academic and personal experiences. Acceptance into a program, solid academic performance, meaningful clinical experiences, professional certification, personal growth, and learning through experience are all key components to setting this foundation. Along the way, I am an advocate of seeking out and learning from mentors who have been where you want to be. Listen, process information, and take the advice from those who have dedicated themselves to educating and providing care for others. Advice is defined as an "opinion about what could or should be done about a situation or problem; counsel." At the very heart of the word *advice* we find possibility and direction (what could or should be done). Advice is not always designed to "tell you what to do." More often than not, good advice is designed to help you make your own decisions. Counsel runs deeper than just opinion—it implies something more thoughtful.

The thoughtful comments below are offered as general advice for students pursuing a career in athletic training.

You can never have enough education. Continue to attain the terminal degree in the profession. Attend seminars and workshops as regularly as you can fit it into your schedule. Read and Read and Read in your field. Never let it be said that you were not well trained. Seek out brilliant professors, physicians, and others who can mentor you.

Ronnie P. Barnes, MS, ATC

Head Athletic Trainer, Vice President for Medical Services

National Football League—New York Giants

Know yourself and don't sell yourself short. It's important to understand the difference between a profession and professionalism. Professionalism is defined by behaviors and attitudes and that is something you define. It can either hurt or enhance the profession accordingly.

Sandra J. Shultz, PhD, ATC, CSCS

Associate Professor and Program Director

University of North Carolina–Greensboro

It's important to find and maintain the right balance between your professional life and your personal life. I can't think of a field where that is any more relevant than ours.

David H. Perrin, PhD, ATC

Provost

University of North Carolina–Greensboro

(continued)

Advice and Wisdom for the Athletic Training Student (continued)

Take in the breadth of the profession, explore all the areas, and as you continue as a professional find those that you wish to concentrate on. Don't get too fixed on the fact that you are at a college and that college has an athletic team that happens to have athletic trainers. It is much more than that. Explore the breadth of the profession.

Dennis Helwig, LAT

Head Athletic Trainer

University of Wisconsin–Madison

Your athletic training education, and the profession of athletic training, is what you make it. Your athletic training education is a strong foundation to lead you down many paths as an allied health professional, maybe some that we haven't even considered yet.

Chad Starkey, PhD, ATC

Graduate Program Coordinator

Associate Professor

Ohio University

Athletic training is the kind of profession that can give you a great deal of satisfaction. You need to look beyond the material things and really decide what you love about it. My advice to students is to find the aspects of this profession that are most satisfying and pursue them with great passion.

Scott Barker, MS, ATC

Head Athletic Trainer

California State University, Chico

"One Line Wisdom"

I call this section one line wisdom—sayings, thoughts, and phrases provided by athletic trainers I respect that can be passed on to others. Some are simple and short, while others reflect personal philosophies and goals. All of them live up to the definition of wisdom:

- The ability to discern or judge what is true, right, or lasting; insight
- Common sense; good judgment
- The sum of learning through the ages; knowledge
- A wise outlook, plan, or course of action

The following are some of my favorites:

I simply find it unprofessional and unproductive to be anything but direct and forthright with people at all times. Keep your compassion, however; once you lose compassion, you are useless as a health care professional.

Ronnie P. Barnes, MS, ATC

Head Athletic Trainer, Vice President for Medical Services

National Football League–New York Giants

Don't put limitations on yourself or the profession.

Dennis Helwig, LAT

Head Athletic Trainer

University of Wisconsin–Madison

(continued)

Advice and Wisdom for the Athletic Training Student (continued)

You control your mind. You control your body. You control your attitude.

Scott D. Linaker, MS, ATC/L

Athletic Trainer

Canyon Del Oro High School–Tucson, Arizona

Don't be afraid to deviate from the norm, there are many paths to travel.

Denise L. O'Rand, PhD, ATC

Associate Professor and Undergraduate Athletic Training Program Director

San Diego State University

Do the best job you can day in and day out and you will earn the professional respect of the people around you. Professional respect has to be earned, and the best way to earn it is with the job you do.

Scott Barker, MS, ATC

Head Athletic Trainer

California State University, Chico

Nasby Reinhardt told me, "Don't say can't and won't, say I can and I will."

Mike Nesbitt, MS, ATC

Retired, Flagstaff, AR

Be comfortable with your limitations, not everybody knows everything and that's OK. It's not a sign of weakness to ask for assistance, it is a sign of strength.

Chad Starkey, PhD, ATC

Graduate Program Coordinator

Associate Professor

Ohio University

Author's note: The comments gathered for this final chapter and through the entire text come from professionals with years of experience in athletic training. There is a genuine thread of optimism for what is best about the athletic training profession, and most cast an eye toward the future. That is the point of these comments and all of the comments that sprinkle this text. Experiences and lessons learned should be passed along for future athletic trainers to help build a foundation for success.

REFERENCES

1. Board of Certification Inc. *Candidate Handbook*. Available at www.bocatc.org. Accessed August 8, 2008.
2. Prentice WE. *Arnheims's Principles of Athletic Training*. 13th ed. New York, NY: McGraw-Hill Higher Education; 2009.
3. NATA Education Council. Standards and Guidelines for Post-Certification Graduate Education in Athletic Training Available at www.nataec.org. Accessed August 8, 2008.
4. Barker WS. Technology influences ATC's continuing education. *NATA News*. 2002;38.
5. National Association of Colleges and Employers. Guide to résumé writing. Available at www.jobweb.com. Accessed May 26, 2002.
6. East RS, Hastings SL. Certification and résumé writing. In: Sladyk K, ed. *OT Student Primer*. Thorofare, NJ: SLACK Incorporated; 1997:289-310.

BOARD OF CERTIFICATION
STANDARDS OF
PROFESSIONAL PRACTICE

INTRODUCTION

The mission of the Board of Certification Inc. (BOC) is to certify Athletic Trainers and to identify, for the public, quality healthcare professionals through a system of certification, adjudication, standards of practice and continuing competency programs. The BOC has been responsible for the certification of Athletic Trainers since 1969. Upon its inception, the BOC was a division of the professional membership organization the National Athletic Trainers' Association. However, in 1989, the BOC became an independent non-profit corporation.

Accordingly, the BOC provides a certification program for the entry-level Athletic Trainer that confers the ATC® credential and establishes requirements for maintaining status as a Certified Athletic Trainer (to be referred to as "Athletic Trainer" from this point forward). A nine member Board of Directors governs the BOC. There are six Athletic Trainer Directors, one Physician Director, one Public Director and one Corporate/Educational Director.

The BOC is the only accredited certification program for Athletic Trainers in the United States. Every five years, the BOC must undergo review and re-accreditation by the National Commission for Certifying Agencies (NCCA). The NCCA is the accreditation body of the National Organization for Competency Assurance.

The BOC Standards of Professional Practice consists of two sections:

I. Practice Standards

II. Code of Professional Responsibility

I. PRACTICE STANDARDS

PREAMBLE

The Practice Standards (Standards) establish essential practice expectations for all Athletic Trainers. Compliance with the Standards is mandatory.

The Standards are intended to:

✓ Assist the public in understanding what to expect from an Athletic Trainer

✓ Assist the Athletic Trainer in evaluating the quality of patient care

✓ Assist the Athletic Trainer in understanding the duties and obligations imposed by virtue of holding the ATC® credential

The Standards are NOT intended to:

✓ Prescribe services

✓ Provide step-by-step procedures

✓ Ensure specific patient outcomes

The BOC does not express an opinion on the competence or warrant job performance of credential holders; however, every Athletic Trainer and applicant must agree to comply with the Standards at all times.

STANDARD 1: DIRECTION

The Athletic Trainer renders service or treatment under the direction of a physician.

STANDARD 2: PREVENTION

The Athletic Trainer understands and uses preventive measures to ensure the highest quality of care for every patient.

Standard 3: Immediate Care

The Athletic Trainer provides standard immediate care procedures used in emergency situations, independent of setting.

Standard 4: Clinical Evaluation and Diagnosis

Prior to treatment, the Athletic Trainer assesses the patient's level of function. The patient's input is considered an integral part of the initial assessment. The Athletic Trainer follows standardized clinical practice in the area of diagnostic reasoning and medical decision making.

Standard 5: Treatment, Rehabilitation and Reconditioning

In development of a treatment program, the Athletic Trainer determines appropriate treatment, rehabilitation and/or reconditioning strategies. Treatment program objectives include long and short-term goals and an appraisal of those which the patient can realistically be expected to achieve from the program. Assessment measures to determine effectiveness of the program are incorporated into the program.

Standard 6: Program Discontinuation

The Athletic Trainer, with collaboration of the physician, recommends discontinuation of the athletic training service when the patient has received optimal benefit of the program. The Athletic Trainer, at the time of discontinuation, notes the final assessment of the patient's status.

Standard 7: Organization and Administration

All services are documented in writing by the Athletic Trainer and are part of the patient's permanent records. The Athletic Trainer accepts responsibility for recording details of the patient's health status.

II. Code of Professional Responsibility

Preamble

The Code of Professional Responsibility (Code) mandates that BOC credential holders and applicants act in a professionally responsible manner in all athletic training services and activities. The BOC requires all Athletic Trainers and applicants to comply with the Code. The BOC may discipline, revoke or take other action with regard to the application or certification of an individual that does not adhere to the Code.

The Professional Practice and Discipline Guidelines and Procedures may be accessed via the BOC website, www.bocatc.org.

Code 1: Patient Responsibility

The Athletic Trainer or applicant:

1.1 Renders quality patient care regardless of the patient's race, religion, age, sex, nationality, disability, social/economic status or any other characteristic protected by law

1.2 Protects the patient from harm, acts always in the patient's best interests and is an advocate for the patient's welfare

1.3 Takes appropriate action to protect patients from Athletic Trainers, other healthcare providers or athletic training students who are incompetent, impaired or engaged in illegal or unethical practice

1.4 Maintains the confidentiality of patient information in accordance with applicable law

1.5 Communicates clearly and truthfully with patients and other persons involved in the patient's program, including, but not limited to, appropriate discussion of assessment results, program plans and progress

1.6 Respects and safeguards his or her relationship of trust and confidence with the patient and does not exploit his or her relationship with the patient for personal or financial gain

1.7 Exercises reasonable care, skill and judgment in all professional work

Code 2: Competency

The Athletic Trainer or applicant:

2.1 Engages in lifelong, professional and continuing educational activities

2.2 Participates in continuous quality improvement activities

2.3 Complies with the most current BOC recertification policies and requirements

Code 3: Professional Responsibility

The Athletic Trainer or applicant:

3.1 Practices in accordance with the most current BOC Practice Standards

3.2 Knows and complies with applicable local, state and/or federal rules, requirements, regulations and/or laws related to the practice of athletic training

3.3 Collaborates and cooperates with other healthcare providers involved in a patient's care

3.4 Respects the expertise and responsibility of all healthcare providers involved in a patient's care

3.5 Reports any suspected or known violation of a rule, requirement, regulation or law by him/herself and/or by another Athletic Trainer that is related to the practice of athletic training, public health, patient care or education

3.6 Reports any criminal convictions (with the exception of misdemeanor traffic offenses or traffic ordinance violations that do not involve the use of alcohol or drugs) and/or professional suspension, discipline or sanction received by him/herself or by another Athletic Trainer that is related to athletic training, public health, patient care or education

3.7 Complies with all BOC exam eligibility requirements and ensures that any information provided to the BOC in connection with any certification application is accurate and truthful

3.8 Does not, without proper authority, possess, use, copy, access, distribute or discuss certification exams, score reports, answer sheets, certificates, certificant or applicant files, documents or other materials

3.9 Is candid, responsible and truthful in making any statement to the BOC, and in making any statement in connection with athletic training to the public

3.10 Complies with all confidentiality and disclosure requirements of the BOC

3.11 Does not take any action that leads, or may lead, to the conviction, plea of guilty or plea of nolo contendere (no contest) to any felony or to a misdemeanor related to public health, patient care, athletics or education;, this includes, but is not limited to: rape; sexual abuse of a child or patient; actual or threatened use of a weapon of violence; the prohibited sale or distribution of controlled substance, or its possession with the intent to distribute; or the use of the position of an Athletic Trainer to improperly influence the outcome or score of an athletic contest or event or in connection with any gambling activity

3.12 Cooperates with BOC investigations into alleged illegal or unethical activities; this includes but is not limited to, providing factual and non-misleading information and responding to requests for information in a timely fashion

3.13 Does not endorse or advertise products or services with the use of, or by reference to, the BOC name without proper authorization

Code 4: Research

The Athletic Trainer or applicant who engages in research:

4.1 Conducts research according to accepted ethical research and reporting standards established by public law, institutional procedures and/or the health professions

4.2 Protects the rights and well being of research subjects

4.3 Conducts research activities with the goal of improving practice, education and public policy relative to the health needs of diverse populations, the health workforce, the organization and administration of health systems and healthcare delivery

Code 5: Social Responsibility

The Athletic Trainer or applicant:

5.1 Uses professional skills and knowledge to positively impact the community

Code 6: Business Practices

The Athletic Trainer or applicant:

6.1 Refrains from deceptive or fraudulent business practices

6.2 Maintains adequate and customary professional liability insurance

BOC Standards of Professional Practice Implemented January 1, 2006. Reprinted with permission of the Board of Certification. Available at www.bocatc.org. Accessed March 1, 2008 available at: http://www.bocatc.org/images/stories/multiple_references/standardsprofessionalpractice.pdf

NATIONAL ATHLETIC TRAINERS' ASSOCIATION *CODE OF ETHICS*

PREAMBLE

The National Athletic Trainers' Association Code of Ethics states the principles of ethical behavior that should be followed in the practice of athletic training. It is intended to establish and maintain high standards and professionalism for the athletic training profession.

The principles do not cover every situation encountered by the practicing athletic trainer, but are representative of the spirit with which athletic trainers should make decisions. The principles are written generally; the circumstances of a situation will determine the interpretation and application of a given principle and of the Code as a whole. When a conflict exists between the Code and the law, the law prevails.

PRINCIPLE 1

Members shall respect the rights, welfare and dignity of all.

1.1 Members shall not discriminate against any legally protected class.

1.2 Members shall be committed to providing competent care.

1.3 Members shall preserve the confidentiality of privileged information and shall not release such information to a third party not involved in the patient's care without a release unless required by law.

PRINCIPLE 2

Members shall comply with the laws and regulations governing the practice of athletic training.

2.1 Members shall comply with applicable local, state, and federal laws and institutional guidelines.

2.2 Members shall be familiar with and abide by all National Athletic Trainers' Association standards, rules and regulations.

2.3 Members shall report illegal or unethical practices related to athletic training to the appropriate person or authority.

2.4 Members shall avoid substance abuse and, when necessary, seek rehabilitation for chemical dependency.

PRINCIPLE 3

Members shall maintain and promote high standards in their provision of services.

3.1 Members shall not misrepresent, either directly or indirectly, their skills, training, professional credentials, identity or services.

3.2 Members shall provide only those services for which they are qualified through education or experience and which are allowed by their practice acts and other pertinent regulation.

3.3 Members shall provide services, make referrals, and seek compensation only for those services that are necessary.

3.4 Members shall recognize the need for continuing education and participate in educational activities that enhance their skills and knowledge.

3.5 Members shall educate those whom they supervise in the practice of athletic training about the *Code of Ethics* and stress the importance of adherence.

3.6   Members who are researchers or educators should maintain and promote ethical conduct in research and educational activities.

PRINCIPLE 4

Members shall not engage in conduct that could be construed as a conflict of interest or that reflects negatively on the profession.

4.1   Members should conduct themselves personally and professionally in a manner that does not compromise their professional responsibilities or the practice of athletic training.

4.2   National Athletic Trainers' Association current or past volunteer leaders shall not use the NATA logo in the endorsement of products or services or exploit their affiliation with the NATA in a manner that reflects badly upon the profession.

4.3   Members shall not place financial gain above the patient's welfare and shall not participate in any arrangement that exploits the patient.

4.4   Members shall not, through direct or indirect means, use information obtained in the course of the practice of athletic training to try to influence the score or outcome of an athletic event, or attempt to induce financial gain through gambling.

NATA Code of Ethics. Modified September 28, 2005. Available at www.nata.org.

APPENDIX C

OBTAINING CONTINUING EDUCATION IN ATHLETIC TRAINING

Part of the professional responsibility of the certified athletic trainer is the requirement to remain current in the standards and practices of the athletic training profession. All athletic trainers certified after January 1, 2006 are required to complete 75 continuing education units (CEUs) every 3 years. One CEU is equal to 1 contact hour of educational time.

TYPES OF CONTINUING EDUCATION ACTIVITIES

The breakdown (and maximum allowable) CEUs by category are as follows.

Number of CEUs Required	Category A Maximum	Category B Maximum	Category C Maximum	Category D Maximum
75	75	50	75	20

CATEGORY A—BOC APPROVED PROVIDER PROGRAMS (75 CEU MAXIMUM)

✓ Activities in this category are available through BOC-approved providers.

✓ The BOC determines the number of CEUs awarded for home study programs. Please visit the BOC Web site at www.bocatc.org to verify the number of CEUs being offered for each home study course.

✓ Each individual BOC-approved provider determines the number of CEUs awarded for nonhome study activities in this category.

✓ A list of current BOC-approved providers is available on the BOC Web site at www.bocatc.org.

CATEGORY A ACTIVITIES

Possible Activities	Number of CEUs	Documentation
Workshops, seminars, conferences	As awarded by provider	Certificate or letter of attendance
Home study courses	As assigned by the BOC	Documentation of completion

CATEGORY B—PROFESSIONAL DEVELOPMENT (50 CEU MAXIMUM)

✓ Activities in this category have been defined by the BOC.

✓ The number of CEUs awarded for an activity is determined by the BOC.

✓ Speaking engagements can be counted only once per topic. If an abstract is connected to a presentation, CE credit can only be obtained for one activity or the other (ie, an abstract and presentation on the same topic—only one will be awarded CE credit).

✓ If a poster is connected to a presentation, CE credit can only be obtained for one activity or the other (ie, a poster and presentation on the same topic—only one will be awarded CE credit).

✓ The initial training for EMT (Basic) certification can be used for CE credit. Refresher courses will not receive CE credit in Category B.

CATEGORY B ACTIVITIES

Possible Activities	Number of CEUs	Documentation
BOC qualified examiner or model	5 CEUs per exam (limit 10 CEUs per year)	Report of attendance
EMT	40 CEUs (initial training only)	Certificate and card for "Basic Course"
Speaker at a conference*	10 CEUs per topic	Letter of acknowledgement from the conference coordinator (date of presentation must be included in the letter)
Panelist at a conference*	5 CEUs per topic	Letter of acknowledgement from the conference coordinator (date of presentation must be included in the letter)
Primary author of an article in a nonrefereed journal**	5 CEUs per article	Copy of the article
Author of an article in a referred journal**	Primary = 15 CEUs per article Secondary = 10 CEUs per article	Guidelines for authors and copy of article
Author of an abstract in a referred journal**	Primary = 10 CEUs per article Secondary = 5 CEUs per article	Guidelines for authors and copy of article
Author of a published textbook**	Primary = 40 CEUs per book Secondary = 20 CEUs per book	Copy of title page, including the publication date
Contributing author of a published textbook**	10 CEUs per book	Publication date and table of contents or list of contributors
Author of a poster presentation—peer reviewed or refereed**	Primary = 10 CEUs per presentation Secondary = 5 CEUs per presentation	Letter of acknowledgement
Primary author of published multimedia material	15 CEUs per publication	Copy of the publication (CD-ROM, audio, or video)**
Primary author of a home study course**	As determined by reviewer	Letter of approval
Home study reviewer##	5 CEUs per review (limit 10 CEUs per year)	Disposition letter
Exam item writer@@	5 CEUs per year of active item writing	Letter of acknowledgment from exam company

*The conference/seminar must be intended for an audience of healthcare professionals (ie, ATC, PT, RN, PA, PTA, MD). The actual content presented by a speaker or panelist must pertain to the domains identified in the *Role Delineation Study, Fifth Edition.*

**The following explanations apply to publication activities:

Published: prepared for commercial distribution

Journal: a periodical containing scholarly articles and/or current information on research and development in a particular field

Refereed: the manuscript/document has been reviewed by an editor and one or more specialists prior to publication

##Includes BOC home study reviewers and reviewers of refereed publications

@@Includes BOC exam item writers and exam item writers for other healthcare professional exams.

CATEGORY C—POSTCERTIFICATION COLLEGE/UNIVERSITY COURSEWORK (75 CEU MAXIMUM)

- ✓ CEUs are awarded for successful completion of college/university courses if the content of the course falls within the domains identified in the *Role Delineation Study, Fifth Edition.*
- ✓ The college/university attended must be accredited by an agency recognized by the US Department of Education.
- ✓ In order to be eligible, a course must be assigned credit hours and be listed on an official transcript.
- ✓ Practicum courses, clinicals, and internship experiences are not acceptable for CE credit.
- ✓ 10 CEUs are awarded for each credit hour (eg, a 3-credit course receives 30 CEUs). A credit hour must be equivalent to a minimum of 10 classroom hours.

CATEGORY C ACTIVITIES

Possible Activities	Number of CEUs	Documentation
College/university official course	10 CEUs per credit hour	Official transcript from accredited college/university
Medical residency	25 CEUs per year	Official transcript from accredited college/university

CATEGORY D—INDIVIDUALIZED OPTIONS (20 CEU MAXIMUM)

- ✓ This category includes attendance at a professional program that is sponsored by groups other than BOC-approved providers. The content of the program must fall within the domains identified in the *Role Delineation Study, Fifth Edition.*
- ✓ CE credit is also earned in this category for viewing educational multimedia (eg, videotapes, DVDs). The content of the multimedia must fall within the domains identified in the *Role Delineation Study, Fifth Edition.*
- ✓ 1 CEU is awarded for each contact hour.

CATEGORY D ACTIVITIES

Possible Activities	Number of CEUs	Documentation
Activities by non-BOC–approved providers	1 CEU per contact hour	Verification of attendance and copy of the program
Videos/DVDs/audiotapes/multimedia	1 CEU per contact hour	Receipt of purchase and independent verification (from an immediate supervisor that details title, length, and date of activity)

BOC Recertification Requirements updated February 2008. Adapted with permission from the Board of Certification. Available at www.bocatc.org. Accessed March 1, 2008 available at http://www.bocatc.org/images/stories/athletic_trainers/recertificationrequirements2006-2011.pdf

APPENDIX D

THE MUSCULOSKELETAL SYSTEM

THE SKELETAL SYSTEM

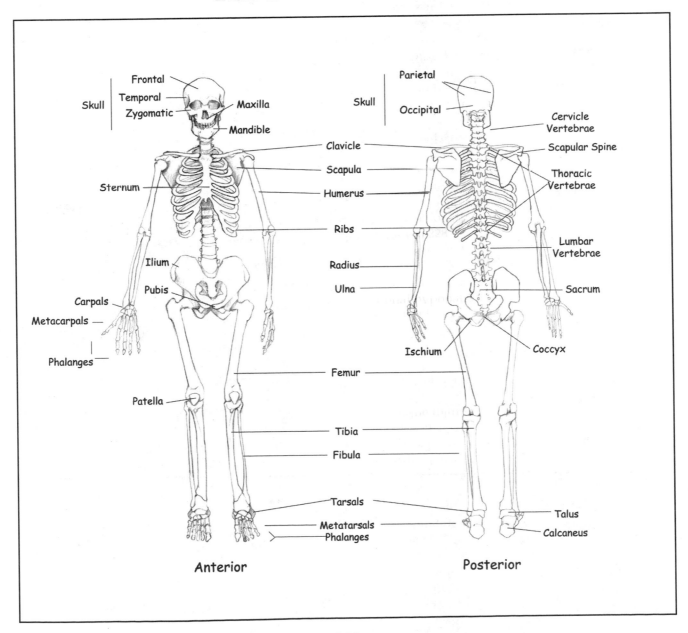

Anterior — Skull (Frontal, Temporal, Zygomatic, Maxilla, Mandible), Clavicle, Scapula, Sternum, Humerus, Ribs, Ilium, Pubis, Radius, Ulna, Carpals, Metacarpals, Phalanges, Patella, Femur, Tibia, Fibula, Tarsals, Metatarsals, Phalanges

Posterior — Skull (Parietal, Occipital), Cervicle Vertebrae, Scapular Spine, Thoracic Vertebrae, Lumbar Vertebrae, Sacrum, Ischium, Coccyx, Talus, Calcaneus

THE MUSCULAR SYSTEM

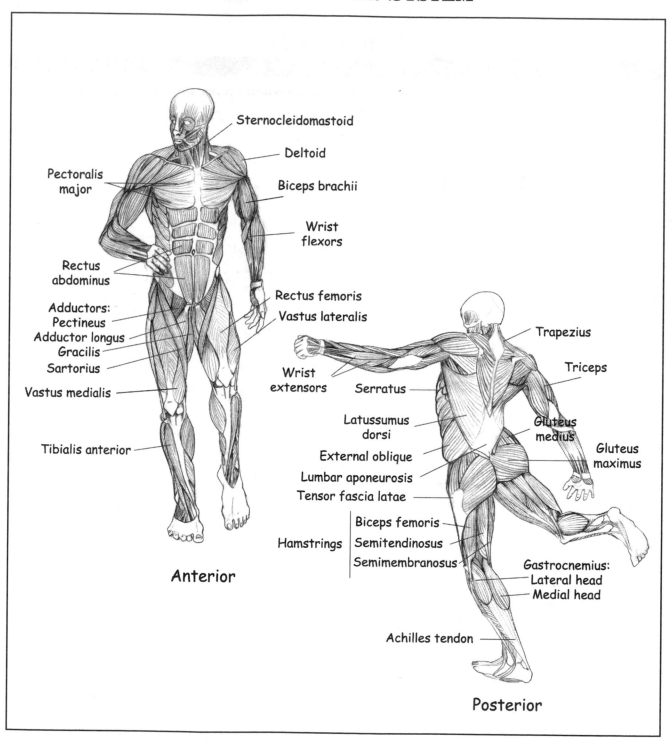

Sternocleidomastoid

Deltoid

Biceps brachii

Wrist
flexors

Pectoralis
major

Rectus
abdominus

Rectus femoris

Vastus lateralis

Adductors:
Pectineus
Adductor longus
Gracilis
Sartorius

Vastus medialis

Wrist
extensors

Serratus

Trapezius

Triceps

Latussumus
dorsi

Gluteus
medius

Gluteus
maximus

External oblique

Lumbar aponeurosis

Tensor fascia latae

Tibialis anterior

Biceps femoris

Hamstrings

Semitendinosus

Semimembranosus

Gastrocnemius:
Lateral head
Medial head

Achilles tendon

Anterior

Posterior

INDEX

WAIT

...There's More!

SLACK Incorporated's Health Care Books and Journals offers a wide selection of products in the field of Athletic Training. We are dedicated to providing important works that educate, inform and improve the knowledge of our customers. Don't miss out on our other informative titles that will enhance your collection.

Administrative Topics in Athletic Training: Concepts to Practice

Gary Harrelson, EdD, ATC; Greg Gardner, EdD, ATC; Andrew Winterstein, PhD, ATC
320 pp, Hard Cover, 2009, ISBN 13 978-1-55642-739-8, Order# 47395, **$63.95**

Administrative Topics in Athletic Training: Concepts to Practice is a dynamic text that addresses important administrative issues and procedures as well as fundamental concepts, strategies, and techniques related to the management of all aspects of an athletic training health care delivery system.

Special Tests for Orthopedic Examination, Third Edition

Jeff G. Konin, PhD, ATC, PT; Denise L. Wiksten, PhD, ATC; Jerome A. Isear, Jr., MS, PT, ATC-L; Holly Brader, MPH, RN, BSN, ATC
400 pp, Soft Cover, 2006, ISBN 13 978-1-55642-741-1, Order# 47417, **$43.95**

Special Tests for Orthopedic Examination has been used for 10 years by thousands of students, clinicians, and rehab professionals and is now available in a revised and updated third edition. Concise and pocket-sized, this handbook is an invaluable guide filled with the most current and practical clinical exam techniques used during an orthopedic examination.

Athletic Training Student Primer: A Foundation for Success, Second Edition

Andrew P. Winterstein, PhD, ATC
250 pp, Soft Cover, 2009, ISBN 13 978-1-55642-804-3, Order# 48049, **$49.95**

Special Tests for Neurologic Examination

James R. Scifers, DScPT, PT, SCS, LAT, ATC
432 pp, Soft Cover, 2008, ISBN 13 978-1-55642-797-8, Order# 47972, **$43.95**

Quick Reference Dictionary for Athletic Training, Second Edition

Julie N. Bernier, EdD, ATC
416 pp, Soft Cover, 2005, ISBN 13 978-1-55642-666-7, Order# 46666, **$39.95**

Athletic Training Exam Review: A Student Guide to Success, Fourth Edition

Lynn Van Ost, MEd, RN, PT, ATC; Karen Manfré, MA, ATR; Karen Lew, MEd, ATC, LAT
300 pp, Soft Cover, 2009, ISBN 13 978-1-55642-854-8, Order# 48548, **$49.95**

Clinical Skills Documentation Guide for Athletic Training, Second Edition

Herb Amato, DA, ATC; Christy D. Hawkins, ATC; Steven L. Cole, MEd, ATC, CSCS
464 pp, Soft Cover, 2006, ISBN 13 978-1-55642-758-9, Order# 47581, **$42.95**

Principles of Pharmacology for Athletic Trainers

Joel Houglum, PhD; Gary Harrelson, EdD, ATC; Deidre Leaver-Dunn, PhD, ATC
440 pp, Hard Cover, 2005, ISBN 13 978-1-55642-594-3, Order# 45945, **$48.95**

The Athletic Trainer's Guide to Psychosocial Intervention and Referral

James M. Mensch, PhD, ATC; Gary M. Miller, PhD, NCC
336 pp, Hard Cover, 2008, ISBN 13 978-1-55642-733-6, Order# 47336, **$46.95**

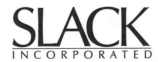